Table of Contents

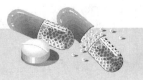

Advances in Women's Reproductive Health

Women's reproductive organs must be cared for outside of pregnancy. The art and science of this care is called *gynecology*. Reproductive diseases range from the trivial (such as the all-too-familiar yeast infection) to the life-endangering (such as cancer or uncontrollable bleeding). Some are "mechanical" problems that are the end result of child bearing, such as a prolapsed uterus whose ligaments have stretched to a point where they cannot properly support it.

Gynecologists nowadays stress wellness and preventive medicine by encouraging annual examinations to identify and treat problems before they become full-blown. The best known of these is the annual Pap smear, an examination of cells taken from the cervix to check for cancer or precancerous changes. This simple test has provided a major contribution to women's health by permitting early diagnosis of cervical disease. Because of it, far-advanced, invasive cervical cancer is rarely seen these days in the United States. By contrast, far-advanced cervical cancer in Third World countries is by no means a rarity because they do not have widespread Pap smear screening.

Another significant contribution to women's health is the technology of mammography, which has improved enormously in the last 5 years. Mammography, x-ray of the breasts, can help physicians diagnose breast cancer 2 to 3 years before any lump can be felt. When a suspicious finding appears on a mammogram, the physician can pinpoint the lesion with a fine needle inserted under local anesthesia to assist with biopsy of the suspicious tissue and early diagnosis of breast disease. The amount of radiation used in mammography is now so low that women can safely have a breast x-ray every year of their lives after age 50. We also recommend that a woman have at least one breast x-ray between 35 and 40 and then one every two to three years until age 50 when the annual exam should begin.

Nowadays a major tool for maintaining wellness after age 50 is estrogen replacement therapy. Estrogen replacement has been available for more than 40 years (it was sold over-the-counter for many decades in Canada!), but some physicians ridiculed it. We now realize that estrogen replacement greatly enhances the well-being of women's lives in many ways, and most gynecologists advocate its use after the menopause.

Consider this: Human females are the only mammals that live a long time beyond their child-bearing years. Current statistics estimate that at least one-third of a woman's life will extend beyond the menopause. Estrogen replacement helps allay uncomfortable menopausal symptoms such as hot flashes, vaginal dryness, urine leakage, and mood swings. It also prevents osteoporosis, a devastating fragility of the bones that is especially serious in elderly women. Recent evidence indicates that estrogen may lower cholesterol and other blood fat levels and thus decrease the chance of fatal heart attack by as much as 50%.

Estrogen replacement may not be appropriate for everyone, but we believe the majority of women should receive it after menopause to maintain good health in their later years. Once started it can be maintained for many years unless a contraindication intervenes.

In 1960 oral contraceptives were approved for use by women. Their most important effect was to allow women to control the spacing of children. Many fringe benefits followed: correction of anemia; prevention of premenstrual syndrome; and a decrease in ovarian cancer and cysts and other ovary-related problems, due to the fact that oral contraceptives give the ovaries a rest by preventing ovulation.

Oral contraceptives have changed lifestyles. Unless there are specific health risks, such as smoking or deep vein blood clot formation, women can safely take the current low-dosage contraceptives through their child-bearing years all the way to the menopause. Within the next five years, at least four exciting new kinds of contraceptives will become available: (1) a birth control pill containing newly formulated progestins with fewer side effects; (2) a vaginal ring with time-released progesterone; (3) new IUDs with fewer side effects; and (4) modified subdermal implants with only two tubes instead of six.

These important advances have greatly improved women's lives. One more thing is necessary, however, and that is a commitment on the part of women to schedule an annual gynecologic examination. Annual exams identify problems before they become big problems. They make available all the advances in women's health technology. Finally, they promote wellness and a high quality of health for a lifetime.

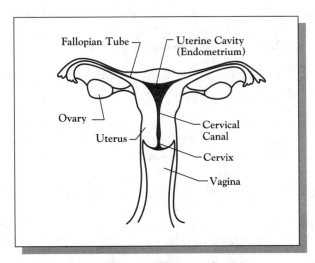

Female Reproductive Organs

Menstrual Cramps and Chronic Pelvic Pain: Treatment Alternatives

Cramps and other pelvic pain can be unpleasant and often debilitating. It may be of some small comfort to know that almost no woman goes through her reproductive years (ages 12 to 50) without some episode of lower abdominal or pelvic pain. Such discomfort may be rare, occasional, frequent, or unrelenting. It may occur only around the time of the menstrual period, or it can come and go at any time. Pelvic and lower abdominal discomfort is one of the leading causes of absenteeism from school and work. The cash value of time lost on the job, at home, and in the community due to such problems problems is enormous, in the millions of dollars. The toll it takes on women themselves is immeasurable, but surely very great.

Premenstrual symptoms such as fatigue, backache, abdominal swelling, and "the blues" can be extremely incapacitating. The extent of incapacitation both with cramps and premenstrual syndrome varies greatly and is often unpredictable. Severe symptoms during the week before menstruation have been associated with an increased rate of suicide attempts, acute psychiatric illness, violent crimes, and accidental deaths *(See Chapter 2, Premenstrual Syndrome)*.

Chronic pelvic pain poses another set of problems. Unsuccessful medical treatment, frustration, and loss of sleep can lead to desperate measures, such as hysterectomy, which, many times does not help. Years of disability, suffering, unemployment, divorce, and social withdrawal can go by while relief from pelvic pain remains unattainable.

Menstrual Cramps
History of Menstrual Pain Treatment

Pain associated with menstruation has challenged physicians throughout the ages. The ancient Greeks described the painkilling effects of sweet wine, fennel root, and rose oil when applied to the external genitals of menstruating women. Hippocrates, the father of modern medicine, said that obstruction of the cervix and retaining of menstrual fluids caused painful menstruation. For a long time many physicians believed this concept and practiced dilation of the cervix to relieve menstrual pain. Chinese women were treated with moxibustion, a technique in which a cone of wormwood was rolled into a giant cigar, placed on a ginger slice at a specific point on the abdomen, ignited, and allowed to burn until the skin became reddened and heated.

In the mid 1800s removal of both ovaries became a popular remedy for menstrual distress. At the turn of the century a number of plant extracts and synthetic chemicals were used, with opium being the most popular.

Not until 1930 did physicians begin to get some idea of what really caused menstrual distress: they noted the connection between menstrual pain and ovulation and shortly after that began to treat dysmenorrhea (painful menstruation) with estrogens to block ovulation. Following their introduction in the late 1950s, oral contraceptives became the favored treatment for menstrual disorders. It wasn't until the mid 1960s that another breakthrough occurred - the discovery of the relationship between prostaglandins and menstrual pain.

Prostaglandins are a kind of hormone produced in certain parts of the nervous system and many other areas of the body, including the lining of the uterus, where they are found in abundance. In the early 1970s researchers realized that aspirin and similar compounds inhibited prostaglandin formation. Women had been taking aspirin to relieve menstrual distress for years, and research revealed that it had some effectiveness as a prostaglandin inhibitor. Many new drugs that were developed in the 1970s proved to be much more effective than aspirin. Currently, doctors feel that further refinement of these prostaglandin-inhibiting drugs will provide an even better means of controlling dysmenorrhea in the future.

The Cause of Menstrual Cramps

From time to time most women will have episodes of dull, intermittent lower abdominal cramps just prior to or during the first few days of their period. The pattern does not appear to change, even after pregnancy, but it does diminish with age.

The uterus is continually contracting, and menstrual cramps are simply stronger, more frequent versions of these same contractions. What causes the contractions to intensify during menstruation? The culprits are the prostaglandins discussed above. Prostaglandins concentrate in the uterus after ovulation and reach their peak at the onset of menstruation, after which they are discharged in the menstrual flow. By causing the muscle of the uterus to tighten, the prostaglandins inhibit oxygen supplied to the uterus through the blood vessels. Any muscle that is deprived of oxygen will be painful, as long-distance runners and cramp sufferers know only too well.

The discovery of prostaglandins shifted much of the thinking about menstrual pain and cramps. Before that many physicians and lay people thought menstrual pain was a psychological problem as much as anything. Now the physical cause of dysmenorrhea is established. Psychological factors cannot be entirely discounted, however, because menstruation is so intimately connected with a woman's sexuality and, by extension, her relationship with her primary sexual partner or mate.

Menstrual cramps caused by prostaglandin production have a fairly specific pattern of occurrence. Usually they start shortly after release of the egg from the ovary and get worse until the menstrual flow begins. They are most intense just before the onset of a period. Menstrual pain that seems more erratic or can be related to emotional upsets may have its roots in psychological disturbance. Of course, diseases often start because of emotional stress but perpetuate themselves because certain physiological processes become established. Situations like these require a dual approach, with both the emotional origins and the physical problems being treated.

Current Drug Therapy

Many drugs are currently available to relieve the physiologically-based symptoms of dysmenorrhea. They act in different ways: to inhibit ovulation, to decrease prostaglandin production, or to slow down the force and frequency of uterine contractions. Side effects from these drugs must be considered along with the relief from menstrual cramping they provide.

Drugs that stop the production or synthesis of prostaglandins are called prostaglandin synthetase inhibitors (PGSIs). They are considered to be effective in 60% to 85% of women. Since prostaglandins are produced in other cells in the body, the PGSIs may prevent their production in other tissues besides the uterus, with relief of symptoms such as bowel difficulties, headache, and backache. Certain gastrointestinal side effects of these drugs do, however, limit a person's tolerance to them. The PGSI products currently marketed in the United States are listed in Table 1-1. These drugs must be taken when menstrual cramps begin. Some require a prescription; aspirin, acetaminophen (Tylenol), and ibuprofen (Motrin, Advil) do not. Aspirin and aceta-

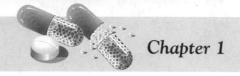

Chapter 1

minophen are not as effective in their action on the uterus as are the other PGSIs. Ibuprofen is the most effective over-the-counter drug sold for menstrual cramp relief. If over-the-counter products are not effective, a physician can write a prescription for a stronger PGSI drug.

Table 1-1	
Drugs to Treat Menstrual Pain	
Drug	**Dosages for Treatment of Dysmenorrhea**
Indolacetic acids	
indomethacin (Indocin)	25-mg capsules 3 x daily, then 50-mg capsules 3 x daily
Propionic acids Naproxen (Naprosyn)	250 mg x 2 to begin, then 250 mg every 4-6 hours
Naproxen sodium (Anaprox)	275 mg x 2 to begin, then 275 mg every 6-8 hours
Ibuprofen (Motrin)	400 mg 3 x daily
Fenoprofen (Nalfron)	200 mg every 4-6 hours
Fenamates	
Mefenamic acid (Ponstel)	250 mg x to begin, then 250 mg every 6 hours
Meclofenamate (Meclomen)	100mg 2 x daily

Women often describe severe menstrual cramps as being similar to labor pains. Extreme sufferers can be treated with the same drugs used to stop premature labor, such as terbutaline or ritodrine. Unfortunately, most of these drugs have side effects that offset their value in relieving menstrual discomfort. For example, some women may use alcohol for temporary relief of cramping and end up being addicted to it after prolonged and excessive use. We favor the prostaglandin-inhibiting drugs discussed above over these other options, because they are less likely to cause unfavorable side effects or dependencies.

Evidence suggests that a deficiency of magnesium accounts for some cases of menstrual cramps. Taking magnesium oxide pills in doses of 100 mg four times per day corrects magnesium deficiency. We suggest that the mineral be taken through two full menstrual cycles before you decide whether it is the answer to your menstrual cramping problem. Pyridoxine (vitamin B6) is advocated by some doctors for cramps. It should be taken in daily doses of 1 to 8 25-mg pills throughout the entire menstrual cycle. If necessary, you can increase your intake to 800 mg per day immediately before or during the menstrual period. Magnesium and vitamin B6 are considered harmless in the dosages we have recommended; on the other hand, their effectiveness is not guaranteed, and more research needs to be done on their role in relieving menstrual pain.

The drugs that relieve menstrual cramps most predictably, for the longest amount of time are the oral contraceptives. By stopping ovulation (See Chapter 12), they prevent the formation of high levels of prostaglandins because the lining of the uterus is thinner. Birth control pills that contain higher amounts of progestin and lower quantities of estrogen are the best to use. A progestin-only pill sometimes helps but may cause more menstrual irregularities than do pills that also contain estrogen. A woman should allow at least a 3-month trial on any pill she uses for menstrual problem relief before deciding whether it is effective. Understandably, most women are reluctant to take hormone pills for menstrual discomfort unless their problem is severe. The same guidelines that are outlined in Chapter 12 apply in this situation: if a woman is otherwise in good health, not substantially overweight, and a nonsmoker, she stands to gain much more than she loses by using oral contraceptives to relieve menstrual pain, regardless of her age.

Other Types of Menstrual Cramp-Like Pelvic Pain

Menstrual cramps due to prostaglandin overload are by no means the only source of pelvic-reproductive organ discomfort. Disorders that tend to be long-standing or chronic include endometriosis - discussed in detail in Chapter 3 - (islands or clusters of endometrial tissue that have somehow escaped the interior of the uterus and migrated to other areas of the abdomen where they swell and recede along with with hormone changes); ovarian cysts or tumors; uterine tumors; adhesions (thin, fibrous bands around the fallopian tubes or ovaries caused by prior pelvic infections or surgery); retroflexed uterus (backward displacement of the uterus); congestion or engorging of the uterine blood vessels; or persistent infections of the uterus, tubes, and ovaries.

Each of these forms of pelvic discomfort represents a different kind of challenge both to the woman, her nurses, and to her doctor. With the tools and drugs available to physicians today, most of them can be diagnosed and treated satisfactorily. In a few cases, surgery may be the best choice, particularly when all other options have been exhausted.

Chronic Pelvic Pain

A large proportion of women visiting gynecologists seek relief from pelvic pain that has been present for months or even years but has eluded medical diagnosis (the number ranges from 2-15% of all gynecologist's visits). If this problem exists, the doctor will need to take a thorough history to find out if the pain has been continuous or intermittent, where it is located, how it relates to urination and bowel movements, whether there have been any vaginal infections, if it occurs during sexual activity, and how it relates to different kinds of stress. Along with a review of past medical, obstetrical, and surgical history, he or she will perform a complete abdominal and pelvic examination. Such an examination, which is done under anesthesia in the operating room, could very well include the technique called *diagnostic laparoscopy*. This slender tube, which is inserted into the abdomen, functions as a kind of telescope that can uncover problems which otherwise might elude the doctor. It is often used when other kinds of diagnostic tests have failed to reveal a specific problem.

Non-specific chronic pelvic pain is often given as the reason for performing a hysterectomy (surgical removal of the uterus), but in many such cases, the uterus turns out to be normal and, sadly, the problem does not go away. We believe that a woman who complains of chronic pelvic pain needs a comprehensive and systematic approach to her problem that addresses the many complexities that can contribute to chronic pelvic pain, before she resorts to surgery. Following is a list of the problems that are often associated with chronic pelvic pain and can either cause or contribute to it:

- Previous nongynecologic surgery in the abdominal area
- More frequent than normal history of spontaneous abortion (miscarriage)
- Multiple sexual partners

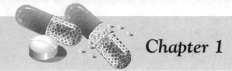

- Seven times more likely to have experienced sexual abuse in childhood
- Co-existing gastrointestinal disease
- Co-existing urinary tract disease
- Presence of abdominal wall "trigger points"(sensitive nerves outside the abdomen around its muscles)
- Infection
- An ovary that is fixed and immovable at the top of the vagina

Drug Treatment

Management of chronic pelvic pain of uncertain origin can be difficult, but it is not impossible. One of the first approaches we recommend is a program of scheduled dosages of prostaglandin inhibitors (i.e., Motrin, Advil, Naprosyn, Ponstel). This is in contrast to using these drugs for control of menstrual discomfort, which is based on a response to the appearance of symptoms. In cases of chronic pelvic pain, such drugs may be more effective if they are put to work before symptoms appear. These drugs occasionally create gastrointestinal upsets or even ulcers, but some new products which are easier on the digestive system have reached the market. One of these is a pain reliever called diclofenac sodium (Voltaren). It is also possible to take another drug, called misoprostol (Cytotec), in conjunction with one of the well-known pain-killers; Cytotec decreases the risk of ulcers when you must use one of the pain-killers associated with ulcers.

If they can be localized, abdominal wall neural "trigger points" may be amenable to a variety of treatments. These include transcutaneous electric nerve stimulation (TENS), acupuncture, and injection of local anesthetic agents or steroids or both into the trigger points.

When chronic pelvic pain can be traced to ovulation (and this is done by keeping "pain calendars," where the days of the month when pain occurs are recorded carefully), drugs that suppress ovulation may be helpful. These are the same drugs that are used to treat endometriosis *(See Chapter 3)*.

"Functional" bowel disorders can be the source of severe abdominal pain. Such problems are different from gastrointestinal disease because, although there is actually nothing wrong with the intestinal tract, there can be pain, diarrhea, and constipation, i.e., problems with gastrointestinal function. One way to treat both constipation and diarrhea is by adding fiber to the diet, either in drug form (Metamucil, Fiberall) or in the diet (oat bran, vegetables, legumes). Diarrhea can also be relieved by Imodium or Lomotil. Imodium is now available over-the-counter in liquid form. Since functional bowel disorders sometimes result from emotional stress, counseling or psychotherapy is another avenue of treatment.

Psychoactive drugs can play a role in treating functional bowel discomfort or other types of pelvic pain. Anti-anxiety medications may help with functional bowel problems, while anti-depressants are sometimes effective in helping women cope with pelvic pain. Among the anti-depressant drugs used for pelvic pain, imipramine, amtriptyline, and Doxepin have been found to provide relief. Doctors have discovered that sometimes they can prescribe much lower dosages of these drugs for pain relief (25-75 mg at bedtime) than is needed for control of depression symptoms.

Vulvar vestibulitis is another cause of chronic pelvic pain. Its location is usually on the outside of the mid-vagina, toward the rectum. Biopsy reports from this area yield a 50%

incidence of human papilloma virus *(See Chapter 10, AIDS, Herpes and Warts)*. When vulvar vestibulitis is present, characteristically, the woman cannot have intercourse because it feels like a knife is being inserted in her vagina. Diagnosis of this problem can be made when the doctor looks through a special type of microscope called a colposcope aimed at the external genitals and vulva. He or she will often note a "cobblestone" appearance to the tissue.

Drug therapy aimed at extinguishing the papilloma may help, and if it doesn't, surgery becomes necessary. This consists of taking out the affected tissue, and then pulling down the vagina over the area with special surgical techniques. After 6 to 8 months, the chances of recovery are 70% to 80%.

Chronic urethral syndrome is another unusual - but not unheard of - cause of pelvic pain. This problem may be treatable with antibiotics or with dilation of the urethra (tube through which urine passes from the bladder).

Finally, although not common among women with chronic pelvic pain, subacute (low-level) hidden infections can be responsible for symptoms. If such an infection is present, it is likely to be located high in the reproductive tract (i.e., in the tubes), and caused by chlamydia. This problem is treatable with a course of antibiotics such as doxycycline. Table 1-2 lists drugs recommended for the treatment of chronic pelvic pain.

Table 1-2
Drug Therapy for Chronic Pelvic Pain: Summary of Selected Agents

Indication	Generic (Trade)	Dosage
Analgesia[*]	Ibuprofen (Motrin)	400-800 mg every 6-8 hour
	Naproxen (Naproxsyn)	250-500 mg every 6-8 hour
	Naproxen sodium (Anaprox)	275-500 mg every 6-8 hours
	Mefenamic acid (Ponstel)	250-500 mg every 6-8 hours
Local anesthetic (trigger points)	Bupivicaine (Marcaine)	0.25-0.5%, 5-10 cc
	Lidocaine (Xylocaine)	1.0-2.0%, 5-10 cc
Ovarian cycle suppression[†]	(Demulen 1/50)	"As directed"
	(Ovral 1/50)	"As directed"
	Medroxyprogesterone (Provera)	20-40 mg daily
	Depomedroxyprogesterone (Depo-Provera)	150-300 mg injected every 2-3mos.
Functional bowel, disorders[‡]	Psyllium mucilloid (Metamucil, Fiberall)	2 tbsp daily with water or juice
	Loperamide (Imodium)	2.5-5.0 mg 4 x daily
	Diphenoxylate/atropine (Lomotil)	2 mg every 1-3 hours up to 16 mg daily
Tricyclic antidepressants[§]	Imipramine (Tofranil)	25-75 mg at bedtime
	Amitriptyline (Elavil)	25-75 mg at bedtime
	Doxepin (Sinequan)	25-75 mg at bedtime

* Recommended on a scheduled rather than on as-needed basis.
†May be used cyclically or continuosly as indicated.
‡ Use antidirrheals only after confirming the diagnosis.
§ Dosages are for chronic pain and sleep disorders.

Surgery

Pelvic pain is one of the most frustrating complaints physicians encounter, and when we have exhausted every other possibility, diagnostic surgery may be needed.

Before surgery, while the woman is fully anesthetized, the doctor performs a thorough pelvic examination. If no obvious problem surfaces, he or she usually dilates the cervix and lightly scrapes the uterus. This procedure is the well-known D&C (dilatation and curettage). The long, tubelike laparoscope, is then inserted just below the navel to permit the doctor to actually see the ovaries, tubes, uterus, and the outside walls of the bladder and bowel. At this time the doctor can obtain fluids for culture of any infectious organisms or a piece of tissue for biopsy or break up any scar tissue that might be causing problems.

Sometimes the source of the pelvic pain will be unveiled during exploration with the laparoscope, and more extensive surgery or stronger drug therapy will be indicated.

If no solution is found, then the search must continue, with perhaps another trial period of medications or further examination of problems such as sexual dysfunction, marital discord, fears, or phobias. We do not believe that the nerves which carry pain from the pelvic region should be severed or that organs like the uterus or ovaries should be removed just because no other answer can be found. Experience has taught us that the role of surgery in curing chronic pelvic pain is quite limited, although certain disorders such as vulvar vestibulitis can be dealt with surgically. Occasionally an injection of local anesthetic through the vagina and into the cervix may help with acutely painful episodes. Hypnosis, biofeedback, and relaxation techniques have also been used with varying degrees of success. Nowadays there are clinics that specialize in the treatment of pain, and referrals to such centers may also be another path to follow in the management of this difficult problem.

Case Study

Erin C, a small, serious 22-year-old graduate research assistant, had had nearly incapacitating menstrual cramps and pelvic pain since the age of 13. She suffered nausea, cramping, bloating, and extreme frustration with each succeeding menstrual period. In between periods she suffered episodes of cramping and shooting abdominal pain. Her chronic pain had prevented her from ever becoming involved in a sexual relationship.

For years she used aspirin to relieve the pain associated with her period, but it was not terribly helpful. One of the many gynecologists she had seen prescribed Ponstel for her, and she found the Ponstel to be more helpful than aspirin, although it by no means solved her entire problem.

She finally met a gynecologist who specialized in the treatment of chronic pelvic pain. A pelvic examination revealed a vague tenderness and feeling of fullness near her right ovary. Erin's new doctor suggested birth control pills to see if they would help her discomfort. She refused, saying she was afraid of subjecting her body to synthetic hormones.

Six months later Erin was at the doctor's office again. In the time that had elapsed she had become sexually active, and much of the time found intercourse to be quite painful. Determined to get to the bottom of her problem, she asked her doctor if she would perform a laparotomy, and she reluctantly agreed. With Erin under general anesthesia, the doctor looked into her abdomen with a laparoscope. She saw nothing unusual, except a slightly

---

Key Points for Pelvic Pain

1. Recurring or persistent pelvic pain is a common reason for a young or middle-aged woman to be absent from school or work and ultimately to seek medical attention. Since this can be a complex problem with multiple causes, her medical, sexual, and emotional history should be carefully considered, when addressing the problem.

2. The relationship of pain and premenstrual symptoms to the menstrual cycle is important to determine. Before visiting a doctor one should keep a "pain calendar," a daily diary of these symptoms, noting when they occur, what they occur in conjunction with, and what relieves or worsens your discomfort.

3. At present, the prostaglandin synthetase inhibitor (PGSI) drugs and birth control pills are the most consistently effective ways to relieve menstrual cramps and long-standing pelvic pain. Other drugs used to treat menstrual cramps may include unpleasant side effects, which vary greatly from person to person.

4. Chronic pelvic pain is usually unrelated to the menstrual cycle. It can be caused by a variety of problems, such as scar tissue, tumors, cysts, infection of any of the female organs, diseases of the nearby bowel or bladder, or emotional problems. If painkillers, antibiotics, or hormones do not work, psychotherapy or counseling may be necessary.

5. Pelvic pain is a major reason for a physician to perform a diagnostic laparoscopy procedure. Laparoscopy is a safe, quick operation done while the woman is under general anesthesia. Unless there are very specific medical reasons, removing the uterus or ovaries or cutting the nerve that transmits pelvic pain is not justified in treating it.

6. Women may become discouraged because pelvic pain does not disappear after certain kinds of treatment have been initiated, but they should continue to work with a sympathetic physician toward exploring the cause and finding effective forms of treatment. Problems related to alcoholism, stress, marital discord, or sexual difficulties can play a role and should be discussed openly.

Chapter 2

Premenstrual Syndrome

Once, when women had "moods" or difficulty controlling their emotions, it was attributed to their being the "weaker sex". Our grandmothers retired to their bedrooms, and our grandfathers were taught to be gentlemen and tiptoe around the house during such times. Then the pendulum swung and, during the feminist movement of the 1960s and 1970s, such mood changes were denied entirely. Women declared that they were strong and certainly not the victims of mere hormones. Female anger was due to political outrage, not estrogen.

What a surprise when one day we picked up the newspaper to read about suicides, violent crimes, even murders, committed by women who claimed to be suffering from something called *premenstrual syndrome*. A nagging suspicion held by some women - that at certain times of the month the world took on a blacker and uglier look - was turning out to be headlines.

Premenstrual syndrome or PMS, as it is popularly called, went from being the problem that no one was sure existed to the disease that got blamed for almost everything. Husbands and kids dived for cover when mom had PMS. Colleagues at work marked their calendars so they could stay out of the way on "those days". Women finally began to realize that they weren't crazy, they simply had PMS.

Physicians have now begun to do research on PMS to see just what this mythical disorder is all about. We still don't know a lot about the cause of PMS, but we do know what it does. There is no drug that will cure premenstrual syndrome, but we have some tools for managing the problem. With a little trial and error, we can help many women feel better on those difficult days.

What is PMS?

PMS is a cluster of symptoms that occur at a particular time each month known as the *luteal phase* of the menstrual cycle. The luteal phase comes after ovulation, on or around the fourteenth day before the next period begins. PMS seems to be more common in women between 30 and 50, but it can occur at any age when a woman menstruates. Severe symptoms affect from 5% to 10% of all women of reproductive age. (In the United States alone, this is represents millions of individuals!). At least 20% of women have some annoying symptoms caused by PMS. Some doctors feel that PMS is more prevalent in women who also suffer from depressive illnesses.

PMS goes away temporarily during menstruation and forever upon reaching menopause. It will not occur unless ovulation occurs, so there are no PMS symptoms during the 14 days prior to ovulation. If there are PMS symptoms during this time frame then it's something else, not PMS. The disease has a wide range of intensity, especially when it comes to the emotions. Some women feel mildly grumpy or weepy, while others feel great sadness or anger.

Doctors have identified four major groups of symptoms in premenstrual syndrome:

1. **Physical symptoms**. These include bloating, breast tenderness, fatigue, headaches, backaches, and weight gain.

2. **Emotional symptoms**. Commonly, these include irritability, mood swings, crying, depression, sensitivity, and hostility.

3. **Cognitive symptoms**. These include difficulty concentrating, loss of memory, difficulty making decisions.

4. **Behavioral symptoms**. Typical examples are insomnia, withdrawal, abusive behavior, overeating.

Symptom relief is the major goal in the treatment of PMS. Women with PMS can have several symptoms from any of the symptom groups. For minor symptoms, diet and lifestyle alterations are often sufficient. For major problems, such as ongoing family conflict or the inability to work, drug therapy may be appropriate.

Menstrual Migraines

Physicians have long been puzzled by the markedly increased occurrence of migraine headaches in girls when they reach adolescence. Many in the past have attributed them to sexual anxiety or deep-seated emotional problems.

Now a physical cause has been identified, related to the changing levels of sex hormones. This phenomenon is called the <u>menstrual migraine.</u> Doctors believe that at least 60% of women with migraine headaches can attribute them, at least in part, to fluctuating amounts of estrogen in the system. Menstrual migraines occur not only during the normal menstrual cycle, but in women who are taking estrogen for contraception, menopausal symptoms, or other purposes, as well.

Typically, just before a period starts or, sometimes, about halfway through the menstrual cycle (at ovulation), women will get a migraine headache, along with nausea, mood disturbances, and ultrasensitivity to light and noise. Discomforts such as fluid retention and breast tenderness often accompany these other symptoms.

In the majority of women with menstrual migraines, the headaches can be triggered by additional things such as drinking (especially red wine), certain foods (cheese, nuts, chocolate), irregular eating, stress, or fatigue. Adding these extra "triggers" at the right time in the menstrual cycle often guarantees a menstrual migraine. Most women with menstrual migraines find relief during pregnancy and after menopause (although occasionally they will grow worse, particularly in woman who take postmenopausal estrogen).

Women who suffer from menstrual migraines need to pay attention to activities and occurrences during their menstrual cycle. One way to do so this is by keeping a headache diary. Everytime a headache begins, the victim should record all possible things done or consumed that may have aggravated it. After a few months, the diarist should be able to draw connections between the headaches and her lifestyle and make adjustments.

Physical exercise can help with menstrual migraines because it produces endorphins to offset the stress elements associated with the headaches. Some women believe sexual activity with orgasm can help to avert oncoming headaches.

Diet and Lifestyle

Two hormonal alterations are seen in women with PMS: *(1)* a decrease in the "happy hormones" known as *endorphins*, and *(2)* an increase in stress hormones known as *catecholamines*. Certain substances in foods can trigger the production of stress hormones. These substances are caffeine, nicotine, tyramine, and the amino acids (i.e., proteins) tryptophan and tyrosine.

We have found that, when women eliminate these substances from their bodies during the 7-10 days prior to their menstrual periods, they get relief from PMS symptoms about 90% of the time.

Step number 1: *Stop smoking to eliminate nicotine*. While this is always good advice, it is particularly important to control PMS symptoms because nicotine increases the levels of stress hormones. If a woman can go 10 days without a cigarette, she may be able to give them up completely.

Step number 2: *Stop consuming beverages, foods, or drugs containing caffeine*. This means giving up coffee, colas, and chocolate (unless they are decaffeinated). Check any over-the-counter drugs for caffeine content: cold remedies, "stay-awake" pills, and diet pills frequently contain caffeine.

Step number 3: *Follow the diet outlined in Table 2-1* and keep a monthly calendar of when PMS symptoms occur. The PMS sufferer will want to weigh herself daily and record those numbers on a weight chart.

Some women will find that, even with this diet, their monthly weight gain continues. If that is the case, a physician can prescribe a medication such as aldactazide or spironolactone to help eradicate salt (and thus water) retention by blocking the production of a salt-retaining hormone called aldosterone.

Since this diet leaves out some important nutrients, it should not be used all the time, just during the "PMS danger zone," 7-10 days before the menstrual period begins. In addition, we recommend taking a multi-vitamin and mineral supplement that contains folic acid, iron, zinc, and magnesium on the days the anti-PMS diet is followed. Other nutritional supplements have been recommended by some researchers. These are listed in Table 2-2.

Note: *This diet was developed by Dr. Zuspan. He has noted improvement in emotional and other central nervous system symptoms in up to 90% of cases of PMS he has treated. The diet has never been scientifically tested in a prospective, randomized study.*

Exercise increases your endorphin level. A daily exercise program during the PMS days such as fast walking for 45 minutes, swimming or biking for 30 minutes, jazzercise, low-impact aerobics, or yoga are all good ways to get the endorphins pumping.

Perhaps one of the most helpful hints is to simply be aware of your PMS days and what's likely to happen during them. Knowing that feelings of sadness or resentment are temporary and not really "you," can go a long way towards helping you deal with them effectively.

Avoid situations that generate tension or conflict. An evening at the movies or at the park with the kids rather than subjecting oneself to business and household stress often helps alleviate the pain and discomfort. Fasting has been reported to worsen PMS symptoms, so this practice should be avoided.

Give the diet and lifestyle program four months to work. Keep track of weight, relationships, sleep and work habits. If things don't improve a physician contact is necessary. There are a number of medications that can help PMS symptoms. These are discussed below.

Medical Management of PMS

Research based on recent clinical trials has uncovered a number of drugs with promising results in the treatment of PMS. However, because this research is fairly new, most of the drugs available to treat it may not yet be approved by the Food and Drug Administration for treatment of PMS. However, most of them have been approved for other purposes and are available by prescription. We expect that a number of them will be FDA approved in the near future.

Drugs to Help with Fluid Retention

Fluid retention seems to be among the most common of luteal phase premenstrual symptoms. Although fluid retention has never been carefully researched, diuretics (pills that cause you to urinate, thus helping to remove extra fluids from the body) are among the most widely prescribed drugs for PMS. Among the newer drugs for handling fluid retention are chlorthiazide and spironolactone.

Prostaglandin Synthetase Inhibitors

Prostaglandins are a special type of hormone made by the body's nervous system when it is put under stress. Prostaglandins appear both prior to and during menstruation. When prostaglandin production is inhibited, stress, pain, and other types of discomfort may be relieved.

The prostaglandin synthetase inhibitors include mefenamic acid (Ponstel) and naproxen (Naprosyn), both of which have been widely used in the treatment of menstrual pain. New research has found that these two drugs help with irritability and depression, headache, back pain, cramping, and muscle aches associated with PMS. Ibuprofen (Motrin, Advil, Nuprin) also falls into this category of drugs and is suggested for the treatment of PMS. Ibuprofen is available over-the-counter, but check with a physician for the proper dosage to treat PMS symptoms.

Tranquilizers

The anxiolytic (or anti-anxiety) drug class appears to have beneficial effects in treating the emotional symptoms associated with PMS. Alprazolam (Xanax) and buspirone are two of the drugs that are being tested for anxiety associated with PMS. Buspirone seems preferable because it has fewer side effects, such as drowsiness. Table 2-3 lists more drugs currently being used to treat emotional distress associated with PMS.

Anti-depressants

Several years ago, physicians looked into the usefulness of lithium, a popular drug, for treating mood disorders, such as occur with PMS. Having found that lithium didn't help, they gave up on this drug class. Now two new anti-depressants, nortriptyline (Pamelor) and fluoxetine (Prozac) are showing some promise for treating the depression that comes with premenstrual syndrome. Recent studies on Prozac have reinforced early findings showing it to be helpful with PMS-related depression.

Hormones

In most cases, hormones used to treat PMS stop ovulation, as birth control pills do. With this form of treatment, a woman is unable to get pregnant. However, other types of hormone therapy have been found to be effective in reducing PMS symptoms, usually without preventing ovulation. These include oral micronized progesterone and Danazol. Some physicians believe that progesterone has a kind of sedative effect and acts as both an anti-anxiety and anti-depressant agent. While Danazol (a drug now being used to treat endometriosis) is very expensive, in some women daily 200 mg doses taken after ovulation have helped with aggravating PMS symptoms.

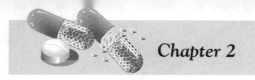

Oral contraceptives are popularly prescribed for premenstrual syndrome. In some cases they seem to help (which is logical because they suppress ovulation), but in other cases, unexplainably, they actually seem to make matters worse.

Medroxyprogesterone (Provera) and megestrol acetate (Megace), two progestins (synthetic progesterones) are sometimes prescribed for PMS symptoms. These drugs have the advantage of being relatively inexpensive, and they are not associated with long-term side effects. Unfortunately, they have not proved to be very effective either.

Danazol, in doses used to suppress ovulation, has been found to significantly reduce breast pain, irritability, anxiety, and grogginess in PMS sufferers. On the down side, Danazol is very expensive, and it also has negative effects on high-density lipoproteins (fats found in the bloodstream). For women who are trying to keep fat and cholesterol levels low, Danazol may not be a good choice. Danazol also causes fluid retention and consequent weight gain.

Gonadotropin-releasing hormone agonist is another new method of ovulation suppression that has shown promise in a small number of women for relieving both the physical and emotional symptoms of PMS. However, this form of therapy must be offset by hormone replacement of both estrogen and progestin, and it is also *very* expensive.

When Should Drug Therapy Be Considered?

PMS does not lead to death or disability. Therefore, doctors are primarily concerned with relieving its symptoms and making women more comfortable. Because any medication prescribed will have side effects on both the body and the pocketbook, we believe that women should try to alter their diet and lifestyle before resorting to drugs to treat PMS. We advise our patients to keep track of symptoms on a calendar for four months before prescribing a particular drug, so that we (and they) know for sure that the source of the problem is PMS and not something else - unless, of course, her symptoms are very severe.

Care is required on the part of the woman and her physician to choose the drug that will most closely address the problems she experiences and to continually assess the effects of the drug therapy to assure that the right prescription has been written. Table 2-3 lists drugs used for treating emotional symptoms of PMS.

Case Study

Janet T was a 36 year-old accountant who had had a tubal ligation following the birth of her second child 7 years previous. For the past three years she had noticed a progressively worsening set of symptoms beginning a week to 10 days before her period. She was irritable and cried at the slightest provocation. She experienced emotional "lows," where she questioned what she was doing with her life. She found it difficult to work during this time, and worried that she was not doing a good job. On the first day of her period, the symptoms rapidly disappeared, and she was fine until the premenstrual period next month.

In addition to the emotional ups and downs, Janet gained 5 or 6 pounds in the week before her period and felt bloated. She and her physician discussed the problem, including its strong impact on her husband and children, and decided something had to be done.

Key Points for PMS

1. Premenstrual syndrome is a cluster of physical, behavioral, and emotional symptoms occurring during the 7-10 day period before menstruation.

2. Some women experience relatively mild symptoms, while others find PMS almost disabling.

3. Diet and lifestyle alterations are the first route for treating the symptoms of PMS. The PMS diet may be very useful, but should be followed only during the 7-10 day premenstrual period and supplemented with vitamins.

4. Physicians are studying the effects of a number of drugs to treat PMS. These include diuretics, prostaglandin inhibitors, hormones, ovulation suppressors, anti-anxiety drugs, and anti-depressants.

5. Before resorting to drugs, women should carefully chart their symptoms to verify that they really suffer from PMS, as well as trying dietary adjustments, exercise, and behavioral modification techniques.

Table 2-1
An Anti-PMS Diet*

Note:
1. Carefully measure the amounts eaten.
2. It's acceptable to use a small amount of salt when cooking, but no additional salt should be used at the table·
3. Avoid processed meats, canned soups, and pickled items.
4. Avoid things that come out of bottles and cans, since they are usually preserved with sodium (salt).

Food Group	Include	Avoid
Milk and Cheese	One small serving a day of: 3/4 cup milk, 3/4 oz. processed cheese, **plus** liquid non-dairy creamer (if desired on cereal or desserts)	Larger amounts of included foods Other cheeses and dairy products, especially aged cheeses

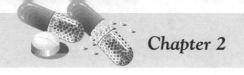

Table 2-1 (continued)		
Meats and Meat Substitutes	**Group I -** 1 choice per day: Cream cheese, 3 tbsp. , Bacon, 2 strips, Peanut butter, 1 tbsp., Egg, 1 small	Chicken, turkey, veal; salted, pickled fish, such as herring; liver; canned meat or fish
	Group II - 1 small serving per day (2 oz): Beef, lamb, fresh pork, Fresh fish (cod, flounder, halibut, haddock, shrimp) Dried beans, 3/4 cup	
Potatoes and Rice	1 serving per day (1/2 cup): 1 medium potato **or** 1/2 cup rice **or** 1 oz. unsalted potato chips	
Fruits and Juices	1 serving (1 fruit or 1/2 juice)	Avocado, bananas, figs, red plums
Vegetables	1 serving (1/2 cup) of: Asparagus, green beans, beets, cabbage, carrots, celery, cucumber, eggplant lettuce, small onion, pumpkin, radishes, summer squash, tomato	Italian broad beans, butter beans, lima beans, broccoli, cauliflower, corn, peas, cowpeas, spinach
Grains, Breads and Cereals	1 serving (1 slice or 1 cup) White bread, crackers with unsalted tops (6), pretzels unsalted (20 sticks), cereal (puffed rice or rice flakes, cornflakes and oatflakes, oatmeal)	Whole grain bread, crackers, whole grain cereals; bread or crackers with cheese; homemade breads with lots of yeast; macaroni, noodles or spaghetti
Fats and Oils	1 serving = 1 teaspoon Butter, margarine, oil, shortening or salad dressing	

Table 2-1 (continued)		
Desserts	Fruit ices using gelatin and juices, plain or fruit-filled gelatin (1/2 cup); shortbread or sugar cookies (3); fruit pie (no eggs); tapioca made with fruit juice, allowed milk or non-dairy creamer (1/2 cup)	Chocolate, nuts, bread, pudding, custard, angel food cake, sponge cake, macaroons, cake, pudding (unless as substitute for milk)
Beverages	Juice, milk (as allowed), water, fruit drinks, lemonade, carbonated beverages (without caffeine)	Coffee, tea, chocolate, alcohol (wine, sherry beer, ale, colas and many soft drinks
Miscellaneous		Meat tenderizer, soy sauce, yeast, concentrate, vanilla, soup cubes, commercial gravies and meat extracts. All foods and beverages sweetened with Nutrasweet. Chinese and Japanese food.

* This diet was developed by Dr. Zuspan, and has been used successfully for relief of PMS symptoms that involve the central nervous system in many of his patients. It has never been scientifically tested in a prospective, randomized study.

Table 2-2
Nutritional Supplements Used for PMS

Supplement	Dosage	Cost per cycle
Calcium	1,000 mg elemental calcium daily	less than $5
Pyridoxine (Vitamin B6)	50-100 mg daily	less than $5
Optivite	6 tablets/day during luteal phase	$20.00
Vitamin E	400 IU daily	less than $5
Evening primrose oil	500 mg, 3x daily during luteal phase	$35.00

Table 2-3
Drugs for Treating Emotional Symptoms of PMS

Name	Dose	Luteal (L) or Daily (D)	Wholesale cost per cycle
Spironolactone	100 mg/day	L	$2-$11
Mefenamic acid	500 mg/3x per day	L	$24
Naproxen	550 mg/3x per day	L	$38
Micronized progesterone	100 mg in a.m., 200 mg in p.m.	L	$22*
Danazol	200 mg	L	$22-$29
Alprazolam	.25 mg/3x per day	L	$17
Buspirone	10 mg/2x per day	L	$22
Nortriptyline	75 mg at night+	D	$45
Fluoxetine	20 mg in a.m.	D	$47

+ The initial dose should be 10 to 25 mg and then increased by 25 mg until relief of symptoms is achieved.
*Retail price

Notes

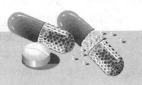

Endometriosis: Old and New Drug Therapies

Gynecologists have tried for a long time to understand endometriosis, but what it is, why it happens, and how to cure it remain an enigma. Technically, *endometriosis* is defined as the presence of tissue from the inside of the uterus (such as endometrial glands and surrounding structures called stroma) found outside its normal environment, the lining of the uterus.

Endometriosis is common. We find it in 30% to 50% of women who go in for infertility evaluations. In major operations done on women in their reproductive years, it enters into the diagnosis at least 35% of the time. It is believed to be present in approximately 15% of all women between 15 and 44 years of age, regardless of racial background. Paradoxically, many women with a substantial degree of endometriosis have no symptoms, while others with very little endometrial tissue outside the uterus have severe symptoms. In one large study, only 21% of the women diagnosed with endometriosis complained of uncomfortable symptoms or infertility. Physicians have wondered about this for years but have not been able to explain it.

The cause is still unknown too, although many physicians believe it is caused by retrograde menstruation, that is, menstrual fluids and tissues backing up through the fallopian tubes and working their way into the abdominal cavity rather than exiting through their normal route of escape, the cervix and then the vagina. Endometrial cells are very easy to grow in tissue culture and the warm, nourishing environment of a women's pelvic cavity provides a perfect growth chamber. Endometriosis may also be spread through the bloodstream because it has been found outside of the pelvis in places like the bowel, the lungs, and even the brain.

Although transplanted outside the uterus, endometrial tissue still responds to the same hormonal messages it did when it was inside. When the lining of the uterus goes through certain cyclic changes, then the glands and stroma, regardless of where they are located, also go through similar changes even to the point where they bleed. When gynecologists examine the pelvic cavity of a woman with endometriosis through a laparascope, they can see "powder burn lesions" and "chocolate" fluid, especially on the ovary, which are caused by old bleeds. The bleeding itself causes an inflammatory reaction with some adhesion formation and scar production.

Symptoms and Diagnosis

Endometriosis usually comes to our attention when a woman is suffering severe, menstrual pelvic pain or when she cannot get pregnant. Severe pain may also be associated with intercourse.

The most common location for endometriosis is an area called the *cul-de-sac*, a closed space below the ligaments that hold the uterus in position. Another common spot is in or on the ovaries. When endometriosis invades the ovary, it is called *endometrioma*.

Diagnosis of endometriosis during a pelvic examination is difficult, unless it is very severe and widespread. The gynecologist must normally do a laparoscopy to verify its presence. Since many of the therapy regimens for endometriosis are expensive and time-consuming, it is important that the diagnosis be clear-cut. Recently the use of transvaginal ultrasound has added to the gynecologist's ability to diagnose endometriosis, especially in the ovary. This tool, however, by no means replaces direct inspection of the entire pelvic cavity with the laparoscope, it is merely an addition.

Following these tests, gynecologists often do a biopsy of suspicious-looking tissue, which will reveal endometrial glands and stroma if active endometriosis is present. At times the endometriosis may be old, scarred, and fibrous, in which case the glands will not be seen.

A laboratory test known as CA-125 will show higher values than normal at least 50% of the time when endometriosis is present. This test is also used to screen for ovarian cancer.

Treatment

Treatment of endometriosis can be very complicated and take a long time. The gynecologist must first determine the answers to several questions: Is the woman experiencing pain with her endometriosis? Is she having difficulty becoming pregnant when she wants to? How soon does she want to become pregnant? Should therapy be hormonal or surgical? What are the advantages and disadvantages of both, given the circumstances of the individual patient? If hormonal therapy is chosen, which drug and what dosage should be used, and for how long? Should supplementary surgery be done as well? Is the endometriosis severe enough to even be treated?

The most common first solution, especially when infertility is the complaint, is one known as *expectant management.* Although this sounds to some like watching and doing nothing, what it really means is that a careful search for other things that might cause infertility is made before any specific therapy for endometriosis is given. Studies have indicated that minimal or mild endometriosis does not really affect a woman's ability to get pregnant, and that neither hormone therapy nor surgery targeted at allaying endometriosis is very effective in these circumstances. Expectant management is not appropriate in cases where the woman has moderate to severe endometriosis or if she is suffering pain.

Hormones

The goal when giving hormones for endometriosis is to cause the endometrial tissue outside the uterus (also called endometrial implants) to shrink. This happens when the tissue is deprived of the hormone flow it needs to swell and grow. The most common form of hormone therapy for endometriosis is the birth control pill *(See Chapter 12).* Oral contraceptives with a higher progestin-to-estrogen ratio are desirable, especially for young women under 35 who are not complaining about pain. We recommend that oral contraceptive treatment for endometriosis continue for a minimum of 6 months. Table 3-1 lists the various agents used for hormonal control of endometriosis and also cites other forms of treatment.

Progestins (synthetic progesterone) are relatively inexpensive and have fewer side effects than some of the other drugs prescribed for endometriosis. Some women do experience bleeding between periods and depression when using progestins.

Danazol, a drug that creates a kind of artificial menopause, has been used for endometriosis treatment for several years. While it is effective in shrinking the endometrial implants, danazol has some strong side effects because it is made of a synthetic male hormone that suppresses the female hormones. More than 80% of women who take it experience masculinizing effects such as facial hair growth, weight gain, or acne.

New on the market within the last couple of years is a group of drugs called the Gonadotropic releasing hormone (GnRH) analogs. Going under the trade names, Lupron, Lupron Depot, and Synarel, these drugs also create a type of artificial menopause - a medical equivalent of having the ovaries removed. These drugs have side effects too, but they are more like menopause (i.e., hot flashes, palpitations, dry vagina, mood swings), and women may be more willing to put up with menopausal-type symptoms than with the problems created by danazol. The latest medical studies indicate that the GnRh analogues are just as effective as danazol in the treatment of endometriosis. Not yet available for prescription is a new GnRH analog called Zoladex that can be implanted under the skin of the abdomen to release small, quantities of the drug over a month's time. This convenient time-released method requires that women come in once a month for six months to have their Zoladex implant, a slender 1.5" long rod resembling a piece of spaghetti, inserted rather than having to use nose drops every day.

Finally, tamoxifen, an estrogen-suppressing hormonal drug, presents another option for endometriosis management. While it has few side effects compared with danazol and the GnRH analogs, it sometimes creates a paradoxical effect and overstimulates (instead of understimulating) the ovaries. Tamoxifen is currently being used in the treatment of post-menopausal women with breast cancer, as well.

Surgery

The laparoscope is an instrument used for treatment as well as diagnosis of endometriosis. Sometimes, when he or she sees the endometrial implants with the laparascope, the gynecologist can vaporize them with a laser. In addition, surgically cutting the sacro-uterine ligaments (cordlike structures that help hold the uterus in place) may relieve some of the pain associated with endometriosis, because pain fibers are located in these ligaments. Both of these procedures can be done in an outpatient surgery unit, with the patient going home the same day.

In certain, more severe cases of endometriosis, a woman may have to undergo abdominal surgery to remove her endometrial implants and suspend the uterus if it is tipped backwards (a condition known as retroverted uterus). The last resort for endometriosis which doesn't respond to drugs and which continues to cause major discomfort is a hysterectomy and bilateral salpingo-oophorectomy, meaning removal of the uterus and both ovaries, as well as all the culprit endometrial tissue. This kind of radical therapy is appropriate for women who do not wish to have children.

Adenomyosis

A special kind of endometriosis that occurs within the wall of uterus is called *adenomyosis*. Oftentimes, this problem is not responsive to hormone therapy, and it is seen more in women in their late thirties and forties who have had a lot of children. Usually it does not create major problems, although it can result in heavy bleeding and pain during menstruation that had not been present before.

Oral contraceptives may help if there are symptoms such as those described, but if further symptom relief is needed, the best solution will often be a hysterectomy.

Case Study

Rachel K was a 29-year-old telephone operator who had incapacitating pelvic pain which would begin 2 to 3 days before her menstrual period and last through the second day of her period. She could not go to work during that time, and she had very heavy menstrual flow associated with diarrhea, adding to her misery. Besides that, she experienced bloating for 5 to 7 days prior to her menstrual period with a weight gain of 4 to 5 pounds. During that time she was extremely jittery with feelings of depression and crying. In certain positions with deep penetration, intercourse was exquisitely painful. Her general health had always been good, and she had not suffered any serious illnesses nor had any operations.

When she first consulted a gynecologist about her problem, Rachel was tense and anxious. She seemed extremely concerned about her health. The doctor conducted a physical exam, which was basically normal, although she felt a fairly large mass on one side of Rachel's uterus. The uterus was fixed in place, tilted backwards, and could not be moved.

The doctor suggested that, more likely than not, Rachel was suffering from premenstrual syndrome and possibly endometriosis. However, before putting Rachel on any specific medication, the doctor felt that a laparoscopy was necessary. This procedure showed a small amount of endometriosis in the cul-de-sac (pocket formed where the uterus connects to the intestinal wall). These areas were burned off without difficulty.

Because of Rachel's discomfort, the gynecologist decided to put her ovaries at rest by using danazol therapy. Danazol, 200 mg, was prescribed 3 times a day for 4 months. During this time Rachel noticed that she felt much better, although she gained 8 pounds. At the end of 4 months, the doctor took Rachel off danazol but decided to continue resting her ovaries with a combined oral contraceptive, Ortho-Novum 1/35-28.

Rachel continued to feel better, but at her annual examination a year later still complained to the doctor that intercourse was painful, especially on her left side during deep penetration. The doctor examined her and found a 10 cm swelling to the left of her uterus, which she believed was an ovary. This was confirmed by intravaginal ultrasound, which showed a dense, fluid-filled mass on the ovary. The doctor diagnosed this as an endometrioma (endometriosis of the ovary).

Rachel was scheduled for a laparotomy which was done through a transverse skin incision. The 10 cm endometrioma was confirmed at the time of surgery. Fortunately the gynecologist was able to shell out the endometrioma and to preserve a portion of her left ovary. She found the uterus to be tilted backward and adhered to some scar tissue in the cul-de-sac where the previous endometrial tissue had been destroyed. The doctor repaired this and suspended her uterus and ovaries up out of the pelvis.

Postoperatively, all of Rachel's symptoms were relieved, and she did very well. A year-and-a-half later she returned for additional counseling because she was not able to get pregnant. The doctor speculated that endometriosis might be at work again, but, after utilizing basal body temperature charting, she found that Rachel was not ovulating. A sperm

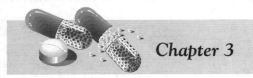

Case Study (continued)

count done on Rachel's husband proved to be normal, so the doctor put her on a course of Clomid to induce ovulation. She eventually conceived, carried through with a successful pregnancy, and delivered an 8 pound boy vaginally during the next year.

Key Points for Endometriosis

1. Pelvic pain from endometriosis responds well to a variety of medical and surgical therapies, none of which is necessarily more effective than the other. Cost, comfort for the woman in terms of side effects, and safety are the main considerations. Oral contraceptives would be the first choice of therapy, using these guidelines.

2. Newer medications such as danazol, the GnRH analogues, or tamoxifen may help with endometriosis by causing a temporary, artificial menopause. Side effects from these drugs can be uncomfortable, and for some women, may be too high a price to pay. All of these new drugs are expensive and need to be administered over a period of several months. A specific diagnosis should be made by laparoscopy before these expensive forms of therapy are begun.

3. Neither medical nor surgical therapy is very useful in women with minimal or mild endometriosis. Surgical therapy is probably necessary for women with advanced disease.

4. Expectant management, i.e., investigating other causes of infertility before starting endometriosis treatment, is preferable for women with minimal or mild endometriosis who cannot conceive.

5. Minor surgery for endometriosis may be effectively performed through a laparoscope on an outpatient basis.

Table 3-1
Treatment for Endometriosis

Management	Comments
Expectant management	Detailed infertility investigation needed to rule out other causes of failure to conceive.
Hormonal therapy	
Oral contraceptives (Progesterone-dominant type of oral contraceptive with minimum therapy period of 6 months):	
Ethinyl estradiol/norgestrel (Ovral)	1 tablet per day.
Ethinyl estradiol/ethynodiol diacetate (Demulen 1/50)	1 tablet per day for 21 days, off 7 days
Ethinyl estradiol/levonorgestrel (Tri-Levlen)	1 tablet every day or 1 tablet every day for 21 days, with 7 days off.
Progestins	
Oral medroxypro-gesterone acetate (Provera)	10 mg 3 times a day for 3 months
Depomedroxyproges-terone acetate (Depo Provera)	Intramuscular injections, 150 mg every month; should not be used if woman is trying to become pregnant.
Megestrol (Megace)	40-80 mg per day for 3 months.
Danazol (Danocrine)	Derived from testosterone. Creates a "pseudomenopause." Starting dose is 200-300 mg twice a day. Increase dose by 200 mg per day if amenorrhea does not occur. Minimum therapy, 4 to 6 months.

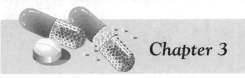
Table 3-1 (continued)

GnRH analogues (Synarel, Lupron, Lupron Depot, Zoladex)	Seen as medical ovary removal. May be given as nose drops daily or as a skin injection daily. New forms include time-released skin implants that can be inserted once a month.
Tamoxifen (Novaldex)	An estrogen-suppressing drug. One or two 10 mg tablets two times a day.
Surgery	
Laparoscopy	Usually done on an outpatient basis. Lesions can be destroyed with a laser. Other procedures may also be done, such as ablation of sacro-uterine ligaments.
Radical hysterectomy	The last and most definitive route of therapy. Uterus, ovaries and surrounding tissue with endometrial implants are removed.

Notes

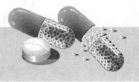

Menstrual Irregularities and Dysfunctional Uterine Bleeding

Everyone needs those elements in their lives that they can depend upon - things that go like clockwork, predictably, reliably, regularly. Many women feel that way about their menstrual periods. The monthly menstrual cycle is a sign that the body is working the way it should be, while reassuring a woman that her hormone status is normal. When the menstrual cycle doesn't follow its normal course, it can be very upsetting. Women often respond with fear and worry that something is wrong - a disease, a cessation of their feminine functions, or an unwanted or complicated pregnancy.

First of all, we want to reassure women that almost no one goes through a lifetime of menstruation without some variation in the pattern. This can be caused by any number of things which do not necessarily mean a problem: a hormone fluctuation, stress or excitement, or a change of diet or environment. Before she starts to worry, a woman should allow herself to go through at least two succeeding menstrual cycles, watching carefully for symptoms and notable occurrences to report to her doctor, if it becomes necessary to see a physician.

A menstrual cycle occurs approximately every 28 days, with normal variations being 7 days, more or less. Menstrual flow will generally be moderately heavy on the first 1 or 2 days and then begin to taper off. Again, there is quite a degree of normal variation from woman to woman in the amount of flow, but a moderately heavy menstrual period will require a change of pad or tampon about every 2 hours. Most women do not menstruate for less than 3 days or more than 7 or 8 days; five days is probably an average length for a period.

When using the term *menstrual irregularities*, we are basically talking about these problems: vaginal bleeding that occurs either too frequently or too infrequently and bleeding that is too light or too heavy.

Irregular Menstrual Flow

The most common menstrual difficulty women encounter is irregular menstrual flow due to inconsistent or no ovulation. This can result in menstrual flow that is either too frequent or not frequent enough, that is every 5 to 7 weeks.

Menstrual periods can be regular, meaning that ovulation is occurring, but still result in very heavy flow. This usually indicates a problem with the reproductive organs themselves rather than a hormone imbalance.

Unpredictable and uncontrollable bleeding suggests a hormone imbalance. It is usually painless and rarely associated with any physical discomfort. It can, however, lead to anemia that causes great fatigue.

After a woman has had a baby, she will experience at least five weeks of bleeding and discharge known as lochia. This, too, is hormone related. Ovulation does not usually occur until at least 2-4 months after delivery. Typically, unless she is breast-feeding, a woman can expect postpartum discharge for at least five weeks after delivery. Within 3-4 months she should revert to a normal menstrual cycle. Breast-feeding delays ovulation and the return to an early normal menstrual cycle. Women who nurse their babies may have to wait 6-9 months before having a normal period.

The years immediately preceding the menopause (called the perimenopausal period) are another time when women may experience irregular and heavy bleeding. Because the reproductive system is getting ready to shut down, the delicate balance of estrogen and progesterone that guide the ovaries and uterus through the fertile years sometimes tips. The ovaries slow their production of estrogen and progesterone both. The most common reason for bleeding abnormalities at this time of life is the lack of progesterone, since ovulation does not occur with regularity any longer.

Another cause of heavy or frequent bleeding is "fibroids." Officially, fibroids are benign growths of fibrous tissue that appear as hard whorls in the wall of the uterus. Their medical name is *leiomyoma*. When the uterus contracts during the menstrual period, it serves the purpose of clamping down on the blood vessels and controlling bleeding at the same time. Fibroids seem to impede this process, possibly by increasing or changing the surface area of the endometrium (uterine lining) and preventing the uterine muscle from contracting properly. Fibroids are not life-threatening, but they can cause trouble. They seem to grow under the influence of estrogen. Submucosal fibroids that grow into the uterine cavity and lining are most often responsible for heavy, progressively worsening menstrual flow. Once menopause sets in, fibroids tend to shrink by about 25% as estrogen production decreases. Heavy bleeding will also diminish.

In addition to those near menopausal age, adolescent girls sometimes visit the doctor because of excessive vaginal bleeding. Between the ages of 12 and 16 the ovaries are frequently not sufficiently stimulated by the hormones from the pituitary gland to release an egg and produce progesterone. Ovulation usually begins to occur somewhere between 2 and 3 years after the first menstruation. Once it does, irregular bleeding tends to clear up. If it doesn't, the doctor must begin to consider other sources of the problem, and they are listed in Table 4-1.

Extent of Bleeding

The extent of bleeding may be estimated by recording the number of pads used each day and the degree of pad saturation. If a woman needs to change pads more often than every 2 hours and if her pads are 80% or more saturated, she is probably bleeding excessively. It is better to use pads than tampons when attempting to determine how heavily you are bleeding because many tampons are extra-absorbent and will conceal the true picture of what is happening.

Women who are concerned about irregular, heavy, or continuous bleeding should have a physical examination to determine where the bleeding comes from: a vaginal laceration, the cervix itself, or the uterus. At that time the doctor may be able to determine if there are any tumors growing in the cervix, uterus, or ovaries or any foreign bodies in the reproductive tract. With this examination a woman should have a Pap smear and a complete blood count. If symptoms persist without a specific diagnosis, the gynecologist may consider testing bloodclotting ability, pituitary gland function, thyroid gland function, and ovarian function. He or she may wish to perform a biopsy (removal of a small piece of tissue) of the endometrium or cervix.

Initial Therapy for Excessive Bleeding

If no other medical disorder is involved and the cause of bleeding is anovulation with hormone imbalance, the primary form of treatment involves the use of supplemental hormones. A woman with heavy active bleeding usually responds to a combination of high-dose estrogens and progestins or a high dose of progestins. Either combination taken four times daily will usually decrease the bleeding within the first few days. In cases of anovulation with resulting lack of progesterone, replacement progesterone is usually given in pill form or sometimes by injection.

Intravenously injected estrogens may be necessary to stop uterine bleeding and are used for several days followed by several weeks of oral estrogen (pills). Common problems associated with this initial therapy using high-dose hormones are nausea and vomiting. Once bleeding is well controlled, the woman will usually be placed on a contraceptive pill that contains both estrogen and progesterone.

The monthly treatment cycle should be continued for at least 3 cycles. If the uterine lining becomes very thin after a prolonged period of bleeding, a conjugated estrogen tablet may be necessary to reestablish this lining. When uterine bleeding has stopped or decreased sufficiently, the doctor may prescribe a lower dose oral contraceptive so that the period of bleeding may be planned and limited.

Further Management of Excessive Bleeding

Once a woman's bleeding has come under control after the 4-month drug course, recurrence of the problem depends upon whether she resumes ovulation (egg production). If she does not plan to become pregnant, she can continue taking an oral contraceptive, either a regular dose or low-dose birth control pill or a progestin only pill. Medroxyprogesterone acetate (Provera), 5=10 mg per day for 5=10 days every 6 weeks will allow predictable withdrawal bleeding to take place. If regular, cyclic menstrual periods begin, hormone pills may no longer be necessary.

In some cases gynecologists have successfully managed bleeding caused by fibroids through prescription of a new group of drugs, the GnRH analogues, including leuprolide acetate and histrolin *(See Chapter 14, Fertility Drugs for a more detailed description of the GnRH analogues)*. These compounds usually produce shrinking of fibroids from 30-60% by 60 days after therapy. Unfortunately, the fibroids tend to increase in size rapidly after the drug is stopped. Regrowth in the fibroid does not, however, always result in renewed bleeding, and thus the GnRH analogue drugs can solve the problem of bleeding for some women. This class of drugs is not commonly prescribed prior to surgery, such as a myomectomy (removal of a fibroid from the wall of the uterus).

Bleeding that continues after a course of drug therapy as just described may require the doctor to perform a dilatation and curettage (D&C) of the uterus or an endometrial biopsy. This is especially true if a woman is aged 35 or older. Other means for evaluating the lining of the uterus include a hysterosalpingogram, a procedure in which a dye is injected into the uterus to allow an x-ray view of it, and a hysteroscopy, in which a telescopic instrument is inserted up the vagina, through the cervix, and into the uterus to permit the doctor to see its internal structures.

Another method of therapy used to control bleeding from fibroids after use of either injection or progesterone or GnRH analogues to shrink their thickness is laser therapy of the endometrium. This procedure, called *rollerball laser therapy,* eliminates most of the endometrium.

Many times, women will become frustrated with heavy or unpredictable bleeding and simply opt for a hysterectomy. This may be an appropriate solution, especially if a woman is approaching menopause or has no further plans for childbearing.

If medical evaluation determines that their heavy bleeding is not dangerous, there are some self-help tools that women can use to minimize its consequences:

Vitamin therapy. Iron and B-vitamins lost through bleeding can create fatigue and weakness. If these are replaced through nutritional supplements, such weakness and fatigue may not seem as debilitating. Gynecologists can recommend or prescribe such supplements.

Diet and exercise. In addition to eating a diet with iron and B vitamins to replace nutrients lost through bleeding, women may find that a very low-fat diet, weight loss, and regular exercise help too. They should drink plenty of water and healthful liquids such as fruit juice and skim milk to replace the fluids lost in bleeding. We caution women against using very high dose iron supplements, however, since new research indicates a possible relationship between iron-rich blood and cardiovascular disease.

Avoiding fatigue and stress. Excessive bleeding tires women out, while stress can serve to worsen any medical problem. During times of heavy bleeding women may find they need more sleep and rest than usual. They should also try to avoid stress-ridden encounters that further drain their energies. The message is, be good to yourself by taking it easy.

Body consciousness. Women should pay attention to body signals and heed them. Fatigue and lack of energy may signal anemia. Pain may mean that an infection or additional medical problem is developing. Watch for signs of pregnancy. When the menstrual cycle becomes irregular, it's harder to know where you are and easier to lose track of important signals.

Frequent checkups. Women should visit a gynecologist at least once a year if their problems are stable and not serious. We recommend more frequent visits if they are concerned about their condition, uncomfortable, or if bleeding or any other symptom is worsening.

Light or Infrequent Menstrual Flow

Light or infrequent menses are usually associated with menopause, use of certain drugs, disturbances of the central nervous system, certain tumors, very strenuous exercise, or emotional problems (Table 4-2). Each one of these causes has a different origin and requires specific treatment by a physician, particularly if the infrequent or scanty bleeding goes on for several months.

Most women can expect to have light or infrequent menstrual flow on occasion. Ovulation and pregnancy still can occur if one is sexually active. Even over 40, effective contraceptive techniques are still mandatory.

Unless there is a particular medical problem that explains persistent irregularity or light flow, the most common reason for this to happen is that the ovaries do not produce an adequate amount of estrogen and progesterone. If the gynecologist decides to treat the problem with drugs, the therapy should be directed toward replacing the hormones that are low, such

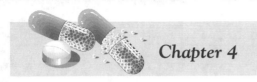

as estrogen and progestin pills. Fertility pills and injections to stimulate the ovaries should be used only when a woman wants to become pregnant and lack of ovulation is the ascertained cause of menstrual irregularity.

Some women with light, irregular periods also suffer the embarrassment of <u>hirsutism</u> (excess facial or body hair). This is caused by excessive amounts of the male hormone, testosterone, in the body and is also related to ethnic background. Spironolactone, ketaconazole, birth control pills, depilatories, and electrolysis are measures that can be used to alleviate hirsutism.

Most women with scant or infrequent menstrual bleeding do not wish to become pregnant and therefore prefer to take an oral contraceptive or sequential estrogen and progesterone replacement. If a woman is perimenopausal, we usually recommend a conjugated estrogen tablet such as Premarin in strengths of 1.25 mg or 17 beta estradiol (Estrace), 1 mg. These should be taken each day from day 1 to day 24 of the menstrual cycle. Then a progestin tablet, usually 5-10 mg of Provera, should be taken from days 20 to 24. Menstruation should begin by day 27 and last for the remainder of the month. This regimen should be adequate not only for regulating periods but also for dependable contraception in most adult women. Adolescents with less sexual development (very small breasts, for example) may benefit from a higher dose estrogen pill.

Case Study

Martha H, a 38-year-old homemaker and mother of three children, had been in good health for years. She had had a tubal ligation 5 years previously, after the birth of her third child. Her only complaint was that she carried 30 extra pounds that she couldn't seem to get rid of. Then she began to notice irregularities in her menstrual cycle. Sometimes her periods would come twice in one month and sometimes not at all. Her bleeding had become very heavy, and she found that, even when wearing a super tampon and a max-ipad, she had to change at least every 2 hours. The period she was having when she arrived at her gynecologist's office had been going on for 2 weeks.

On examination the doctor observed that her uterus was enlarged to about the size of a three month pregnancy, but was not soft. Her thyroid gland was of normal size. He found nothing else of note. He suspected a hormone imbalance and decided to prescribe Provera. She took 10 mg of Provera twice a day for the first 5 days of her monthly cycle to control when her monthly periods would begin. She also began taking iron pills because blood tests revealed that she had become anemic. Her Pap smear report was negative for cancer.

Two months later on a Saturday night Martha found herself in the emergency room, bleeding heavily. The gynecology resident on call gave her an intravenous injection of high dose estrogen which he told her should slow the bleeding until she could visit her own doctor.

Martha's gynecologist scheduled her for a D&C the next day after he saw her. After she was put under mild general anesthesia, he gently scraped her uterine lining, discovering two noncancerous endometrial polyps in the process. With the polyps removed, Martha's bleeding problems disappeared. She no longer had to take hormones, and her menstrual periods resumed a regular cycle.

Key Points for Menstrual Irregularities

1. Most women have a strong psychological need for regular and predictable menstrual cycles, so the need to treat irregularities is important.

2. Abnormal menstrual bleeding is most commonly represented by painless and heavy or more frequent flow. This additional blood loss is often perplexing, since it is often unpredictable and may be difficult to control.

3. Excessive, irregular, or frequent uterine bleeding occurs most commonly during adolescence or around menopause. Many physical and psychological conditions are associated with menstrual irregularities, but the most common is a hormone imbalance resulting in lack of ovulation with associated absence of progesterone.

4. Women experiencing heavy or irregular bleeding should schedule a thorough physical, including a Pap smear. Further testing may be necessary if certain medical conditions, such as a thyroid problem or bleeding disorder, are suspected. Samplings of the uterine cavity can usually be done in the office.

5. Choosing a treatment for excessive bleeding is not always easy. Unless a specific medical disorder is found, the physician will usually prescribe estrogen and progestin pills to temporarily correct any hormone imbalance.

6. Women with heavy bleeding that is not dangerous may be able to help themselves through those times by taking iron and B vitamin nutritional supplements, drinking plenty of fluids, eating a very low fat diet, and getting adequate rest and exercise.

7. Surgical procedures such as a D&C or hysterectomy are rarely necessary but may be required if bleeding continues after use of the hormone pills. Other procedures, such as a hysterosalpingogram or hysteroscopy, may be performed to visualize the inside of the uterus so the doctor can pinpoint precisely the source of the bleeding.

8. A woman with persistent scanty or infrequent menstrual bleeding should be evaluated by a physician for pregnancy or a chronic disorder requiring medical attention. In many cases her menstrual cycle may be safely regulated with oral contraceptives or a monthly schedule of sequential estrogen and progestin tablets.

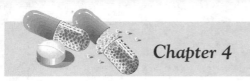

Table 4-1

Conditions Related to Excessive or Frequent Menstrual Bleeding

Lack of ovulation	Stress
Excess weight gain	Underactive thyroid
Early menopause	Polycystic ovaries
Medications	Overactive adrenal glands
Sex hormones	Central nervous system disorder
Tranquilizers	Intrauterine device
Some high blood pressure medications	Cancer of the cervix, uterus or ovaries
Fibroid tumors	

Table 4-2

Conditions Related to Light or Infrequent Menstrual Bleeding

Pregnancy; ectopic pregnancy	Medications, especially use of low-dose oral contraceptives, cessation of oral contraceptives, or use of long-acting progestin injections.
Threatened miscarriage	
Chronic medical illness	
Menopause (older women)	
Lack of ovulation (young women)	Lean muscular bodies, strenuous exercise, and high stress
Underactive pituitary gland	
Central nervous system	Anxiety, stress, or other problems
Scarred or inactive uterine lining	Drastic weight change
Genetic disease	

Notes

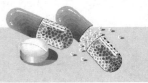

Chapter 5

Menopause and Estrogen Replacement

At one time menopause was not discussed in polite company, but that has changed. Menopause is now the subject of feature articles in major magazines, TV talk shows, and social gatherings. And why not? Female baby boomers are rapidly approaching the "change of life," and in the next two decades, nearly 40 million American women will pass the age of 50. The health-conscious women of this generation will live, on average, thirty years beyond the cessation of menstruation, and they want to feel good doing so!

Medical research on menopause done over the past 30 years and continuing on through the 1990s has provided physicians with much-needed information about drug therapy, specifically hormone replacement therapy, for the symptoms women experience before, during, and after menopause. We now believe, that for a substantial number of women, hormone replacement therapy will help avert cardiovascular disease and osteoporosis, a devastating fragility of the bones in the years following menopause. It will also alleviate many of the uncomfortable symptoms women experience at this very important time of their lives.

Estrogen replacement therapy is not a panacea, however. Some women shouldn't use it. In addition, there are other things a woman can do to reduce the risk of heart attack or osteoporosis, and we will discuss some of those in this chapter.

What is the Menopause?

Technically speaking, the term *menopause* refers to the time of the last menstrual period. The five to eight years preceding this time is known as *the climacteric* or, more popularly, the "change of life." Though the normal climacteric can start as early as age 35 or as late as age 60, most women reach it in their late forties and early fifties, with 51 being the average age of the last period. Terms such as *pre- or perimenopausal* (referring to the years before menopause) and *postmenopausal* (after menopause) are also commonly used.

Human beings are the only mammals that outlive their reproductive years, and historical evidence indicates that living past menopause is a phenomenon of the 20th century. A mere 100 years ago, at the turn of this century, white women lived to 47 years of age, on average, and black women only to age 38. Estimates for 1992 indicate that 120 million women living in the United States will survive to about 78 years of age, on average. Of these, 35 million have no ovarian function (that is, have passed menopause, or in a few cases have had their ovaries surgically removed). Yet only about 20% of all these women are on some form of hormone replacement therapy.

Menopause results when estrogen and progesterone production begin to slow down. This can be a long, slow process characterized by many fluctuations in hormones, but ultimately the ovaries stop producing the hormones needed for reproduction. The decline of reproductive hormones may be nature's way of allowing the bodies of aging women to avoid the hazards of childbearing, which becomes risky past the age of 45.

Why Women Need Estrogen

It is the lack or irregular supply of estrogen, in particular, that is responsible for the irregular periods, hot flushes (also known as hot flashes), vaginal dryness, urinary problems, and emotional ups and downs. While probably the most talked about, these symptoms are not the most serious consequences of estrogen shutdown. A precipitous increase in heart and blood vessel disease occurs among women after the menopause. This increase is evidenced by the fact that women have many fewer heart attacks than men between the ages of 40 and 55. However, by age 60 or 65 their rates are just about the same if women are not on estrogen therapy, which tends to lower their cholesterol and raise their good blood fats known as high-density lipoproteins (HDLs).

Estrogen works with the calcium metabolism of the body to keep bones healthy and to prevent brittleness caused by demineralization (depletion of calcium and other minerals). Without estrogen, in the years following the menopause, women lose from 1 to 1.5% of their bone mass *per year,* and over the course of 15 years or more many post-menopausal women may lose 3 or more inches of their original height. They may develop problems with bone fractures and arthritis, due to osteoporosis, which is particularly common in older women. This bone loss starts at least 5 years before menopause. We recommend non-hormonal therapy during this period.

During the fertile years, estrogen's main function is to stimulate the release of eggs for conception, but it plays an important part in many other vital functions of the body *(See Table 5-1).* Estrogen has a major role in cell growth and maintenance of cell vitality. Thus, many women will notice a difference in skin tone and the moisture and flexibility of the vaginal tract after menopause.

Estrogen has numerous other effects on various regions of the body such as the liver, the bladder and bladder outlet, the clotting factors of the blood, the breasts, and the pituitary gland and hypothalamus, important glands that help regulate body temperature. The well-known hot flushes (or flashes) of menopause are thought to result from blood vessel instability and the metabolic control mechanisms of the pituitary and hypothalamus responding to decreasing levels of estrogen.

Many women find that sexual intercourse is painful because of the dryness of the walls of the vagina; some develop urinary tract problems such as painful urination or incontinence (leaking of urine; *See Chapter 6).*

Scientists have recently noted a connection between lack of estrogen and deterioration of nerve cells in the brains of experimental animals. This has led to speculation that lack of estrogen could be associated with Alzheimer's disease or similar neurological disorders.

Oftentimes a lack of estrogen will result in physical and emotional discomfort. Women need to know that it is possible to replace their naturally occurring estrogen and relieve these problems without significant threat to their overall health and well-being.

In summary, the "big three" reasons for needing estrogen replacement are:

- To decrease the incidence of heart and blood vessel disease, in particular heart attacks.
- To prevent or halt the progress of osteoporosis.
- To alleviate the uncomfortable symptoms of insufficient estrogen in the body.

Symptoms of Menopause

Changes in Menstrual Periods

Some women are lucky. They menstruate regularly throughout their reproductive years, and then one day they simply stop having periods. Most women, however, notice that their periods become unpredictable. They may skip periods, have very light or heavy periods, have between-period spotting, or find the time between periods lengthening. This becomes annoying and worrisome, with fears of pregnancy or disease cropping up. When this begins to happen, even if it really means the onset of normal menopause, a trip to the gynecologist's office may be in order.

Specifically, we recommend that a woman consult a doctor if she experiences any of the following:

- Bleeding more often than every 2 to 3 weeks
- A period that lasts more than 9 to 10 days
- A period that starts again after 12 months without a period

Hot Flushes

Almost 75% of women experience hot flushes during the menopausal years. Hot flushes create a sensation of heat spreading over their chest, arms, neck, and face. This is sometimes accompanied by heavy perspiration, which may cause awakening in the night. Hot flushes usually are not serious and tend to go away after awhile.

In the meantime we suggest some simple methods to cope with them when they occur:

- Control ventilation in the home and office, so windows may be opened and closed when necessary.
- Layer clothing with removable pieces. Silks and wools are not as comfortable as cotton or cotton and synthetic blends after intense perspiration.
- Invest in a personal fan, which can be placed discreetly on a desk or work table.
- Learn how to stay calm during a hot flush. Most people are not paying close enough attention to realize when they occur and probably only you will notice your distress.
- Investigate stress relief and relaxation techniques through classes and tapes. These can help with control of hot flushes and also reduce related anxiety.
- Exercise regularly. This can tone up the cardiovascular system, which is responding to estrogen fluctuations during a hot flush.
- Keep weight down. Heavier women tend to have more ups and downs with estrogen production and seem to suffer more with hot flushes.

If hot flushes create great difficulties for a woman, such as chronic sleeplessness, she should see her gynecologist to discuss estrogen replacement therapy, which will cure the hot flushes.

Vaginal Dryness and Soreness

While vaginal dryness doesn't receive the lip service that hot flushes do, it is of equal or greater concern to women. In the context of a relationship with a sexual partner, vaginal irritation can loom very large and spoil sexual pleasure.

Estrogen deficiency causes a thinning of the lining of the vagina, which becomes dry and loses its elasticity. This can make sexual intercourse very uncomfortable, with irritation and bleeding resulting. In addition to estrogen replacement therapy, there are "home remedies" that can help avoid vaginal soreness during intercourse:

• K-Y, Surgilube, or especially some of the newer water soluble jellies, such as Replens, applied to the penis and vaginal area just prior to intercourse can provide helpful lubrication.

• Irritating bubble baths, gels, or other bath preparations should be avoided when bathing.

• Douche solutions should be avoided because they tend to be drying. If a yeast infection develops, a mild vinegar-water solution for douching may be advisable.

• Loose fitting panties and pants are preferable to panty hose. Women may wish to consider going back to old-fashioned stockings to provide ventilation to their genital area.

• Estrogen cream will improve the tone of the vaginal walls.

• Adequate foreplay prior to intercourse and frequent intercourse will increase vaginal secretions.

Loss of Urine

Women of menopausal age find that sometimes vigorous exercise (especially jumping, such as is done in aerobics), coughing, or hearty laughing can cause them to leak a little urine. This is terribly embarrassing, although neither abnormal nor dangerous. Loss of estrogen also causes the structures around the mouth of the bladder to "loosen," and this, combined with childbearing, can result in a bladder sphincter that is not as tight as it should be.

Estrogen creams applied to the vaginal and bladder entry area may possibly help with urinary incontinence, but an easier method is oral estrogen pills, since the dosage is more accurate. Kegel exercises - repeatedly tightening and loosening the muscles around the bladder and the vagina - can be very helpful in reconditioning those muscles so they hold back urine more effectively. "Kegeling" should be done as a daily routine.

Urinary tract infection or bladder irritation can also be responsible for leakage, and if this is the case, a physician should be consulted.

Other Body Changes

While the body is in the course of changing throughout life, changes seem to accelerate at the menopause and may seem more noticeable. In addition to differences in the reproductive function, *women may notice the following normal changes in their bodies:*

• Change in breast size, coupled with a flattening or drooping of the breasts
• Weight gain
• Skin changes, such as drying, wrinkling, blotchiness, and the appearance of skin tags
• Hair changes, such as thinning and drying or the appearance of facial hair
• Varicose veins in the legs
• Sleep disturbances
• Emotional changes, such as depression
• Loss of concentration and memory

In most cases, a positive, healthful lifestyle with interesting activities will offset the inevitable changes that women in midlife experience. Cosmetic surgery may be an option for women who cannot live with their changing appearance, but they should be aware that all surgical procedures come with risks.

Osteoporosis

While aging can bring a certain amount of bodily discomfort, especially in the joints and the spine, severe bone and joint pain should be evaluated by a physician. Such pains may be the early signs of *osteoporosis*, a disease where the architecture of bone tissue deteriorates, leaving it fragile and susceptible to fractures.

Osteoporosis affects 24 million American women and 200 million women worldwide. It causes 1.3 million fractures a year in elderly American women. Of those, between 20 and 35% die within 18 to 24 months from complications of the fracture.

Certain types of women are more at risk for osteoporosis. These include:

* Women over 50, entering or already in menopause
* Caucasian or Asian women
* Slender, petite women with small bones
* Women who had an early menopause, either surgically (i.e., having ovaries removed) or normally
* Those with grandmothers, mothers, sisters or other close relatives with osteoporosis
* Women with sedentary lifestyles who get inadequate physical exercise
* Smokers (Smoking makes estrogen less effective)
* Women who consume excess alcoholic beverages
* Women with amenorrhea (lack of menstruation) due to anorexia or excessive athletic activity, such as long-distance running
* Women on certain medications such as cortisone, anticoagulants (blood thinners), lithium, anti-cancer chemotherapy, immunosuppressive drugs given to transplant patients, anti-thyroid medications, and certain drugs for diabetes therapy

Osteoporosis is preventable, provided the prevention program begins early enough, and that means before menopause sets in.

As women age, they need to pay more attention to their diet and lifestyle, including substances that they ingest. Therefore the first front in combating osteoporosis is to follow these sensible measures:

* Stop smoking cigarettes and using recreational drugs.
* Minimize alcohol intake.
* Keep weight at levels recommended for your body type and height.
* Eat a balanced diet, low in fat.
* Include adequate dietary calcium (premenopausal women, 1,000 mg per day; post menopausal women, 1,500 mg/day.) If you do not consume dairy products, plan to take calcium supplements.

Tip: Tums and Rolaids are an excellent way to get calcium, with 750 mg of calcium per tablet.

- Exercise regularly, and remember to include some low impact or weight-bearing exercises such as walking, jogging, or dancing, and some exercises to strengthen back muscles.
- Learn to lift heavy objects properly to prevent bone and back injuries.
- Consider taking a baby aspirin daily if there is a significant family history or other risk of cardiac or vascular disease

At about age 45, women should begin to measure their height every year and put a mark on the kitchen door, as is done for children. If loss of height exceeds one-half to three-quarters of an inch, they should assume that compression of the vertebrae may have occurred with the onset of early osteoporosis. We know that it takes a loss of at least 20% of the calcium from bones before osteoporosis begins. Women over 60 who have never had estrogen replacement therapy tend to be the ones developing early osteoporosis.

Studies have demonstrated that estrogen replacement therapy will stabilize the process of osteoporosis or prevent it from occurring. Adequate calcium intake is also important, but after menopause, unless there are sufficient estrogen levels in the body, the calcium will not be well absorbed. Estrogen plus calcium plus exercise has become the name of the game in osteoporosis prevention for women.

Heart and Blood Vessel Disease

Once menopause occurs, cholesterol levels increase and the proportions between the good, high-density lipoproteins (HDLs) and bad, low-density lipoproteins (LDLs) shift, with the latter increasing. Nowadays, doctors believe that cholesterol levels should be no higher than 200 milligrams per milliliter of blood. However, most of the research on cholesterol and heart and blood vessel disease has been done on men up to this point. Major research studies have now started on cardiovascular disease in women, and we have already learned some important things.

We are convinced that estrogen plays a major role in protecting women against heart disease, because it is not until 8-10 years after the menopause that women begin to have heart attacks and other vascular problems at the same rate men do.

Recent studies have shown that estrogen replacement therapy will decrease total cholesterol by approximately 4%, increase high-density lipoproteins by approximately 10% and decrease low-density lipoproteins by approximately 11%. Women on estrogen replacement therapy have 40-50% better protection against acute myocardial infarction (severe heart attack) than those who are not on estrogen. Studies using a special imaging technique for the heart called coronary arteriography have shown that women taking estrogen have significantly less coronary artery disease. Physicians believe that certain other factors also affect whether or not a woman will eventually fall prey to heart disease. These include lifestyle, eating habits (especially dietary fat consumption), smoking, and heredity.

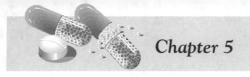

Depression

Studies done on the effects of estrogen on depression are limited. However, all of them present good evidence that women taking estrogen experience less depression.

Drug Therapy During Menopause

Estrogen Replacement

Over the past 30 years a great deal has been learned about the use and action of estrogens in the body. Physicians now know that estrogen compounds combined with progestins given in a pattern that emulates the menstrual cycle seem to yield the best results with the fewest number of problems in postmenopausal women who still have a uterus. In fact, this combination may *decrease* the risk of cancer to the uterus and possibly to the breast. The progestins counterbalance the estrogens so they don't overstimulate the uterus and cause bleeding. Women who do not have a uterus can take estrogens without the added progestins.

Estrogen use basically helps restore the hormonal climate of menopausal women to normal. Pills for estrogen and progestin replacement therapy have much lower doses than birth control pills whose hormone levels are 4 to 6 times higher than necessary for correction of insufficient hormones. Tables 5-2 lists the various types of estrogen products that may be used in replacement therapy. Prior to starting a course of estrogen replacement, a thorough breast and pelvic examination, including a Pap smear, is mandatory. Women who have had breast cancer or active liver disease should probably not take estrogen replacement therapy. Women who still have a uterus require more careful evaluation prior to therapy and during therapy, especially if abnormal bleeding occurs.

There are many different estrogen therapy plans. It is the major therapeutic drug for treating menopause. Doctors will use different regimens, depending upon what their patients want and need. No one therapy is better than the other. The only standard of treatment is that estrogen be used.

If a woman does not have a uterus, therapy decisions are easier since her main drug will be estrogen. Some physicians may add a small quantity of progestogens to the prescription, but to date we are not sure this is necessary. Either way is acceptable.

If a woman does have a uterus, the problem is much more complex and therapy should be tailored to the person. Age and time since the date of menopause are critical factors since dosages of both estrogen and progestogens will vary depending upon the patient and her own peculiarities. The basic ingredient is still estrogen, but the question is, how much? Also, will it be taken intermittently or continuously? When will progestogens be added?

We have found that most menopausal women do not wish to continue having menstrual periods, and this becomes a major challenge during the first one or two years of therapy. Our preferred therapy regimens usually result in no more menstruation for 90% of women after 6 to 9 months. This regimen is based upon the use of some form of progestogen to counteract the effects of estrogen on the uterus. If enough progestogens are used, the endometrium undergoes atrophy resulting in no bleeding. This can be tested with a larger dose of progestogens.

Hormone replacement therapy regimens include the use of estrogen and progestogens as listed below. Each company producing these products thinks their product is best. Different doctors prefer to use different drugs. The important part is that estrogen is the key to preventing osteoporosis and elevating cholesterol, which will reduce the chance of a myocardial infarction.

Forms of Estrogen and Treatment Plans

Estrogen comes in many forms, such as tablets to be taken orally (Table 5-2), vaginal creams (Table 5-3), tiny pellets implanted in the skin, injections (Table 5-4), and skin patches (Table 5-4). Oral medication is the least expensive, and many different types are available.

Oral estrogens. The following treatment programs are currently being used:

1. Estrogens designed to eliminate bleeding after 6-9 months. (For example, Premarin 0.625 mg; Estrace, 1 mg; Ogen, 0.625 mg; Estinyl, 0.05 mg; Estraval, 0.1 mg) each to be taken Monday through Friday, stopping on Saturday and Sunday. A progestogen such as Provera (2.5mg) or norethindrone (0.3mg) is taken with each estrogen tablet. (The two days off help prevent over stimulation and tenderness of the breast and endometrium and reduce fluid retention.) Provera is added in dosages of 10 mg daily for at least 7-10 days every 2-3 months to see if the uterus can still be stimulated to bleed 3-5 days after the large dose of Provera is stopped. Either bleeding or no bleeding is normal, as long as there is no bleeding between periods.

2. Estrogens designed to create menstrual cycles every month. (For example, Premarin, 0.625 mg; Estrace, 1 mg; Ogen, 0.625 mg). These are taken from Day 5 of the menstrual cycle to Day 25 of the menstrual cycle, and, from the 15th through 25th day, add a progestogen, such as medroxyprogesterone acetate (Provera) 10 mg a day, stopping all medications after Day 25, with the expectation of a bleed 3 to 5 days later. Both regimens do basically the same thing, that is, they provide estrogen. Different treatment plans work better for different women, and they should be individualized.

Transdermal estrogen. This is a relatively new form of estrogen therapy given by applying hormone-containing skin patches containing 0.05 or 0.1 mg of estradiol to the lower abdomen, twice a week. While transdermal estrogen has not been studied for a long time, early evidence indicates that it is similar in effect to oral estrogen. It may, however, not affect the HDL cholesterol as positively as oral estrogen, and thus may provide slightly less protection against cardiovascular disease. Transdermal estrogen offers an advantage to women who have had liver or biliary tract disease, in that it avoids going through the liver and gastrointestinal tract on its initial entry into the body. If a woman still has her uterus, she must also take 2.5mg of Provera daily.

Percutaneous estrogen. Percutaneous estrogen comes in the form of pellets placed just under the skin of the abdomen. The pellets last for 6 to 9 months and are gradually absorbed from the subcutaneous fat. Usually two pellets of 25 mg each are inserted through a minor operation under local anesthesia. Often a small testosterone pellet (75 mg) is also inserted. Currently these percutaneous estrogen pellets are not available in the U.S. market, but they may become available in the near future. If a woman still has her uterus, addition of progestogens is still necessary.

Vaginal estrogen. For women whose major complaints are dryness, tightness and tenderness of the vagina, or urine leakage, vaginally applied estrogen may be helpful. (Oral estrogen, however, still works better). Both estradiol and estrone are rapidly absorbed by the walls of the vagina. The recommended daily dose of 1 to 2 grams of estrogen cream contains 0.625 to 1.25 mg of conjugated estrogens. The cream should be used in 1 gram doses, once or twice a week.

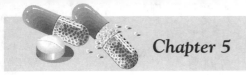

Monitoring Estrogen Replacement Therapy

Women should be carefully monitored when they are undergoing estrogen replacement therapy. Those who still have a uterus should see their gynecologist at least every six months to a year. As with oral contraceptives, the estrogens must be processed by the liver after absorption in the gastrointestinal tract and before they enter the bloodstream. Since much of the hormone will be lost during this process, the amount of hormone contained in conjugated estrogen tablets is as much as five times higher than what would normally be produced by the body.

Women using the vaginal estrogen creams must be cautious to apply the correct dosage at the right intervals. The drug is readily absorbed through the vagina and can produce blood levels less than those of the oral estrogen tablets. Their effects will still be systemic.

Cost

The cost of oral estrogen replacement-progestogen therapy is probably less than $100 per year, using generic brands (although it could be two or three times that much using "name brand" products.) Transdermal, percutaneous, and vaginal estrogens are more expensive and could run between $135-$250 per year. Supplementary calcium and Vitamin D tablets, for example Os-Cal 500 + D, would run approximately $75-80 per year. Used in the form of TUMS or Rolaids, it should cost substantially less than that per year.

Other Drugs Used to Treat Symptoms of Menopause

If estrogen replacement therapy is contraindicated after menopause, there are some new alternatives on the market that offer protection, particularly against osteoporosis.

One of these is *calcitonin,* a hormone that is naturally secreted by the thyroid gland in humans and other mammals and salmon. Calcitonin by injection helps prevent bone tissue loss. Injections must be given frequently, however, since the effects are temporary. Calcitonin has recently become available in inhalers and can be taken through the nose. Indications are that this product may be as effective as the injections.

Another drug that has attracted the attention of physicians treating postmenopausal women is *calcitriol* (Vitamin D3). Calcitriol is believed to increase absorption of calcium in the digestive tract. Studies have shown that women taking calcitriol have fewer fractures than women taking conventional calcium supplements.

Etidronate is another bone-strengthening product that can be given to menopausal women. Studies have shown that it increases mineral content in the vertebrae and decreases fractures. Women who have taken etidronate have tolerated it well and experienced few side effects. *Fluoride* is also known to strengthen bone tissue, and may have an application in the prevention of post-menopausal osteoporosis. However, fluorides have side effects and can be toxic if dosages are not carefully monitored.

Risks versus Benefits of Drugs Used During Menopause

Although the benefits of estrogen replacement therapy are clear, controversy about its use for menopause continues. Specifically, there is a definite correlation between estrogen replacement therapy and endometrial cancer, and there is some evidence (although not conclusive) that estrogen therapy may slightly increase the risk of breast cancer. This, unfortunately, has caused many people to shun the use of estrogen replacement therapy. Research indicates that balancing the estrogens with progestogens greatly lowers the risks in endometrial and maybe breast cancer. Women taking estrogen replacement hormones who do not have a family history of breast cancer and who undergo regular mammographic screening probably run no higher risk of breast cancer than anyone else.

Spotting may occur under estrogen replacement therapy, more often when continuous rather than interrupted doses are given. This situation should be monitored with an occasional endometrial biopsy (sampling of the endometrial tissue), once a year or less.

Many studies have taken place, and results consistently show that women taking estrogen after age 50 have a sharply lowered rate of heart attacks compared to those not taking estrogen. In a large Harvard research study of 121,700 nurses that began in 1976, with all other factors being equal, *the group taking estrogen replacement therapy had 61% the rate of fatal heart attacks* of nurses who didn't take estrogen.

The absolute risk of a woman over 50 with no special cardiovascular risk factors dying of heart disease is 31%. The absolute risk of dying of breast cancer is 2.8%; the absolute risk of dying of a hip fracture caused by osteoporosis is 2.8%; and the absolute risk of death from endometrial cancer is 0.7%.

In other words, the likelihood of dying of a heart attack appears to be much greater than the likelihood of dying of any of the other three diseases. Due to the fact that estrogen reduces the incidence of heart attack so drastically, we conclude that the cancer risk associated with estrogen replacement therapy is greatly outweighed by the preventive effects it provides against heart disease. (This is of course assuming that a woman is not in a high-risk category for breast cancer or endometrial carcinoma.) While we don't recommend estrogen replacement therapy for women with a prior history of deep venous thrombosis (blood clots in the legs), research indicates no increase in blood clots in women who have never had clots who take post-menopausal estrogen.

In conclusion, we recommend that all women undergoing the menopause consult with their gynecologists to assess their needs and eligibility for estrogen replacement therapy. Healthy women with no particular risk factors who are carefully monitored may be able to use estrogen replacement therapy for the rest of their lives and greatly enhance its quality.

Case Study

Alice C was a trim, well-dressed woman of 51 who worked as a managing editor for a large publishing house. With an embarrassed look on her face, she told her doctor, "I'm afraid my age is starting to catch up with me. My hot flushes are getting so bad I have to have the windows wide open even when it's 20 degrees outside. To make matters worse, I have arthritis in my knees and ankles and I have to wear leg warmers so the cold air doesn't bother them. The people in my office think I'm going bananas." She paused. "What's more, my sex life with my husband has really deteriorated lately. My vagina is very dry, and most of the time I don't have much interest, I just want to get it over with. We've tried K-Y Jelly, but it's messy and really doesn't help much. My arthritis just adds to the whole problem because my legs are so sore."

Case Study (continued)

Alice's doctor examined her and took a careful medical history. His only concern was that she had some benign fibrocystic breast changes on her recent mammogram. Even so, because Alice was having so many difficulties, he decided to put her on low dosage estrogen-progestogen therapy (Premarin 0.625 mg and Provera 2.5 mg). Alice took her estrogen and progestogen pills Monday through Friday each week, then took a larger dose of the Provera every 2 months for seven days. She also began to exercise three times a week by walking and playing golf.

Three months later Alice's spirits were much higher. Her hot flushes were improving steadily, and her vagina was once again lubricated. She was also taking a calcium supplement, and a regular aspirin every day for her arthritis. Her arthritis seemed to bother her less, and that may have been a result of her regular exercise program as well as the drug therapy.

Key Points for Menopause

1. Most women experience some response to the body's gradual decline in female hormone production during menopause. Hot flushes, skin inelasticity, osteoporosis, and urinary difficulties are examples of changes occurring from a loss of tissue stimulation by estrogen.

2. Lifestyle changes may help a woman cope with the symptoms of menopause, and also improve the quality of her life as well as prolonging it. These include stopping smoking and recreational drug use; minimizing alcohol and recreational drug intake; eating a nutritious, low-fat diet; taking supplementary calcium; exercising regularly; and, if cardiovascular disease is a risk factor, taking a baby aspirin every day.

3. Estrogen replacement treatment to relieve these symptoms and to prevent further osteoporosis usually consists of a low-dose tablet that is taken either Monday through Friday or daily. If a woman still has her uterus, she needs progestogen medication to counteract the effects of estrogen on the uterus.

4. Most of the hazards associated with the estrogen in birth control pills do not apply in menopausal women because the dosage of estrogen is at least four times lower. There are no problems associated with increased heart disease, blood clots, or breast, ovarian, or endometrial cancer.

5. Local treatment using a vaginal estrogen cream once or twice weekly may be all that is necessary to relieve local discomfort such as vaginal dryness, painful sex, or burning while urinating.

6. Progestins (Provera 10 mg, twice a day) alone are an alternative for treating hot flushes if estrogens must be avoided for certain medical reasons. Although they are considered safe, they sometimes cause unpleasant side effects such as irregular vaginal bleeding, weight gain, and mild depression.

7. The benefits of using estrogen replacement therapy must be weighed carefully against the risks. Women with certain medical conditions such as chronic liver disease or venous blood clots should not take estrogen. In otherwise healthy women, the benefits in preventing cardiovascular disease appear to outweigh the risks of endometrial or breast cancer, especially if progestin therapy is used along with the estrogen.

Table 5-1
Actions of Estrogens

Genital tract
Stimulation of endometrial glandular and stromal compartment
Stimulation of myometrium
Proliferation of vaginal and urethral epithelium
Increase in vascular flow to genital tract
Increase in cervical gland secretions
Stimulation of production of receptors for progesterone and luteinizing hormone

Breast
Stimulation of ductular growth

Skin
Increase in moisture content
Reduction in breakdown of collagen
Decrease in sebum production
Decrease in epithelial proliferation

Bone
Decrease in bone resorption
Increase in parathyroid hormone concentrations

Liver
Stimulation of production of multiple binding globulins (i.e. steroid-binding globulin
  cortsol-binding globulin, thyroid-binding globulin)
Increase in concentration of bile salts

Pituitary-hypothalamus
Suppression of vasomotor symptoms
Suppression and stimulation of gonadotropin secretion
Increase in prolactin secretion

Coagulation
Stimulation of factor VII, VIII, IX, X, and prothrombin
Depression of antithrombin III
Increase in platelet adhesiveness

Lipids
Increase HDL cholesterol or decrease LDL

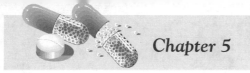

Table 5-2
Oral Estrogens

Name	Estrogen	Dose (mg)	Manufacturer
Premarin	Conjugated estrogens	0.3 0.625 0.9 1.25 2.5	Ayerst
Estrace	Micronized estadiol	1.0 2.0	Mead Johnson
Ogen	Esterified estrogens	0.3 0.625 1.25 2.5 5.0	Reid-Rowell
Estinyl	Ethinyl estradiol	0.02 0.05 0.5	Schering
Estrovis	Quinestrol	0.1	Parke-Davis

Table 5-3
Estrogen Vaginal Creams

Name	Estrogen	Dose	Manufacturer
Premarin Vaginal Cream	Conjugated estrogens	0.625 mg	Ayerst
Estrace Vaginal Cream	17 β-Estradiol	1 g	Mead Johnson
Ogen Vaginal Cream	Estropipate	1.5mg	Abbott
Ortho Dienestrol Cream	Dienestrol	0.01%	Ortho
Estraguard Cream	Dienestrol	0.01%	Reid-Rowell

Table 5-4			
Other Forms of Estrogen			
Name	*Estrogen*	*Dose (mg/mL)*	*Manufacturer*
Depo-Estradiol	Estradiol cypionate	1 5	Upjohn
Delstrogen	Estradiol valerate	10 20 40	Squibb
Estraval	Estradiol valerate	10 20	Reid-Rowell
Estraderm	Transdermal estradiol	0.05 mg/day 0.1 mg/day	Ciba-Geigy

Notes

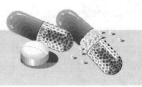

Chapter 6

Drugs for Urinary Tract Problems

Although they are not reproductive organs, the bladder and other lower urinary tract structures are located directly in front of the vagina, cervix, and uterus, and the two organ systems often affect each other (Fig. 6-1). Women frequently consult and get treated by their gynecologists when they are troubled with urinary tract problems. In fact urinary tract complaints are a leading cause of unscheduled visits to a physician's office. Problems related to difficult urination occur frequently and usually involve either an infection or an inability to control urination. Fortunately, doctors now have much better diagnostic tools to use when they try to pinpoint one of the numerous causes of urinary tract distress.

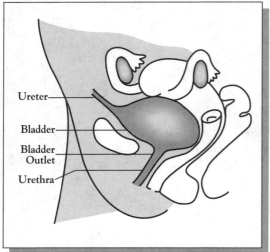

Figure 6-1

Relation of lower urinary tract structures to the vagina, cervix, and uterus.

Urinary Tract Infections

Urinary tract infections, sometimes jokingly referred to as "honeymoonitis," are in fact a very unamusing problem for women.

Women are more prone to urinary tract infections than men because they have a much shorter urethra (tube that brings urine out from the bladder), and bacteria can easily ascend the short urethra into the bladder to multiply.

These infections are much less common in women who have not begun to engage in sexual activity, and an initial urinary tract infection often accompanies the first intercourse, hence, the term honeymoonitis. The thrusting motion of the penis traumatizes the urethra and pushes bacteria from the outer genitals into the urethra, where they can begin to grow and move quickly up into the bladder. One way to prevent this is to empty the bladder soon after intercourse to flush out any bacteria that might have entered. If you notice urinary tract symptoms after initial intercourse or after frequent intercourse, see a doctor for treatment so the problem does not become chronic.

There are several other causes of urinary tract infections too. Among them are surgery, pregnancy, catheterization of the bladder, improper hygiene, abnormal anatomy, restrictive clothing, and even failure to urinate frequently enough. (To protect themselves against urinary tract infections, women ought to urinate no less often than every three to four hours.)

Pregnant women are prone to urinary tract infections because their urine collecting systems are somewhat slowed down due to the influence of hormones, as well as the mechanical pressures caused by the growing fetus. From 5% to 8% of all pregnant women have a urinary tract infection with no symptoms. This problem should be treated quickly because it can turn into a kidney infection, which is more serious. Inflammation of the kidneys can precipitate premature labor, among other things. Such kidney infections tend to occur during the fifth to seventh month of pregnancy, when the uterus moves out of the pelvis and puts more pressure on the right ureter (urine collecting tube), causing poor drainage. This then makes the kidney vulnerable to bacteria, if there are any in the urinary tract. Fortunately, it is usually easy to clear up urinary tract infections quickly with antibiotics.

Symptoms

The symptoms of a urinary tract infection are often extremely uncomfortable. They include: the feeling of needing to urinate all the time; cramping pain and burning on urination; very little actual urine production; dark concentrated urine; and, at times, bleeding. Women who suffer these symptoms can start helping themselves by drinking large amounts of fluid, particularly water or orange or cranberry juice. The high acid content of the latter two beverages has an antibacterial action. If the infection does not clear up quickly, a trip to the doctor's office is in order.

Treatment

Along with taking a careful medical history, the doctor will thoroughly examine the abdomen and pelvis. He or she will look for white blood cells and bacteria in the urine, a relatively simple procedure that can be done in the office. A urine specimen may be sent to a laboratory so that a culture will identify specific organisms. Probably the doctor will not wait for the results to prescribe an antibiotic, such as ampicillin, one of the sulfa drugs such as sulfisoxazole (Gantrisin) or possibly trimethoprim/sulfamethoxazole (Bactrim, Septra) or nitrofurantoin (Macrodantin) (Table 6-1). Immediate treatment is necessary to relieve the discomfort of symptoms and to prevent the infection from spreading further into the kidneys. Fortunately, these drugs rapidly achieve high concentrations in urine and usually relieve symptoms within 24 hours. Drinking large amounts of fluid - 6 or more glasses of water per day - is important along with the antibiotic therapy.

Nowadays, some physicians often prescribe a single large dose of antibiotic medication for acute urinary tract infection (Table 6-2). This method is less expensive and has fewer side effects than a longer course of therapy on a drug. Single dose therapy doesn't seem to be as effective for women who are pregnant, have upper urinary tract diseases, or have diabetes or conditions with lowered immunity, caused by things such as AIDS or anti-rejection drugs for transplants.

In 95% of bladder infections the microorganism involved is *Escherichia coli*, which responds quite successfully to the drugs cited in Tables 6-1, 6-2. *E. coli* bacteria are found in the bowel, where they play a normal rather than an infectious role. They can find their way into the bladder when women are not careful about wiping or cleaning themselves after bowel movements or simply because the vagina and the anus are close to one another

Recurrent Infection

Most bladder infections can be successfully treated without further difficulty. Occasionally they persist or recur for the following reasons: women fail to take the prescribed quantity or course of antibiotics; the drug prescribed was not effective against the specific organism causing the infection; the length of antibiotic therapy was inadequate (stubborn infections may need to be treated longer); or an incorrect diagnosis was made and the real problem was related to an upper urinary tract infection, menopausal changes, noninfectious inflammation, or kidney stones.

Further efforts must then be made to determine the problem. The urine culture should be repeated and perhaps an x-ray examination of the kidneys, bladder, and urine collecting tubes done. This x-ray examination is called an intravenous pyelogram, or IVP. Blood tests should be performed to analyze kidney function and, if indicated, a cystoscopy performed. A cystoscope is a long, narrow, hollow tube with a tiny light on the end of it that allows the doctor to look at the inside of the bladder and urethra.

Women who are beyond menopause may notice irritation on urination, resulting from a loss of estrogen support for the bladder, bladder outlet, and vaginal tissues. Oral estrogen pills or an application of estrogen cream in the vagina may help to strengthen the bladder tissue. The bladder lining and surrounding tissue respond in a positive way to estrogen therapy.

Prevention

Because urinary tract infections are so common, all women should take measures to prevent them. The most important of these is to urinate at least once every 3 to 4 hours. Retaining urine causes it to concentrate, and the likelihood of infection becomes greater. A full bladder also puts pressure on the pelvic organs, causing irritation.

Next, wearing clothing that permits air circulation around the bladder and vaginal openings can prevent problems. Bacteria thrive in warm, moist cramped environments created by tight jeans, stretch pants, or pantihose, particularly if they are made of synthetic fabrics rather than cotton. Panties with cotton crotches are by far the best choice of underwear. Some women find that pantyliners or minipads are good substitutes for undergarments that do not come with cotton crotches.

Good personal hygiene is essential. This includes daily bathing with mild soap and water and proper cleansing after urination or bowel movements. It is inadvisable to add bathing gel or bubble bath to bath water if recurrent urinary tract infections are a problem. Substances in these products are irritating to the delicate tissues in the female genital area. After bowel movements, women should always remember to wipe from front to back to avoid contaminating the bladder and vaginal outlets.

Finally, adequate fluid consumption, that is, 6 or more glasses of water per day, is wise to promote frequent urination and keep urine from becoming too concentrated.

Urinary Incontinence

Urinary incontinence is the involuntary loss of urine. This embarrassing and distressing situation occurs most frequently in elderly women in whom the nerve pathways from the brain or spinal cord to the bladder have begun to deteriorate. Another cause in older women is a stretching or slipping down of the opening to the bladder because of inadequate elasticity.

Younger women tend to suffer more from what is called *stress incontinence*, urine leakage usually associated with hearty laughing, running, jumping, lifting, bending, coughing, vomiting, or late pregnancy. They may also suffer from a particular kind of neurological problem that produces uncontrollable bladder contractions, termed *urge incontinence*.

Sanitary napkins, diapers, or some other form of protection should be worn until effective medical treatment can be found for the particular form of incontinence from which a woman suffers.

Diagnosis of Urinary Incontinence

Doctors now have sophisticated tools at hand to help them determine the cause of incontinence. They can determine different pressures in the urinary tract and at what point they override the body's normal ability to hold back urine. They can detect nerve disorders that might cause poor communication between the central nervous system and the bladder. They can pinpoint fine details related to urine flow.

In addition to these high-tech medical diagnostic procedures, however, physicians also must rely on some of the older and simpler methods for diagnosis of urinary incontinence. These include a woman providing a detailed medical history that will give clues to causes, particularly factors such as nervous system disorders, diabetes, and psychological disturbances. Any medications being taken should be reported, and caffeine and alcohol consumption habits should be mentioned also. The relationship of urinary tract problems to previous pregnancies or surgery will be a consideration.

The doctor will also need to conduct a physical examination that includes inspection of the top of the vaginal wall and a search for any fistula (opening or connection between two structures that would not normally be there) between the bladder and the vagina or for an outpouching of the urethra. Muscle tone and sensation surrounding the vagina and lower bladder region must be assessed.

A woman may be asked to urinate into a special receptacle from which the doctor can determine how quickly urine is expelled and how much is retained in the bladder. A catheter (a slender tube) is then inserted to measure the amount of urine left. The doctor may then fill the bladder artificially using colored water. Once the bladder is full, the catheter is removed, and the vaginal canal is inspected for any staining. The presence of stain suggests a fistula.

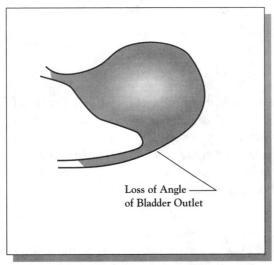

Loss of Angle of Bladder Outlet

Figure 6-2

A common cause of urinary incontinence is a distortion or loss of the angle of the bladder outlet.

The patient may then be asked to bear down so the doctor can observe any leakage. Finally, a clean cotton swab is placed in the urethra. Stress incontinence (Fig. 6-2) is suspected if the swab is deflected upward during the process of bearing down. Urine may also be lost at this time. Additional tests that might be made are an intravenous pyelogram, urine culture, blood tests to check for diabetes, and possibly cystoscopy, a slender tube inserted into the bladder with a light on the end of it to help the doctor visualize the bladder interior.

Therapy for Incontinence

Treatment depends on cause. In most cases of incontinence, there is a distortion of the bladder outlet, and women affected by this problem require an operation to lift up the bladder outlet and restore normal anatomy. Under less extreme circumstances or when the cause is not related to a distorted outlet, certain drugs may prove useful (Table 6-3). These medications partially inhibit the nerves that cause contractions of the bladder and thus prevent the loss of urine. Occasionally, these drugs cause dryness of the mouth, blurred vision, constipation, and weakness. The main consideration is whether an anatomic defect or bladder hyperactivity or both are present. Each requires different therapy.

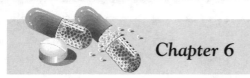

Chapter 6

Among the newer drug approaches to controlling urinary incontinence due to overactivity of the bladder are phenylpropanolomine/chlorpheniramine maleate (Ornade) and phenyl-propanolomine/guanefesin (Entex LA). These drugs, which have been commonly used to control cold and allergy symptoms in the past, seem to help in controlling stress incontinence. Propranolol (Inderal), a drug used in heart patients and people with high blood pressure is sometimes used in cases of stress incontinence. It may be especially desirable for women with heart disease or high blood pressure who could not tolerate some of the other drugs.

Calcium channel blockers, which have also been used to treat heart disease, can suppress some of the urinary tract muscle activity involved in cases of incontinence. Drugs such as terodiline are under study for this usage. Physicians are also studying the use of indomethacin (Indocin) for incontinence. Indocin has been used for several years in the treatment of gout.

In menopausal women, estrogen therapy may improve the condition of the bladder outlet by improving its blood supply and increasing its muscle tone *(See also, Chapter 5)*.

Occasionally, women benefit from the insertion of pessaries, vaginal support devices that, when inserted in the vagina, push the bladder, urethra, and vagina into a more normal position, which helps restore normal control.

Women in all age groups can often help themselves with urinary incontinence by practicing Kegel exercises. "Kegeling" is the voluntary tightening and relaxing of the muscles surrounding the vagina and bladder. Women can work these muscles almost anywhere at any time. We recommend working up to a schedule of 25 contractions and relaxations at least four times a week. Added benefits are the strengthening of all the organs in the lower pelvic region and more satisfying sexual intercourse.

Difficult Urination

The most hazardous condition discussed in this chapter is the inability or near inability to urinate. Although losing urine through incontinence is embarrassing, it does not pose a major threat to health. If a person does not urinate, she can become ill very rapidly. Difficulty in urinating can be caused by a bladder infection, swelling of the bladder outlet after the birth of a child or after a pelvic operation, nerve damage, or a tumor blocking the outflow of urine. Diagnosing the problem involves similar procedures to those used for both infection and incontinence.

Drugs that are helpful in stimulating urination are listed in Table 6-4. Medications such as bethanechol and phenoxybenzamine, which promote bladder contractions and relax the bladder outlet, act directly on the nerves in the vicinity of the bladder. Drugs such as diazepam (Valium) and dantrolene act indirectly by reducing muscle tension or anxiety. Because these drugs often have side effects, women using them must be under close observation by a physician.

Prazosin (Minipress), one of the newer drugs to aid in urination, is an antihypertensive agent (high blood pressure medication), relaxes the muscles in the urinary tract with fewer side effects than some of the older forms of therapy.

If drug therapy does not work, women with difficulty urinating will have to be catheterized or learn to catheterize themselves.

Case Study

Jeannette B, a small, frail-looking 62-year-old widow, had led an active and demanding life. She owned a highly successful real estate agency and spent what free time she had left helping her two daughters with their five children.

Ever since her teens she had had back problems stemming from a swimming accident. The pain and numbness that also involved her left leg had become almost incapacitating. Her doctor had prescribed Motrin for pain relief for her back problem and also for osteoarthritis that had developed at the back of her neck. Jeannette could not seem to obtain the pain relief from the Motrin that she needed.

Her doctor ordered a myelogram, an x-ray examination of the nerves of the spine, and it revealed that Jeannette's arthritic vertebrae were putting pressure on specific spinal nerve roots. A neurosurgical operation was suggested, but the doctor warned her that the operation was somewhat risky and did not always produce the desired results. Unable to tolerate her pain any more, Jeannette decided to go ahead with the operation anyway.

Postoperatively, Jeannette found herself unable to urinate. She had to be catheterized for 8 days. Because of the repeated catheterizations, she developed a urinary tract infection that required a 10-day course of ampicillin. She was also given bethanechol tablets to help stimulate urination.

The spinal root surgery was moderately successful; her shooting pains became much less frequent. However, about 2 weeks after the operation, she suddenly lost all control over her urination and bowel movements. Jeannette was at her wits end when she consulted the doctor about her lack of control. He prescribed Probanthine, which minimized the uncontrollable urine loss caused by involuntary bladder contractions. However, she found that the Probanthine produced constipation and an uncomfortable dryness in her mouth, so she switched to Ditropan, a drug similar to Probanthine but with fewer side effects.

With the assistance of drugs and a newly manufactured adult diaper, Jeannette learned to adjust to her unfortunate surgical complications. She continues to need Ditropan, but her bowel function has returned almost to normal, so she has one less problem to contend with.

Key Points for Urinary Tract Infections

1. Lower urinary tract problems in women of reproductive age are most commonly due to infection. In women beyond menopause the major problem is urinary incontinence.

2. Most urinary tract infections can be easily and permanently treated with an appropriate course of an antibiotic that concentrates well in urine.

3. Pregnant women are especially susceptible to urinary tract infections because of hormonal and anatomical influences. These infections should be treated quickly to prevent spread to the kidneys, which can precipitate premature labor.

4. Recurrent or persistent symptoms of urinary tract infection require a more detailed history and physical examination, with urine culture, and, possibly, x-ray examination, blood tests, and cystoscopy.

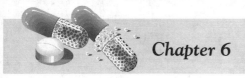
5. If urinary incontinence, an involuntary loss of urine, persists for long periods, it is probably due to a distortion of the bladder outlet. Surgery is usually necessary to correct it, but in mild cases or instances where surgery won't help, drugs may be of value.

6. Difficulty in urinating, with retention of urine, must be treated quickly. Drugs that stimulate the nerves around the bladder or that relax the muscles may be useful, but women using them must be carefully monitored. Catheterization may be the only effective solution.

7. In women at or beyond the menopause, conditions that suggest urinary tract infection or incontinence may relate to lack of adequate support from estrogen in the tissues. Estrogen pills or vaginally-applied estrogen creams may relieve these symptoms.

Table 6-1
Single-Dose Therapy for Uncomplicated Bladder Infections

Medication	Dose
Trimethoprim	400 mg
Trimethorprim plus sulfamethoxazole	320/1,600 mg
Nitrofurantoin	200 mg
Amoxicillin	3g
Amoxicillin plus clavulanate	500 mg
First-generation cephalosporin	2 g
Sulfisoxazole	2 g
Ciprofloxacin	250 mg
Norfloxacin	400mg

Table 6-2
Multidose Oral Therapy for Acute Bladder Infections

Medication	Dose (mg)	Interval (hr)
Trimethoprim	100	12
Trimethorprim plus sulfamethoxazole	160/800	12
Nitrofurantoin	100	6
Amoxicillin	500	8
Amoxicillin plus clavulanate	500	8
First-generation cephalosporin	500	6
Ciprofloxacin	250	12
Norfloxacin	400	12
Sulfisoxazole	500	6
Tetracycline	500	6

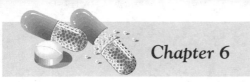

Table 6-3
Drugs That May Aid in Urine Storage

Generic Name	Mode of Action
Propantheline (Pro-Banthine)	Inhibits parasympathetic nervous system
Methantheline (Banthine)	Inhibits parasympathetic nervous system
Oxybutynin (Ditropan)	Inhibits parasympathetic nervous system, local anesthetic, local anesthetic, smooth muscle relaxant
Dicyclomine (Bentyl)	Inhibits parasympathetic nervous system, smooth muscle relaxant
Flavoxate (Urispas)	Very weak parasympathetic inhibitor, local anesthetic, smooth muscle relaxant
Imipramine (Tofranil)	Anticholinergic α-and β- adrenergic agonist, smooth muscle relaxant
Ephedrine	Adrenergic stimulation
Phenylpropanolamine (Propadrine)	α- Adrenergic stimulator
(Ornade)	α- Adrenergic stimulator (antihistamine)
(Entex LA)	α- Adrenergic stimulator (expectorant)
Propranolol (Inderal)	β- Adrenergic blocker
Estrogen	Trophic hormone for urethral mucosa and submucosal vascular plexus; enhances α -adrenergic effects

Table 6-3 (continued)

Dosage	Adverse Reactions
15-30 mg by mouth two to four times a day	Dryness of mouth, blurred vision, constipation, tachycardia, mydriasis, drowsiness
50-100 mg by mouth three to four times a day four times a day	Anticholinergic effects as above
5 mg by mouth two to four times a day	Anticholinergic effects as above (less severe and less frequent)
10-30 mg by mouth three to four times a day	Anticholinergic effects as above but less frequently
100-200 mg by mouth three to four times a day	Anticholinergic effects as above are rare. Not a potent drug
25-50 mg by mouth three to four times a day	Sweating, weakness, fatigue, headache, and anticholinergic effects as above (but all are rare) withdrawal
15-50 mg by mouth three to four times a day	Central nervous system stimulation, palpitations, gastrointestinal disturbance, hyperexcitability, nervousness, hypertension, insomnia
25-50 mg by mouth three to four times a day	As above
One capsule (75 mg) two times a day	As above plus drowsiness
One capsule (75 mg) two times a day	As above
10-40 mg po three to four times a day	Bradycardia, hypotension, depression, gastrointestinal disturbances, bronchospasm. Not potent
Oral or vaginal replacement dosage	Those associated with estrogen replacement therapy

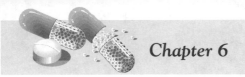

Table 6-4

Drugs That May Aid in Urine Evacuation

Agent	Mode of Action	Dosage	Adverse Reactions
Bethanechol (Duvoid,) Myotonachol, Urecholine	Stimulates parasympathetic nervous system	10-100 mg po three to four times a day	Lacrimation, flushing, sweating, gastrointestinal disturbances, headaches, visual disturbance
Phenoxybenzamine	α-Adrenergic blocker	2.5-10.0 mg SC three to four times a day 10-20 mg po one to three times a day	Postural hypotension, miosis, nasal stuffiness, sweating, dryness of mouth, tachycardia, Animal study: carcinogenesis
Prazosin (Minipress)	Postsynaptic α-Adrenergic blocker	1-5 mg po three to four times a day	Postural hypotension (may be severe with first dose), tachycardia headaches, drowsiness, nausea, dry, mouth
Diazepam (Valium)	Centrally acting skeletal muscle relaxant; anti-anxiety agent	2-10 mg po three to four times a day	Sedation, ataxia, fatigue
Dantrolene (Dantrium)	Skeletal muscle relaxant	25-150 mg po two to four times a day	Generalized weakness, severe hepatotoxicity

Notes

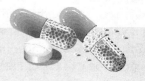

Rx for Depression, Anxiety, and Insomnia

More than 20 million people in the United States have symptoms of anxiety and depression that are serious enough to warrant treatment. Twice as many women as men are clinically depressed long enough and deeply enough to need to see a doctor. Why is this so? Women are known to be more willing to come in for treatment, so it may be that the true depth of depression in men just hasn't been documented in official medical histories.

Anxiety is something virtually everyone experiences from time to time, especially considering the stresses of modern living. The past 25 years have seen major changes in women's social roles, especially in the workplace. Some have taken added responsibilities without relinquishing those at home, undoubtedly a major cause of stress with resulting depression or anxiety. In addition, recent studies of premenstrual syndrome have shown that hormonal changes during the menstrual cycle may cause temporary symptoms of depression and anxiety. Women who are not aware of the physical basis of premenstrual syndrome symptoms may have developed more profound and lasting depression because they have believed all along that there was something wrong with them.

Depression

How does one identify a major depression and distinguish it from what is simply an unhappy but passing mood that results from conflicts in a personal or family relationship, job- or school-related pressures, or hormonal shifts? If the answer to five or more of the following questions is yes, chances are the person is suffering from depression and should seek help:

1. Have you felt a general loss of interest or pleasure in your normal activities over a period of 2 weeks or more?

2. Have you felt restless, uneasy, and uncomfortable without being able to explain why?

3. Have you noticed an appetite or weight change with no apparent physical cause?

4. Are you sleeping much more or much less than you normally do?

5. Are you more easily agitated or more sluggish in responding to others?

6. Are you considerably less energetic than usual and do you tire easily?

7. Do you feel worthless, guilty, or angry at yourself for something you think you have done?

8. Do you have trouble concentrating on things?

9. Do you often think of death or suicide?

What should a woman do about depression? Probably the most common reaction is to do nothing, to let it happen and simply live with it until it goes away. Between 50% and 85% of the people who experience real depression recover spontaneously after perhaps 6 to 12 months of symptoms. Unfortunately, depression has a tendency to recur; even if it doesn't, up to a year is a long time to wait for recovery. If a woman is depressed, it can be very hard on family members and others around her, besides being difficult for the woman herself. Depression can foster hostility, chaos, less productive work, and even suicide attempts.

Some people are willing to seek counseling from a psychiatrist, psychologist, social worker, clergyman, or other individual skilled in handling emotional problems. This type of support can be valuable, but it usually takes a long time to uncover the cause of the depression. This is where the use of drugs may be of assistance. Drugs used to treat depression and other forms of emotional illness are called psychoactive drugs. When used appropriately, they can quickly relieve the symptoms of depression, thus allowing a counselor to work with the person more effectively. In many cases drug treatment is all that is necessary to overcome an episode of depression.

A problem in recent years has been not the underuse of psychoactive drugs, but rather their indiscriminate use without thorough understanding of their power and their potentially beneficial and harmful effects. Women should use psychoactive drugs only under the watchful eye of a physician who understands their application and who is not willing to write an endlessly renewable prescription without frequent evaluation of the patient. The lowest effective dose is desirable.

Tricyclic Antidepressants

The tricyclic antidepressants are used to control major depression. In common terms tricyclics are "uppers," since they elevate your mood and restore your energy and willingness to do things. Several brands of tricyclic antidepressants are currently available in the United States (Table 7-1). These drugs are similar, although different people may have different reactions to each one. A knowledge of their side effects is important when choosing the correct drug. The most common side effects involve sedation and anticholinergic effects (dry mouth, blurred vision, constipation). Elderly patients may also have other anticholinergic effects such as urinary retention, psychosis (a form of mental derangement), low blood pressure, and certain other heart and blood vessel problems.

It is wise to start a course of tricyclic antidepressants with the smallest effective dosage. If results are not obtained quickly, for example, improvement in sleep habits or energy, the dosage can be increased every 24 to 48 hours. By the end of 2 weeks a woman should feel noticeably better; if she does not, she may need psychiatric help along with the antidepressant drug. Drug use can continue for 3 to 6 months if her symptoms do improve. After 6 months she should have her condition reevaluated, and if her symptoms continue to lessen in intensity, the drug dosage should be decreased gradually.

Some physicians hesitate to prescribe these drugs to pregnant women. The drugs pose no known danger to the unborn baby, but as is the case with so many other pharmaceutical agents, not enough studies have been conducted to conclusively rule out any problems. They should therefore be used cautiously during pregnancy, with the lowest possible dosages given over the shortest effective time and preferably under a psychiatrist's supervision.

Overdosing, either deliberate or accidental, is a concern with the use of these drugs. Although the tricyclic antidepressants are of tremendous benefit, they can be fatal when taken in sufficient quantities. An overdose can cause high fever, high blood pressure, seizures, and ultimately coma. If a woman overdoses on a tricyclic drug, she should be immediately attended to by paramedics or emergency room personnel. Induction of vomiting by syrup of ipecac or insertion of a stomach tube through the nose may be necessary. If she

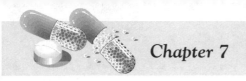

can swallow activated charcoal, it may absorb some of the drug, but this should be done under the supervision of medical personnel even if she is still conscious.

Table 7-1 Antidepressant Drugs		
Generic Name (Brand Name)	**Oral Preparations (mg)**	**Average Daily Dosage (mg)**
Tricyclics		
Amitriptyline (Elavil. Endep. others)	10, 25, 50, 75, 100, 150	150 to 300
Desipramine (Norpramin, Pertofran)	25, 50	150 to 250
Doxepin (Adapin, Sinequan)	10, 25, 50, 75, 100, 150	150 to 300
Imipramine (Presamine, Tofranil)	10, 25, 50; PM: 75, 100, 150	150 to 300
Nortriptyline (Aventyl, Pamelor)	10, 25	50 to 150
Protrityline (Vivactil)	5, 10	10 to 60
Trimipramine (Surmontil)	25, 50	150 to 250
Monoamine oxidase (MAO) inhibitors		
Hydrazines		
Isocarboxazine (Marplan)	10	10 to 50
Phenelzine (Nardil)	15	15 to 75
Nonhydrazine ,		
Tranylcypromine (Parnate)	10	20 to 40
Fluoxetine (Prozac)	20	20 to 80
Combination agents		
Amitriptyline/perphenazine (Etrafone, Triavil)	2/10, 4/10, 2/25, 4/25, 4/50	
Amitriptyline/chlordiazel)oxide (Limbitrol)	12.5/5, 25/10	

Monoamine Oxidase Inhibitors

If tricyclics are not effective, there are alternative drugs to combat depression. Monoamine oxidase inhibitors have been found to be particularly effective in younger people with depression characterized by anxiety accompanied by many body symptoms, hypochondriasis (obsession with imagined physical illness), irritability, agoraphobia (fear of leaving the house or being in an open space), and other types of phobias (aversions or fears). The three best known monoamine oxidase inhibitors are the hydrazine phenelzine (Nardil), nonhydrazine tranylcypromine (Parnate), and fluoxetine (Prozac).

Major side effects, especially with tranylcypromine, include insomnia, restlessness, irritability, and agitation. Women should keep in mind that these drugs can cause problems if used in conjunction with meperidine (Demerol), alcohol, and most other central nervous system depressants. They will react with tyramine-containing substances, such as chocolate, red wine, cheese, nuts, coffee, and pickled herring, to produce severe hypertension. If the hypertension is severe, the drug should be discontinued. If the blood pressure remains elevated, it should be treated with phentolamine (Regitine).

Anxiety

Anxiety is most commonly caused by life stresses, which range from interpersonal conflicts, to financial crises to natural catastrophes. The list is endless, and it seems to increase daily as life grows more complicated. Normal anxiety usually disappears when the source of the problem is resolved. Another type of anxiety, more complex and more remote in origin, stems from fear, apprehension, and nervousness without certainty of the source of these feelings. This condition is termed free-floating anxiety. Persons with either form of anxiety may require treatment because the symptoms are just as uncomfortable. Persons suffering from free-floating anxiety may also need prolonged psychiatric therapy to determine its ultimate source.

If the answer to five or more of these is yes, a woman may be suffering from anxiety, and you need to find relief:

1. Do you feel keyed up, tense, and apprehensive much of the time?

2. Do you experience fear, dread, or fright without knowing why?

3. Do you have unexplainable aversions to certain things or situations?

4. Are you ever overcome with panic in public places?

5. Do you constantly feel worried and overly concerned about situations around you?

6. Do you experience breathlessness, tightness of the chest, or dizziness without any apparent cause?

7. Does your heart race, and do you have sweaty palms, shakiness, and flushing?

8. Do you get uncontrollable urges to urinate or move your bowels?

9. Do your muscles get very tense, including those in your throat? Do you sometimes feel like you're choking?

10. Do you lie awake at night with thoughts racing through your head, unable to fall asleep?

Certain drugs or medical conditions listed in Table 7-2 may cause anxiety-like symptoms. When you consult a doctor because you are suffering from anxiety, he or she should be certain to rule out nonemotional conditions as the source.

Several types of tranquilizing drugs are used to treat anxiety. They fall into the categories of benzodiazepines, barbiturates, propanediols, β–blocking agents, certain antihistamines, and the tricyclic antidepressants. A more comprehensive list of tranquilizers or antianxiety agents, including the benzodiazepines, appears in Table 7-3.

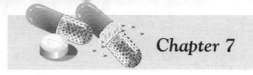

Benzodiazepines

The benzodiazepines are the most commonly prescribed drugs for anxiety. In everyday language they are called "downers," and their brand names are familiar: Xanax, Valium, Librium, Tranxene, Centrax, Serax, and Buspar. These drugs are best prescribed only when anxiety interferes with the ability to function normally, provided that a medical condition or use of an anxiety-producing drug such as caffeine has been ruled out. Benzodiazepine drugs are particularly valuable when a person is under sudden but short-lived stress or is about to undergo a medical or surgical procedure. Stress-provoking situations should be assessed before the prescription of these medicines. The lowest possible dosage should be taken over the shortest time needed to achieve results. Women need to understand that the use of these medicines has special applications; they should not become a daily habit, accompanying the morning coffee. Physicians should closely monitor their patients who take benzodiazepines to see that the drugs are being used correctly.

The benzodiazepines are remarkably free from side effects when used alone. In dosages higher than normally prescribed, drowsiness and problems with coordination may develop. Elderly persons have more problems with side effects. They may also become dizzy or confused and have trouble speaking clearly and coordinating their eye muscles. These drugs must not be taken with narcotic painkillers, sleeping pills, or alcohol because they may cause dangerous drowsiness and even unconsciousness. Unpredictable side effects such as irrational rage sometimes occur.

Table 7-2	
Conditions That May Create Anxiety Symptoms	
Drug overdose	Heartbeat irregularities
Drug withdrawal	Pheochromocytoma (adrenal gland tumor)
Caffeine overuse	Premenstrual tension
Organic brain syndromes	Lung clot
Epilepsy	Angina or heart attack
Hypoglycemia (low blood sugar)	Hyperthyroidism
Chronic lung disease	Mitral valve prolapse of heart (floppy mitral valve)
Inner ear problems	Depression
Pain	Schizophrenia

We recommend that pregnant women not take these drugs. Their effect on the unborn baby's brain is unknown. These medications may also accumulate in high levels in nursing infants as well, so we believe they should also be avoided when a woman being treated for anxiety is breast-feeding.

Table 7-3
Antianxiety Drugs

Generic Name (Brand Name)	Oral Preparations (mg)	Average Daily Dosage (mg)
Benzodiazepines		
Alprazolam (Xanax)	0.25, 0.50	0.75 to 1.50
Chlordiazepoxide (Librium)	5, 10, 25	15 to 100
Clorazepate dipotassium (Tranxene)	3.75, 7.5, 15	15 to 60
Clorazepate monopotassium (Azene)	3.25, 6.5, 13	13 to 52
Diazepam (Valium)	2, 5, 10	5 to 60
Lorazepam (Ativan)	1, 2	2 to 10
Oxazepam (Serax)	10, 15, 30	30 to 120
Prazepam (Centrax)	5, 10	20 to 60
Alternatives		
Propanediols		
Meprobamate (Equanil, Miltown)	200, 400	600 to 2000
Tybamate (Solacen, Tybatran)	250, 350	750 to 2500
Antihistamines		
Diphenhydramine (Benadryl)	25, 50	75 to 300
Hydroxyzine (Atarax, Vistaril)	10, 25, 50, 100	75 to 400
Tricyclic antidepressants		
Doxepin (Adapin, Sinequan)	10, 25, 50, 75, 100, 150	50 to 150
Buspirone (Buspar)	5, 10	15 to 60

Other Drugs

The propanediol drugs, such as meprobamate (Miltown, Equanil), seem to hold no advantages over the benzodiazepines in relieving anxiety and often produce more problems. They have greater potential for tolerance and dependency, and withdrawal reactions can be very severe. Nor do we recommend the B-adrenergic blocking agents such as propranolol (Inderal) for control of anxiety. We feel they are being used in inappropriate circumstances, such as when giving speeches or performing or to slow down a rapid heart rate that often accompanies normal anxiety. The appropriate use of B-blocking drugs is for certain heart conditions and hypertension, not ordinary nervousness.

Occasionally antihistamines such as diphenhydramine (Benadryl) and hydroxyzine (Atarax) may relieve anxiety. Although not as effective as the benzodiazepines, they are less habit-forming and are useful when there is a history of drug abuse. The tricyclic antidepressant doxepin (Adapin, Sinequan) may be used to relieve anxiety, but only when depression coexists.

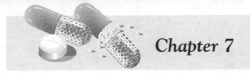

Buspirone (Buspar) is less sedating than most drugs. It has shown no potential for abuse or diversion, and there is no evidence that buspirone causes physical or psychological dependence. Many doctors consider this to be the drug of choice for those with anxiety.

Insomnia

Difficulties in sleeping (insomnia) usually involve an inability to fall asleep, remain asleep, or experience satisfaction after sleep. Insomnia may be the most widespread complaint of people suffering from both anxiety and depression, but it is also probably the one most clearly improved with the use of drugs.

Table 7-4 Hypnotic Drugs		
Generic Name (Brand Name)	**Oral Preparations (mg)**	**Average Hypnotic Dosage (mg)**
Benzodiazepines		
Temazepam (Restoril)	15, 30	15 to 30
Flurazepam (Dalmane)	15, 30	15 to 30
Diazepam (Valium)	2, 5. 10	5 to 20
Triazolam (Halcion)	0.125, 0.250	0.125 to 0.250
Barbiturate		
Secobarbital (Seconal)	50, 100	100 to 200
Halogenated hydrocarbon		
Chloral hydrate (Noctec)	250, 500	500 to 2000
Carbamates		
Meprobamate (Equanil. Miltown)	400	400 to 800
Glutarimide		
Glutethimide (Doriden)	250, 500	500
Quenazolones		
Methaqualone (Quaalude)	75	150 to 300

Anxious women may plead with their doctors to give them a sleeping pill so they can at least enjoy the relief of a good night's sleep. Physicians must, however, be careful to fully understand the cause of sleeplessness before prescribing a hypnotic (sleeping drug), especially for more than a few days. Hypnotics can be difficult to give up once a person has gotten into the habit of taking them. Hypnotics are not advisable in cases of depression or serious emotional disturbances, but antidepressant drugs are usually very helpful under those circumstances.

Hypnotics are useful for the short-term treatment of insomnia resulting from stressful adjustment situations (Table 7-4). Their principal action is depression of the central nervous system. When taken to induce sleep, the benzodiazepines (Halcion, Dalmane, Valium, Serax, Ativan) are considered hypnotics and are probably the safest drugs for this purpose. They produce a better quality of sleep than do barbiturates and narcotics and have less potential for dependency and overdose. Flurazepam (Dalmane), Temazepam (Restoril), and Triazolam (Halcion) are probably the most popular sleeping drugs that have been approved for that purpose by the Food and Drug Administration.

Alternative drugs that may be used as very short-term sleep-loss remedies include secobarbital (Seconal), chloral hydrate (Ioctec), meprobamate (Equanil), glutethimide (Doriden), methaqualone (Quaalude), and antihistamines in certain over-the-counter remedies. Side effects from these medications involve slowing down of breathing mechanisms, but usually only with dosages greater than would be used for sedation. Addiction is possible with long-term use.

Case Study

Mary M, 36, was an assistant manager at a local clothing and department store. She and her husband, Bill, married just out of high school. They quarreled and disagreed throughout the course of their marriage but stayed together for the sake of their two daughters, now 14 and 17. Over the past 4 years Mary and Bill's relations grew even more strained. Bill turned to alcohol and Mary to Xanax. She started to use Xanax innocently enough to relieve her occasional bouts of sleeplessness. When she found out Bill was seeing a secretary at his office, she began to rely much more heavily on the drug to relieve her sadness and pain. No one was surprised when Mary sought and was granted a divorce from Bill.

Relieved to have finally severed her ties with Bill, at the same time she found she missed him and occasionally still had mixed feelings about splitting up with him. Looking at family pictures recipitated crying spells, and despite her now steady use of Xanax, she would often awaken in the middle of the night thinking of him. She had difficulty taking an interest in things around her and most of the time she felt fatigued. She found herself plagued by thoughts of her own worthlessness.

Her family doctor finally decided to treat her problem with Elavil because her low mood had persisted for 4 months. He told her she had to discontinue her use of Xanax before she could start taking Elavil. Her initial dosage was 50 mg per day, but she did not find relief until the doctor increased the dosage to 100 mg per day, taken at bedtime. She improved with the Elavil and soon began to sleep more easily at night. Mary also consulted a psychologist, and he recommended group therapy to her.

Mary now belongs to a close-knit group of six people who meet once a week and under the guidance of a psychologist share their problems with each other. By attending Parents Without Partners she has met people in similar situations, has gained several new friends, and is dating a man she met there. She still uses Elavil but recently decreased her dosage without any ill effects.

Key Points for Depression, Anxiety and Insomnia

1. Anxiety and depression are widespread in the United States. Twice as many women suffer from depression as do men.

2. There are several indicators of depression, the most important of which is loss of interest and enthusiasm in normal activities .

3. Depression will often resolve spontaneously after a period of 6 to 12 months, but drug therapy may shorten this time and reduce some of the stresses it creates in the interim.

4. The tricyclic antidepressants are the most popular drugs for treating depression. They occasionally produce side effects, such as dry mouth, blurred vision, and constipation, especially in the elderly.

5. If after two weeks of using a tricyclic antidepressant a woman does not feel better, she may need to have the drug dosage increased and her condition reevaluated. Psychiatric therapy may be necessary.

6. An alternative to tricyclic antidepressant therapy is treatment with monoamine oxidase inhibitors. They are particularly effective in young people with unusual manifestations of anxiety, such as hypochondria and irrational fears.

7. There are several indicators of anxiety, the most important of which include tenseness, apprehension, fear, inability to sleep, and physical symptoms such as shaking, racing heartbeat, tightness of the chest, and sweaty palms.

8. Certain drugs or medical conditions may cause anxiety, and they should be considered by your doctor before any other drug is used.

9. Most people suffer from anxiety caused by life stress from time to time. A more serious condition, free-floating anxiety, sometimes requires extensive counseling along with antianxiety drugs.

10. Buspirone and the benzodiazepines are the tranquilizing drugs most commonly used to treat anxiety. They include Xanax, Valium, Librium, Tranxene, Centrax, and Serax and generally produce no major side effects.

11. Tranquilizers should be prescribed when anxiety begins to interfere with a woman's ability to function. They should never be used beyond the time actually needed to overcome or lessen symptoms.

12. Insomnia should be treated first by decreasing the intake of stimulants such as caffeine and nicotine and by using relaxation techniques and warm milk at bedtime.

13. Along with the benzodiazepines, other drugs may be prescribed to induce sleep. These medicines are intended for short term therapy when getting a good night's sleep has not been possible. Prolonged periods of insomnia require careful attention to underlying emotional or medical disturbances which are not treatable by these hypnotic drugs alone.

14. The lowest effective dose and avoidance of other psychoactive drugs or chemicals are the best policy.

Notes

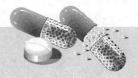

Chapter 8

Treatment of Vaginitis

Ask any woman and she'll tell you, an uncomfortable vaginal discharge can be pure misery and very frustrating. What's more, vaginitis (soreness, itching, and discharge in the area surrounding the vagina) is the most common reason a woman visits her gynecologist or family doctor. It has been estimated that 5% to 10% of all gynecologist appointments are made because a woman has a vaginal discharge - 14 million appointments for yeast infections alone!

Vaginitis is an ancient disease, first described by Hippocrates in the first century A.D. To this day just about every woman alive will experience its symptoms at some time in her life. And, while vaginitis is not usually serious or life-threatening, it can cause a great deal of suffering, on both the physical and emotional level. It can also become very expensive because of the need for repeated medical visits, time lost from work, and money spent on a variety of treatments that sometimes don't work.

Causes and Symptoms

Bacteria, protozoans, funguses, viruses, chemicals, allergic reactions, and foreign objects can all cause vaginitis. One can look at the vagina as a kind of ecosystem, an environment with several components that balance each other out and usually work together harmoniously. When that balance is upset, a woman may begin to have symptoms. These include an increase in vaginal discharge, a change in color and texture from normal secretions, an unpleasant odor, itching, burning, soreness, and swelling in the vulvar area (area surrounding the vagina).

Many different things can be responsible for upsetting the vaginal ecosystem: improper hygiene, therapy with antibiotics or steroids (such as cortisone); sexual contact with an infected person; vaginal douching; immunosuppressive drugs (such as are given to transplant patients); hormonal changes and aging; uncontrolled diabetes; or foreign objects in the vagina.

The vagina is a relatively insensitive organ with rather weak nerve impulses. For example, a foreign object such as a tampon or a diaphragm can be in the vagina and not be apparent to a woman. Thus, if a vaginal infection is present, there are usually no symptoms of pain or irritation, only a discharge. Once the vaginal infection involves the nerve-rich vulvar area, symptoms of pain, irritation, and itching become apparent.

Diagnosis of Vaginitis

Physicians will seldom be able to tell what is wrong in the vagina by listening to a description of the symptoms. They make their diagnosis by examining the woman and analyzing the discharge. For instance, yeast infections are white and lumpy like cottage cheese and *Trichomonas* has a yellow-green color and strong odor. Often the doctor will swab the vagina with a Q-tip and suspend it in normal saline and then look at the material under a microscope to help identify the microorganism responsible for the problem. The doctor may also test the acid-base balance (pH) of the vagina to determine whether or not there is an infection present. The vagina is normally acidic with a pH of 3.5 to 4.5. When this number increases, meaning the vagina is less acidic, it usually indicates a problem.

In difficult cases where a causative agent cannot be easily identified and a woman suffers repeated infections, secretions from the vagina may have to be cultured (grown) in the pathology laboratory for positive identification.,

Common Types of Vaginitis and What To Do About Them

Bacterial Vaginosis

Bacterial vaginosis (an "-osis" is a discharge that does not cause itching or soreness versus an "-itis," which does) is the most common of all the abnormal vaginal discharges. Several microorganisms have been identified in relation to it, including *Haemophilus vaginalis* and *Mobiluncus* species. Bacterial vaginosis goes by other names such as *Gardnerella vaginalis* or non-specific vaginosis.

Women complain of a fishy-smelling or foul odor to their vaginal secretions and, occasionally, some burning with bacterial vaginosis. We don't generally regard bacterial vaginosis as a sexually-transmitted disease, believing instead that it originates with microorganisms in the woman's own gastrointestinal tract. However, women with multiple sexual partners seem to have a higher incidence of bacterial vaginosis.

It is important to know that bacterial vaginosis, left untreated, can have serious side effects. These include mucopurulent cervicitis (inflammation and discharge from the cervix), postoperative cuff cellulitis (an inflammation at the top of the vagina after a hysterectomy), recurrent urinary tract infection, and occasionally pelvic inflammatory disease. In pregnant women, it may be associated with premature membrane rupture and resulting inflammation chorioamnionitis (an inflammation of the placenta or "afterbirth" and membranes around the baby); as well as postpartum endometritis (inflammation of the endometrium).

One of two drugs is usually prescribed for bacterial vaginosis: metronidazole (Flagyl), in a 500 mg oral dose taken twice daily for 7 days, or clindamycin (Clinocin), in a 300 mg oral dose taken twice daily for 7 days or Cleocin vaginal cream. Drugs that are less effective but still useful include ciprofloxacin (Cipro) and triple sulfa cream.

Candidiasis (Yeast Overgrowth)

Yeast overgrowth infections of the vagina are very common. At least 75% of women will experience them at some point in their lives. They seem to be more common during pregnancy. A fungus called *Candida albicans*, has, in the past, been responsible for most yeast overgrowth infections in the vaginal tract. *Candida albicans* is always present to some extent in the vaginal secretions and lives normally without causing problems in many other parts of the body, especially the bowels. *Candida albicans* gets out of control when, for example, a woman takes a course of antibiotic therapy for a respiratory infection, and the antibiotics stamp out many or most of the other microorganisms in the vagina, along with the offenders in the lungs or sinuses. This upsets the natural balance and the yeast-producing fungi grow out of control, creating an itchy and aggravating vaginal discharge. We recommend that women who take antibiotics for more than three days should also use an antifungal suppository in the vagina to prevent yeast infections.

A woman can give herself a yeast infection by careless wiping after bowel movements (i.e., pulling the toilet paper forward and bringing yeast from the rectum into the vaginal area instead of wiping backward) or by not cleaning herself thoroughly after bowel movements. She can also get yeast infections from a sexual partner, particularly if a man is not circumcised, but this is uncommon. Usually, if a woman is being treated for a yeast infection, her sexual partner need not receive the same treatment unless he has a penile infection. Table 8-1 summarizes the drugs used in the treatment of Candidiasis infections.

Currently, treatment for *Candida albicans* yeast infections is a nystatin vaginal suppository or cream (Nilstat, Mycostatin) inserted in the vagina twice a day for 10 days. Nystatin cream may be used on the vulva or spread on the penis of the male partner, as well. Possibly because of the widespread usage of antibiotics, in the last few years several different strains of *Candida* have begun to crop up in yeast overgrowth infections. Nystatin is not as effective against these other types of *Candida*. Fortunately, a new class of drugs called the triazoles has proved effective against them, and two of them, clotrimazole (Gyne-Lotrimin) and miconazole (Monistat), are even sold over the counter as vaginal suppositories. A single 500 mg tablet may be all that is necessary for cure. Alternatively, Monistat may be used in single 200 mg doses for 3 days or 100 mg doses for 6 days.

A caution is in order, however. If, after a course of treatment with Monistat, a yeast infection does not improve, it is time to see a physician. Continuing application of the wrong drug can worsen a problem and make it much more difficult to cure. For stubborn, recurrent yeast infections, ketoconazole (Nizoral) and fluconazole have been prescribed. These drugs are taken by mouth and do have occasional side effects such as nausea and liver toxicity. Boric acid capsule suppositories have also been recommended for these Nystatin-resistant yeast infections. Topical gentian violet applications are quite effective for certain types of *Candida,* but these must be handled in the physician's office and can cause staining of both tissues and clothing. A very small percentage (1%) of people have a severe allergic reaction to Gentian violet, and this must always be considered.

Women who have stubborn, chronic yeast infections might want to consider eliminating yeast-containing foods or other products that aggravate yeast infections from their diets.

These include:

- Brewer's, torula, or other yeasts
- B complex vitamins (unless they are yeast free)
- Peanuts
- Pistachios
- Honey, sugar, and sugar-containing foods
- Yeast breads and pastries
- Alcoholic beverages
- Root beer, cider, fruit juice or any other fermented beverage
- Malt products
- Cereals and candy
- Condiments such as ketchup, mustard, Accent, pickles, relishes, etc.
- Processed and smoked meats
- Dried and canned fruits; melons
- Mushrooms
- Cheese
- Coffee and tea

Trichomoniasis

Fortunately, trichomoniasis (popularly known as "trich") has been on the decline since the 1970s due to better diagnostic techniques and more effective drug therapy, combined with parallel treatment of sexual partners.

Trichomoniasis is a sexually transmitted disease that, in its severe forms, causes symptoms of profuse, bad-smelling, greenish-yellow discharge; pain; sores in the vaginal area; pain during intercourse; spotting between periods or after intercourse; difficulty urinating; and a feeling of fullness in the vaginal area. It is caused by a tiny parasite called a flagellate protozoan, which when seen under the microscope is oblong and, has a characteristic whipping tail. Routine Pap smears are highly accurate in diagnosing trichomoniasis. Doctors also use what is called a wet mount, where a sample of the discharge is taken on a moistened Q-tip and observed under the microscope. Trichomoniasis may also be diagnosed with more sophisticated microscopic techniques such as immunofluorescence studies.

The trichomonas microbe is often found in the urinary tract, and the prostate gland of men. Thus, to avoid reinfection, male sexual partners of women diagnosed with trichomoniasis should undergo simultaneous drug treatment.

Fortunately, metronidazole (Flagyl) is highly effective against *Trichomonas*. A single dose of 2 grams works well for the average person. The alternative is 250 mg three times daily for 7 days, which will prevent early reinfection. It sometimes creates side effects such as nausea, diarrhea, or abdominal discomfort. However, since the single dose is so effective, if these side effects occur, they should not last long. We strongly recommend that a woman avoid alcohol when taking metronidazole, as alcohol seems to aggravate or even create some of the unpleasant side effects of metronidazole.

We are still not absolutely certain of the effects of metronidazole during early pregnancy, but we feel comfortable prescribing it after the second trimester.

Menopausal and Prepubertal Vaginitis

Following menopause, women sometimes experience vaginitis related to estrogen deficiency *(See Chapter 5)*. This type of vaginitis is primarily related to drying and thinning of the vaginal walls and is reversible with hormone replacement.

At the other end of the age spectrum, girls who have not yet reached puberty may also experience vaginal irritation related to lack of estrogen. Teaching better hygiene habits to girls this age, such as careful daily washing with soap and warm water, often solves this problem.

One note of caution: Girls before the age of puberty are sometimes seen in physician's offices with vaginal discharges containing gonorrhea or chlamydial organisms. This is often a sign of sexual abuse, which indicates not only treatment by a physician but intervention by a social service or other governmental agency as well.

Other Causes of Vaginitis

Contraceptive Techniques and Vaginitis

At one time it was thought that women who used oral contraceptives were more susceptible to yeast infections. We no longer subscribe to this theory and find that the rate of yeast infections in oral contraceptive users and non-users is just about the same.

Chlamydia trachomatis seems to be more prevalent in the vaginal tract of oral contraceptive users, but, interestingly, they seem to suffer less from the more serious upper genital infections caused by chlamydia infections. *(See Chapter 9 for a more detailed discussion of chlamydial infection).*

Women who use barrier methods of contraception such as the diaphragm should be careful not to leave the device in place longer than the recommended 8 hours following intercourse, as this can sometimes cause vaginal discharge and even infection. Occasionally, sensitivities to contraceptive creams, jellies, or suppositories can develop, causing vaginal irritation and discharge. In such cases, use of the product should be discontinued and a non-irritating alternative substituted.

Vulvar Vestibulitis Syndrome/Pudendal Neuralgia

Women who continue to have extreme vaginal soreness and irritation after all the other causes discussed above have been ruled out may suffer from one of two rare conditions. *Vulvar vestibulitis syndrome*, which is characterized by severe pain, burning, or rawness to the touch in the area surrounding the vagina, must be managed by meticulous cleaning of the area with plain water at least twice daily. Soaps, detergents, pads, pantyliners, and tight-fitting pantihose must be avoided and loose fitting garments worn instead. At least half of all women with this problem have associated genital warts (human papilloma virus) (*See Chapter 10, also*).

Topical anesthetics may help relieve pain. Topical steroids may relieve the inflammation after any necessary infection control agents have been used. Women who have this problem chronically are sometimes treated with injections of interferon, a biological product synthesized from living tissue. In the most difficult cases, surgery may be necessary to relieve pain with good results in approximately 80% of the cases.

Pudendal neuralgia is an unremitting burning and pain sensation caused by inflammation of the major nerve to the genital area. It is associated with herpes infections, tumors, or previous surgery in the genital area, as well as the human papilloma virus.

Women who complain of pudendal neuralgia have been sometimes unfairly labeled neurotic or hysterical in the past. Physicians believe that the disease is "real" and have had some success in treating it with tricyclic antidepressant drugs or anti-seizure drugs such as phenytoin or carbamazepine. If herpes is involved, acyclovir may need to be taken on a regular basis. Again, in worst case scenarios, surgery may have to be used to relieve unremitting pain. Other treatments such as acupuncture, TENS (transcutaneous electrical nerve stimulation), regional anesthesia blocks, and capsaicin have been used with occasional good results.

Case Study

Deborah T., a 28 year old executive secretary was concerned about a vaginal discharge problem that started about three weeks after she began sexual relations with a new boyfriend. The infection had begun with an itchy, cottage cheese-like discharge, which she had guessed was a yeast infection. She purchased Monistat vaginal suppositories at her local drugstore and used them for three days, as directed on the package.

The infection cleared up temporarily, but a few days later it returned. This time her discharge had a "fishy" odor, and its color had changed from white to grayish. She scheduled an appointment with her gynecologist, nervously explaining that she thought she had a "venereal disease."

The doctor examined Deborah and told her she had bacterial vaginosis, an infection caused by bacteria that could have several sources. After reviewing Deborah's sexual history, the gynecologist reassured her that it was not a serious problem yet, nor had it necessarily been transmitted to her by her new boyfriend. She prescribed Cleocin/cream, a topical antibiotic and also urged Deborah to change contraceptive jelly brands. She advised her to bathe her genital area with mild soap and water daily. She also suggested that Deborah wash her diaphragm carefully with soap and hot water after each usage. Since her boyfriend wasn't circumcised, the doctor recommended that he wash around his foreskin more carefully to avoid the introduction of bacteria into Deborah's vagina.

The bacterial vaginosis cleared up. A few months later Deborah suffered from an itchy white discharge again. This time she went to the doctor who gave her a prescription for Mycostatin cream to clear up the yeast infection. Although she continued to get yeast infections every now and then, neither Deborah or her doctor felt that stronger measures were needed, since the commonly prescribed drugs and over-the-counter drugs always cleared them up.

Key Points for Vaginitis

1. The most common sites of female reproductive tract infections are the vulva, vagina, and cervix. Women's complaints typically include genital sores, vulvar itching, and vaginal discharge, which may have a bad odor. Many viral, bacterial, and fungal infections produce no symptoms.

2. Most infections of the vagina result from either Candida (yeast), Trichomonas, or bacterial vaginosis infections. In their early stages, none of these poses a strong threat to health. They can be uncomfortable and cause itching, burning, and a foul-smelling discharge. Recommended drugs taken for an appropriate length of time should eradicate these infections successfully.

3. Yeast infections can be stubborn and continue to recur. In such cases, stronger drugs or boric acid or gentian violet applications in the doctor's office may be needed. Women with this problem may wish to consider eliminating yeast-containing foods from their diet.

4. Other causes of vaginitis include hormonal imbalances, contraceptive practices, or rare conditions such as vulvar vestibulitis or pudendal neuralgia.

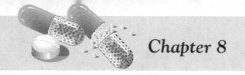

Table 8-1
Drugs Used in the Treatment of Vulvovaginal Candidiasis

Drug Name	Doses	Comments
Gentian violet	Paint vulvovaginal area-repeat 72 hr and weekly as needed	Severe allergy (1%) office procedure; messy
Nystatin (Mycostatin, Nilstat)	100,000 vaginally twice daily x 14 days	Least active antifungal; poor for recurrent infection; oral ineffective to eliminate rectal reservoir
Clotrimazole (Gyne-Lotrimin, Mycelex*)	100 mg/day vaginally x 7 days 200 mg/day vaginally x 3 days 500mg vaginally x 1 day	Suppository, tablet, cream, lotion forms:worsening symptoms suggest drug sensitivity
Miconazole (Monistat*)	100 mg/day vaginally x 7 days 200 mg/day vaginally x 3 days	Same as for clotrimazole
Boric acid capsules	600 mg vaginally daily-twice daily x 14 days	Inexpensive; must be made; topical ointment (Borfax) available
Ketoconazole (Nizoral)	200mg/day orally x 3 days 400 mg orally orally x 3 days 400 mg/day orally x 5 days 400 mg/day orally x 14 days 400 mg/day orally x 5 days each month (intermittent prophylaxis)	For selected recurrent persistent cases; for liver toxicity potential
Butoconazole (Femstat)	5 g of 2% cream intravaginally at bedtime x 3 days 5 g of 2 % cream intravaginally at bedtime x 6 days	Appears as effective as similar intravaginal agents
Terconazole (Terazole)	80 mg suppository intravaginally h.s. x 3 days 5 g of 0.4% cream intravaginally at night or "nightly" x 7 days	Appears as effective as topical clotrimazole or miconazole
Diflucam	100-200mg, orally, once or twice a week	Helps eradicate yeast infection Used in immunosuppressed patients, for example, transplant AIDS patients.

*Available as over-the-counter preparations

Notes

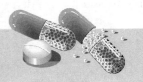

Curable Sexually Transmitted Infections

Virtually all women who have ever been sexually active have had infections related to sexual activity. Some of these, as discussed in Chapter 8, are not officially considered "venereal diseases" or sexually transmitted diseases, while others are. Some of them have no cure, while for others, excellent drug therapy exists.

This chapter focuses on sexually transmitted diseases for which, happily, we have a cure. These include infections caused by bacteria, parasites, spirochetes, and other organisms.

We also suggest a practical approach to dealing with the epidemics of sexually transmitted disease that currently exist. Women do not have to feel "unclean," outcast, or disgraced because they have a sexually transmitted disease. Sexual activity is normal and natural, but like many other aspects of life comes with some risks. Contact with other human beings, sexual or otherwise, can result in disease transmission. This does not mean a women should worry incessantly about contracting a disease. It does mean she should be careful and take certain precautions!

There are three important things to remember with regard to sexually transmitted disease:

1. Prevention is a key point. Unless you know your sexual partner very well, you should protect yourself at all times against the possibility of any sexually transmitted diseases (including AIDS) by using a male condom plus a diaphragm and spermicide or a female condom.

2. If you have symptoms which may indicate a sexually transmitted disease, see your doctor immediately. Early treatment prevents more serious problems from developing and may avoid further accidental spread of the disease.

3. Inform your sexual partner or partners if you have a disease, because they may be the source of your infection to begin with. In any case, all partners should be treated along with you to avoid "ping-ponging" organisms back and forth or spreading the disease further.

Chlamydia

Chlamydia is one of the "newer" sexually transmitted diseases that has been on the upswing for the last 20 years. It is much more common than gonorrhea, but because its symptoms are not always obvious, many people don't know they have it. Women in particular, often will go for an extended period of time without realizing they harbor the chlamydia organism. Therefore, it is important to be aware of subtle clues that the disease is present.

Chlamydia is caused by a bacteria-like organism called *Chlamydia trachomatis.* When symptoms are present, women may notice a yellowish discharge that originates from the cervix, itching, bleeding between periods, painful intercourse, or bleeding after intercourse. An active chlamydia infection may be more obvious in her male sexual partner, where symptoms of burning or itching during urination or need to urinate frequently may be a clue. If a man is diagnosed with chlamydia, then his female sexual partner is very likely to have it too. They should both undergo simultaneous antibiotic therapy.

The preferred drug choice for chlamydial infections is doxycycline, 100 mg, twice daily for 7 days. Tetracycline or erythromycin are also effective. Pregnant women with chlamydia should not take doxycycline or tetracycline, so erythromycin is the best alternative during pregnancy.

Although the symptoms of chlamydia are not necessarily severe, treatment of the disease is very important to avoid a serious upper genital tract infection called pelvic inflammatory disease (PID), which can result in infertility. *(See below)*

Gonorrhea

In contrast to chlamydia, gonorrhea is a very old sexually transmitted disease, that still continues on an epidemic scale. Teenagers with multiple sexual partners seem to be at especially high risk for gonorrhea. Known as "clap," "drip," or "the dose," medical texts and other literature going back hundreds of years, refer to this hardy disease and its impact on the human race.

Gonorrhea is caused by *Neisseria gonorrhoeae*, a gonococcal bacterium. Detecting and controlling it is, once again, difficult in women because symptoms may be subtle or absent. Sometimes it causes a whitish or yellowish vaginal discharge or burning during urination. Most of the time it confines itself to the cervix, the vagina, or the bladder. If it goes untreated for too long, it may move up into the pelvic organs where it can do great damage by causing pelvic inflammatory disease in the fallopian tubes (See below).

Men, on the other hand, will often have obvious symptoms, such as a yellowish-green discharge from the penis, swelling and redness at the tip of the penis, difficulty urinating along with the urge to urinate frequently. Thus, women should take their clues from their male sexual partners. If a man has symptoms such as those described, *both the man and woman should be tested for a sexually transmitted disease, such as gonorrhea.*

Gonorrhea during pregnancy is cause for concern. If the gonococcal organism contacts the baby's eyes during delivery, the bacteria can cause a severe infection called conjunctivitis. For this reason, state laws require that silver nitrate drops or erythromycin be put routinely in the eyes of newborn babies.

Table 9-1 lists drugs used successfully in treating uncomplicated gonorrhea in the doctor's office. Penicillin is still a standard treatment for ridding the body of gonorrhea organisms. Initially the doctor will inject penicillin in each buttock and concurrently prescribe oral probenicid, a drug that prolongs the effectiveness of penicillin.

In recent years, some strains of gonorrhea have developed resistance to penicillin. If a person finds herself dealing with recurring bouts of gonorrhea, she may be harboring one of these mutant strains of the organism. People who are allergic to penicillin comprise another challenging treatment group. Ceftriaxone (Rocephin) is the favored drug for penicillin-resistant gonorrhea treatment these days. It is given as a single 250 mg intramuscular injection. Following that, physicians will prescribe doxycycline (Doryx) capsules, 100 mg, twice a day for one week. Single dose injections of spectinomycin or tetracycline may be substituted for penicillin when people are allergic to penicillin or the cephalosporins (a drug class that includes ceftriaxone). We strongly recommend that individuals be tested for penicillin allergies before a decision is made on drug treatment for gonorrhea, since most people do not have a true allergy. Both (or all) sexual partners must be treated simultaneously to eliminate the disease.

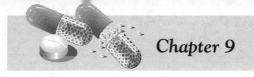

After a week of drug therapy, the couple should return to the doctor's office for a culture of the cervix and rectum to determine if the drug course was effective. Sometimes women will have chlamydia as well as gonorrhea. We routinely check for both diseases, when one or the other is diagnosed.

Pelvic Inflammatory Disease

Pelvic inflammatory disease (PID), a major infection of the upper reproductive tract in women, is indeed a serious condition. It can result from inadequately treated gonorrhea, chlamydia or other infections. If infection reaches the fallopian tubes, a woman may be left sterile for life because of tubal blockage and scarring. She may experience appreciable and lasting pelvic pain, as well.

While inflammation of the tubes and ovaries can be caused by a variety of organisms, both sexually and nonsexually acquired, gonorrhea is the most common cause. Other bacteria that cause pelvic infections are *Escherichia coli* (the organism most commonly found in the bowel) and streptococcal bacteria. Tuberculosis is known to cause pelvic inflammatory disease, and, although it is not as frequent in the United States as it was 40 or 50 years ago, it is on the upswing in people with AIDS.

Women are most vulnerable to pelvic inflammatory disease after their periods, after having a baby, or after a D&C. The cervical mucus barrier is gone at these times, and bacteria may ascend more easily into the uterus and fallopian tubes. Menstrual blood and tissue are ideal media for the growth of bacteria.

Extensive infection of the uterus, ovaries, and especially the fallopian tubes causes marked pelvic tenderness, fever, and an abnormal vaginal discharge. Complete blood count and appropriate cultures must be taken. It may be necessary to insert a long needle through the upper vagina to withdraw any pus within the lower pelvis for culture. As with many other genital infections, sexual partners should also be evaluated and treated to prevent reinfection.

Intrauterine devices appear to have a slight correlation with pelvic inflammatory disease in women with multiple sexual partners. The device itself somehow renders conditions in the uterus more susceptible to infection by causing an inflammation (not infection) in the uterine lining. Women with IUDs who contract pelvic infections should receive antibiotic therapy and then have their IUDs removed.

Because the bacteria causing pelvic inflammatory disease are inside the fallopian tubes, it is much more difficult for the doctor to obtain culture specimens and identify the specific organism to be treated. Diagnosis may be more firmly established using sophisticated techniques such as ultrasound, magnetic resonance imaging (MRI), laparoscopy, or computed tomography (CT scanning). When an abscess is present, surgery may be necessary.

A broad-spectrum intravenous antibiotic or several antibiotics may be necessary to rid a woman entirely of her infection. The primary antibiotic for treating pelvic inflammatory disease is penicillin, either with or without another broad-spectrum antibiotic.

A woman will need to be hospitalized if she does not improve after two days of drug treatment or if she has a pelvic mass, a temperature exceeding 100 degrees Fahrenheit, or marked pelvic tenderness.

Most of the time antibiotics are effective against pelvic inflammatory disease. They relieve symptoms and eradicate the organisms at the source of the infection. Some women continue to have persistent or recurrent pelvic infections, a process that occasionally goes on for months or even years. The antibiotics evidently do not attain high enough concentrations in the tissues to destroy all the bacteria present, or the bacteria become resistant to the antibiotic. As a result, women feel persistent pelvic pain, especially during sexual activity. Laparoscopy may be necessary to better assess the nature of the chronic pain and to determine whether there are other abnormalities involving the ovaries or tubes.

Syphilis

Syphilis is another ancient sexually transmitted disease, still with us and still dangerous. In fact, it seems to be once again on the rise in the United States. It is caused by *Treponema pallidum,* a spiral-shaped bacterium called a *spirochete*. Men often notice painless sores on their genitals when they have syphilis, but woman may see absolutely nothing, since their sores can be inside. The primary or first-stage ulcers of syphilis are painless and can develop in the vulva, vagina, or cervix. Without treatment, these ulcers subside, and in its place, the raised red rash of secondary or second-stage syphilis appears on the body. The disease is highly contagious during either of these stages. From there the disease enters an inactive or latent period, in which there are no symptoms, and the only way to detect its presence is through the VDRL or RPR blood tests.

Early syphilis is easily treated with penicillin using a 4.8 million unit dose of benzathine penicillin given as an intramuscular shot. This should be followed by a week's course of doxycycline, 100 mg, twice daily. In the advanced stages, the disease becomes more stubborn, and more penicillin shots and doxycycline are necessary. Intravenous penicillin may be necessary. If left untreated, it can cause blindness and severe brain damage in both the mother and the fetus. Alternate drugs that can be used instead of penicillin include erythromycin during pregnancy and tetracycline or erythromycin when a woman is not pregnant.

Pubic lice

Although not dangerous, pubic lice (also known as "crabs" or "cooties") are the source of discomfort and embarrassment. The lice are tiny "animals" that live and multiply on the skin's surface. Pubic lice target the pubic hair for their habitat. They cause intense itching and some bleeding because they burrow into the skin. Lice eggs or "nits," tiny white specks, attach themselves to the pubic hair and provide another clue that public lice are present. Normally pubic lice are transmitted through sexual contact, but they can be picked up from fabrics such as bedsheets.

The treatment for lice is either lindane (Kwell) or gamma benzene hexachloride applied once a day for two days, in shampoo, cream, or lotion form. Application may be repeated in 10 days to destroy any nits that survive, but prolonged application of these rather toxic drugs should be avoided, as they can cause dermatitis on the genitals. At the same time treatment is given, all clothing and bedclothing must be washed with detergent to get rid of possible sources of infestation. Sexual partners must be treated at the same time to break the tenacious life cycle of the pubic louse.

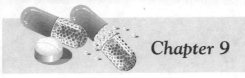

Chapter 9

Case Study

Keisha B., 18, went to Planned Parenthood because she wanted to begin using birth control pills. She was sexually active, but she had found the men she met reluctant to use condoms. When the clinical practitioner at Planned Parenthood examined her, she noticed a yellowish discharge and suggested to Keisha that they test her for sexually transmitted diseases.

Keisha tested positive for chlamydia and gonorrhea, both of which were apparently in the early stages because she showed no symptoms of pelvic inflammatory disease. Her pregnancy test was negative. She also requested an AIDS test. Planned Parenthood referred her to a private physician but told her that they themselves would be doing AIDS testing in the near future.

After the doctor determined that she was not allergic to penicillin, he gave her an injection of penicillin and a prescription for one week's worth of doxycycline capsules. However, after the second day on doxycycline, she felt nauseated and had heartburn and gas. The doctor changed the prescription to erythromycin tablets and she was able to tolerate those long enough to finish the prescribed 10-day dose. She also notified her sexual partners that she had gonorrhea and encouraged them to see a doctor.

After discussions with the Planned Parenthood counselors, Keisha decided to try using a diaphragm and spermicide because of the protection they offered her against sexually transmitted diseases. She received suggestions on how to persuade her sexual partners to use condoms and purchased a low-cost supply of them from Planned Parenthood for herself.

Key Points for Curable STDs

1. Prevention, early treatment, and simultaneous treatment of sexual partners are the keys to managing sexually transmitted disease.

2. The cornerstone of preventing spread of any sexually transmitted disease, including AIDS, is use of condoms, both male and female, and the diaphragm and spermicide in conjunction with male condoms.

3. Chlamydia and gonorrhea, although not always serious, initially, are hard to detect in women. An unusual vaginal discharge may be one of the few clues. Symptoms in male sexual partners may also be a clue, as men have more clear-cut symptoms with these diseases.

4. Doxycycline is the drug of choice for treatment of chlamydia; penicillin or ceftriaxone are the primary drugs for treatment of gonorrhea. Tetracycline is an alternate choice option for treatment of both diseases. Erythromycin may be used to treat chlamydia in pregnant women.

4. If left untreated, chlamydia and gonorrhea can move deeper into the reproductive system to cause pelvic inflammatory disease. This is a very serious problem, which can result in sterility and lasting pelvic pain.

5. Syphilis, although less common, is still very serious because it can produce blindness and central nervous system destruction. Penicillin is the number one drug used to treat syphilis.

6. Skin testing for penicillin allergy is necessary if a woman thinks she may be allergic to penicillin. Most people are not truly allergic to the drug.

7. Sexually active people will often carry more than one sexually transmitted disease, and they should be tested for all of them. After treatment, they should return to the doctor to verify that the diseases have been eradicated.

Table 9-1
Treatment of Vaginal Gonorrhea Infections
Treatment of choice Aqueous procaine penicillin G, 4.8 million units intramuscularly, with 1 gram probenecid orally **plus** Doxycycline, 100 mg orally, two times
Slightly less effective therapy Ampicillin. 3.5 gm, with 1 gm probenecid orally **or** Amoxicillin, 3.5 gm, with 1 gm probenecid orally per day for 7 days
For penicillin treatment failures Ceftriaxone, 250 mg, single intramuscular injection **plus** Doxycycline, 100 mg, 2x daily for 7 days
For people with penicillin allergies Spectinomycin, 2 gm intramuscularly (one dose) **or** Ciprofloxacin, 500 mg, one dose, orally

AIDS, Herpes, and Warts:
The Sexually Transmitted Viruses

The era of carefree sex came to an end in the early 1980s. While unwanted pregnancy could be effectively prevented, people discovered that the same was not true for sexually transmitted diseases. Slowly it dawned on people that they were not only having sexual relations with an individual, but by extension, all the individuals he or she had contact with and all the individuals those people, in turn, had contacted. After years of disfavor, the idea of sexual monogamy (restricting sexual activity to one partner) once again become popular. Unfortunately, more lip service than actual practice is probably paid to sexual monogamy.

Epidemics of sexually transmitted disease cropped up, in the United States, Europe, Asia, and Africa. The most frightening of these were the viral diseases - AIDS, herpes, and warts. Unlike gonorrhea and chlamydia, which could be cured with antibiotics, the viral diseases had no cure. Herpes and warts, while not necessarily fatal, recur unpredictably, sometimes producing great pain or discomfort. AIDS of course, has no known cure, but we are finding ways to prolong the lives of AIDS patients and better treat their many symptoms.

Right at this moment researchers worldwide are working hard to unlock the secrets of the AIDS, herpes, and wart viruses. Drugs which provide relief from or a temporary halt to these viral diseases have come on the market. However, none of these infections can be "cured" in the traditional sense of the word, nor has anyone produced a vaccine to immunize people against them. Because of their ability to mutate (change their genetic structure) and because they are difficult to isolate, viruses have eluded science's best attempts to conquer them.

This chapter will address three important areas related to sexually transmitted viruses:

• Protection against initial infection and prevention of spread to others
• Drug and other therapy available, once diseases are contracted
• Lifestyle guidelines for disease management

Acquired Immune Deficiency Syndrome (AIDS)

AIDS is now the sixth leading cause of death in Americans under age 65 and the worst is yet to come. In 1992, about 45,000 people died from AIDS. An estimated 1 million Americans are currently infected with HIV (human immunodeficiency virus), the presumed cause of AIDS, and a large proportion of them don't even know it.

When a person has full-blown AIDS, they may actually be suffering from several diseases simultaneously, including *Pneumocystis carinii* pneumonia, Kaposi's sarcoma (a type of cancer that affects the skin and the internal digestive organs), tuberculosis, and severe diarrhea. To date, we believe that AIDS (which stands for acquired immune deficiency syndrome) is caused by the human immunodeficiency virus (HIV). HIV, possibly in combination with other factors, destroys very important white blood cells that combat infections and other diseases in the body. HIV is a special type of virus, known as a retrovirus, which means it carries an enzyme called reverse transcriptase. Researchers working on drugs to combat AIDS have attempted to "defuse" the reverse transcriptase enzyme by blocking its ability to reproduce, but so far they haven't met with great success.

Around the world, at least 13 million people are currently infected with HIV or they have full-blown AIDS. HIV and AIDS are spreading very rapidly in Africa, Asia, and India. By the turn of the century, some experts predict that 120 million people will have AIDS. These frightening statistics can lead to only one conclusion: individuals must take every step available to protect themselves and those around them against AIDS.

Fortunately HIV is not highly contagious, and can only be transmitted in a limited number of ways, i.e., through blood-to-blood contact and semen-to-blood contact. Thus, in order to get AIDS, someone must transmit HIV in his or her blood or semen into someone else's bloodstream.

HIV may be passed on in the following ways:

- Reusing needles that someone else has already used for intravenous injections (injections into the blood)
- Transfusion of contaminated blood products
- Vaginal sexual intercourse
- Oral sex
- Anal sexual intercourse
- Breast feeding
- During pregnancy, from the mother to the fetus through the placenta and umbilical cord

Although the epidemic in the United States started among homosexual men, women are now catching the virus just as often as men. Recent studies have concluded that women are actually more vulnerable to HIV than men. The reason for women's special susceptibility is that they are more likely to have small open sores in the vaginal tract or surrounding areas where a virus can easily enter the bloodstream. The lining of the uterus also becomes a viral entry port when a woman has her period. Many women infected with HIV pass the virus along to their unborn babies through the placenta and then through the blood supply of the umbilical cord, which just adds to the tragedy of the epidemic.

Protection

Knowing your partners' sexual history is the first line of defense against getting HIV. Table 10-1 presents an HIV/AIDS assessment risk questionnaire. The questionnaire lists different situations where people are likely to have contracted the AIDS virus.

To protect themselves against HIV infection, women must insist that their sexual partners wear condoms, especially if they are new partners or if the woman is not completely familiar with her partner's sexual history. Some people insist on HIV testing before they enter into a sexual relationship with a new partner.

It is a good idea to use a diaphragm with a spermicidal jelly containing nonoxynol-9 (for example, Ortho-Gynol jelly or cream), *in addition to the male partner's use of a condom*. For awhile it was thought that nonoxynol-9 killed HIV, but recent information has discredited that theory. However, nonoxynol-9 is still believed to be effective against other sexually transmitted organisms, and people who are sexually active with multiple partners often have more than one sexually transmitted disease.

A female condom has recently been developed, which provides better protection against HIV because it covers the entire genital area *(See Fig. 10-1)*. The vaginal condom is a large, lubricated, polyurethane adaptation of the men's version. It is about 7 inches long, has flexible rings at both ends, and is inserted like a diaphragm. The female condom was developed in Switzerland, but at this writing was not yet widely marketed in the United States. In Europe it sells for about four times as much as male condoms.

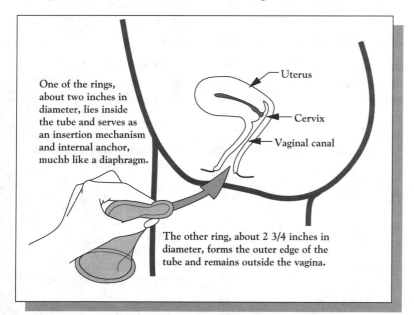

One of the rings, about two inches in diameter, lies inside the tube and serves as an insertion mechanism and internal anchor, muchb like a diaphragm.

Uterus

Cervix

Vaginal canal

The other ring, about 2 3/4 inches in diameter, forms the outer edge of the tube and remains outside the vagina.

Figure 10-1
Female Condom

The condom, about seven inches long, consists of a soft polyurethane tube and two flexible polyurethane rings.

Condoms should always be worn during anal sex and oral sex because small open sores in the rectum and the mouth may allow HIV viruses in semen to enter the bloodstream.

If a woman injects any kind of drugs with a needle, she must remember to use new, sterile needles each time. Sharing needles with someone else is dangerous and risks disease transmission not only of AIDS, but of other dangerous diseases like hepatitis.

Women who are HIV positive or who have full-blown AIDS have a high risk of transmitting the disease to an unborn baby. Getting pregnant poses great dangers to the infant - the risk that it will be born with HIV infection and die at a young age and that it will have a sick mother who will not be able to care for it or who will die before it is grown. We therefore counsel HIV-positive women to think twice before allowing themselves to become pregnant, so they do not worsen an already difficult situation. HIV-positive women who bear children *should not breastfeed these babies*, since the virus is also transmitted through breast milk. Breast milk after all, is just "white blood," proteins and other nutrients taken from the mother's own blood and given to the baby as food.

Drugs for People with AIDS

A wide variety of drugs are given to AIDS patients to help them with their many symptoms. Antibiotics can treat some of the numerous infections that occur. Immunoglobulin transfusions (processed blood proteins that fight infection found in human blood) also help with infections, especially in babies and small children with AIDS. Unfortunately, people with AIDS often develop infections that resist all drug therapy. Tuberculosis, which was virtually eliminated a few years ago, is on the rise again in a form that seems to resist treatment from currently available drugs, especially in AIDS sufferers.

Thus far, three antiviral drugs have been approved to actually combat HIV: Zidovudine (going under the trade name Retro and formerly called AZT), DDI, and DDC. Basically, the approach with Zidovudine, DDI and DDC is to give substantial dosages of these drugs as soon as possible after HIV positivity is identified in attempt to delay, as long as possible, the appearance of AIDS. These drugs slow the progress of the virus, but they do not destroy it. After a period of time, they seem to lose their effectiveness.

Zidovudine is given to pregnant women who are HIV positive because it is believed to reduce transmission of the virus from mother to fetus. Recent studies have indicated that zidovudine is not harmful to the fetus, and it may help prolong the mother's life. Recently the Upjohn Company began clinical trials with BHAP-E, a drug that attacks an enzyme vital to reproduction of the HIV. While no conclusions can be drawn yet, clinical researchers hope that this drug will prove to have more combative power against the virus.

Lifestyle Considerations

Although the outlook for HIV-positive people is not good, some of them remain healthy for a long time before falling prey to AIDS. Doctors believe that a healthy lifestyle contributes to this longevity.

If a person is HIV-positive and not yet sick with AIDS, we recommend that she put herself on a program of good nutrition, exercise, adequate rest, and positive thinking. Smoking, alcohol, and recreational drug use should be abandoned or minimized. Stress reduction activities such as yoga, meditation, or positive visualization can be very helpful. A support system of family and friends helps to induce the positive thinking so necessary at this time. Many people with HIV have become active in the AIDS movement and have thus channeled their energies in a way that helps others and at the same time lets them feel better about themselves.

Above all, if a person knows that she is HIV positive and continues to be sexually active, she should protect her partners by assuring that they use a male condom in combination with a diaphragm or a female condom. We strongly recommend that HIV positive women not become pregnant.

Herpes

Most women we see in our clinics who have genital sores have nothing more remarkable than a skin abrasion, a blemish, or an infected hair follicle. If the sore is blistered or bleeding and craterlike, then we suspect something more serious like herpes or even cancer. This is why genital sores of any type should be seen by a physician, even if they turn out to be minor or, as in the case of herpes, not really curable.

Herpes is a highly contagious, recurring, intracellular virus disease that produces painful, infected sores on the labia (skin folds surrounding the vagina), the anus, and the perineal area. *Herpes* became almost a household word in the eighties. TV and print media interviewed people with herpes, examining in detail not only their symptoms, but the destructive impact herpes had on their lives. Singles groups and dating services matched up male and female herpes sufferers so they wouldn't have to inflict themselves on the rest of society. Today, we realize that people with herpes do not have to be treated like lepers. They can fit into the social order very well, and even mate with herpes-free people, provided they take precautions when an outbreak of blisters occurs.

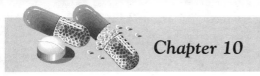

The incidence of herpes infections in the United States is estimated to be between 15 and 20 million. A half million new victims add to these statistics each year. Men outnumber women in the ranks of people with herpes, and among both sexes, most of these people are between the ages of 18 and 45. This epidemic is assumed to reflect the sexually liberal attitudes of the seventies and eighties. It is probably also related to the post-World War II baby boom, reflected in this age group.

Two types of herpes viruses infect people. The first, herpes simplex type I, usually does not affect the reproductive organs, but instead causes cold sores around the mouth and lips. The other, herpes simplex type II, appears on the genitals and is usually transmitted sexually. Although the two viruses are very closely related, the type II strain is more worrisome. Not only does it tend to cause greater pain and discomfort, women who have type II herpes show a higher incidence of cervical cancer than those who have never contracted the infection.

Herpes can break out any time from 2 days to 2 weeks after contact with a carrier. The typical attack begins with a burning or itching sensation in the genital area followed by the appearance of small, slightly raised bumps. Blisters form and then rupture, leaving tiny ulcers or clusters of ulcers that weep fluid. Most herpes infections run their course between 3 and 6 weeks after breaking out if it is the primary, or first, infection. Secondary infections last about 7 to 10 days. These must be kept very clean and as dry are possible to prevent them from becoming contaminated with bacteria, resulting in a bacterial infection as well as the herpes viral infection.

Unfortunately, once contracted, the herpes virus remains in the body and may appear again and again over the years. After a herpes infection has healed, the virus ascends the nerve pathways that lead to the genitals and hides within the nerve roots near the spine until something causes its reappearance. Scientists can only speculate on how herpes is able to keep itself alive like this, but one theory holds that the herpes mutates or changes just enough after each infection that the antibodies formed by the person with herpes cannot destroy it.

Although the first infection is usually the worst in terms of physical symptoms, it is probably the recurring outbreaks that most distress its victims. Repeated outbreaks seem to have some causal relationship to stress and anxiety. Psychologists have identified a herpes-related syndrome in which people with the disease feel rejected by society, become very depressed, and withdraw from social contact. They recommend that people contact a herpes support group in their area. Some feel that reducing consumption of caffeine, alcohol, and recreational drugs keeps down the number of repeat attacks of herpes. The average person with herpes has about 3 or 4 outbreaks a year, and these seem to become less frequent and less severe as the years go by.

Protection

Except during the initial and recurrent outbreaks of blisters, people with herpes need not withdraw from the rest of the world. Women with herpes don't necessarily have to restrict themselves to partners who also have herpes, but at the first sign of blistering, they should refrain from all sexual contact until the blisters are completely healed. It is only fair to inform sexual partners that one has herpes and to give them the facts about contracting the disease. Women who live with an uninfected person should not share towels or clothing with them during outbreaks. They should wear underwear when sleeping so virus particles are not shed on the bedclothes.

The common occurrence of herpes is just one more reason women should protect themselves when having relations with new sexual partners whose sexual histories they don't know. The same suggestions made for AIDS apply to herpes: Use of a male condom combined with diaphragm and spermicidal jelly or a female condom is mandatory for each sexual contact.

Managing Herpes

Some people suffer no more than minor itching and burning with herpes, whereas others experience an agony of pain. For women in particular, urination can often burn intensely, and mere contact with fabrics can be unbearable. Home remedies suggest things such as: blowing air from a hair dryer on the blisters; bathing them with a diluted iodine (Betadine) solution; using a topical anesthetic such as lidocaine (Xylocaine); rinsing them with baking soda, Burow's solution, or Epsom salts dissolved in cold water.

Virtually everyone agrees that women should avoid tight clothing such as pantihose (or cut out the crotch) and tight jeans to give the blisters as much "breathing room" as possible. Drinking extra fluid helps too because it dilutes the acidity of urine and makes it less painful to urinate past any open sores.

Other home remedies that may reduce the discomfort of herpes include:

- Applying petroleum jelly (Vaseline) over the sores before urinating to prevent burning and stinging
- Applying Vitamin E, Neosporin, Campho-Phenique, or zinc oxide to the sores
- Taking zinc or lysine monohydrochloride tablets (These are available in health food stores).
- Using herbal preparations on the blisters such as golden seal, myrrh, ground comfrey root, aloe vera or peppermint tea bags.

A major concern with herpes arises during pregnancy, when the virus may be transmitted to the unborn baby. At the time of delivery, after the membranes have ruptured, approximately half of the infants delivered vaginally to mothers with herpes will become infected. About 1,000 babies per year are born with herpes. Half of these infected infants will and the other half are likely to become severely brain damaged. Any pregnant woman with a history of herpes, especially if she is near term, must watch herself for signs of recurring blisters. Her physician may wish to culture the cervical mucous, since impending infections sometimes show up in culture before they can be seen on the body. The pregnant woman's partner should be carefully watched at the same time. If a herpes infection occurs at or near delivery, the baby should be delivered by cesarean section, before the membranes rupture.

Many drugs have been used to treat patients with herpes, with little success. Cortisone, which is found in over-the-counter creams, such as Cortaid, is one of these. We believe cortisone-containing drugs should be avoided, since the infection could be worsened by their application.

Medications shown to be of some use in treating herpes are listed in Table 10-2.

Acyclovir (Zovirax) has become the mainstay of treatment for vulvar herpes. It is available in ointment, capsule or intravenous forms. Both topical and oral forms are effective for otherwise normally healthy people during the first outbreak of herpes. The intravenous forms are appropriate for people with low immune resistance, resulting in severe outbreaks of herpes, for example, people with AIDS.

Acyclovir contains a chemical that is thought to interfere with the way the herpes virus multiplies. During the first outbreak, it reduces the amount of virus shedding, thus rendering the

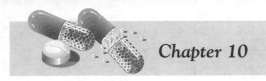

disease less contagious. It reduces the number of new lesions and the length of time new lesions remain blistery and sore, thus shortening the healing process and the period of painfulness.

In second outbreaks, oral acyclovir seems to be more effective than topical acyclovir, even in people with normal immunity, in about 50% of cases. We are also using long-term doses of oral acyclovir to suppress herpes outbreaks. Unfortunately, along with the intravenous form, it seems to have more side effects than the topical form. These include nausea, vomiting, headache, diarrhea, dizziness, and achiness. Oral and intravenous acyclovir are also very expensive.

Table 3 outlines a treatment plan for genital herpes using acyclovir.

Warts

Human papillomavirus (HPV), the cause of genital warts, is believed to be the most common of the sexually transmitted viral diseases. Some studies indicate that 10-15% of all apparently healthy women have an HPV infection that isn't visible to the naked eye. Furthermore, HPV and genital warts are sometimes predecessors of genital cancers, so it is important that they be eradicated.

The wartlike growths, called *condyloma acuminata*, appear on the vulva and the perineum (area between the vaginal opening and the anus). They range from a single wart to an extensive, warty "carpet" that hides the underlying skin cells. They are highly infectious and easily transmitted by sexual partners and can cause itching and burning. In their milder forms, they are painless, and in about 20% of women they regress spontaneously. Left untreated, however, they can increase in size and number, causing discomfort and distress. Their tendency, in some cases, to continue on to precancerous lesions and even cancer is all the more reason for swift and appropriate treatment.

During routine Pap smears we often see a condition under the microscope called *koilocytosis*, which means the presence of certain cells suggesting HPV infection. This occurs in many women who have never, to their knowledge, had a wart. When we find these cells, we do another test using acetic acid, which clarifies whether the cervix needs treatment because it has developed an abnormal or precancerous condition. If we do find this dysplastic or precancerous condition, we remove the abnormal cells with trichloroacetic acid, laser therapy, or electro-coagulation of the cervix.

Many women have koilocytosis, and it is not necessarily dangerous or something that should cause great worry. Its presence does indicate that women should have a Pap smear annually, so their physicians can keep an eye on the situation.

Management of Genital Warts

As initial treatment for external genital or perianal (warts around the rectum), we recommend cryotherapy (freezing) with liquid nitrogen or the use of a cryoprobe to accomplish the freezing. Cryotherapy is not toxic, does not require anesthesia, and should not cause scarring.

Following this, our choice for drug therapy would be trichloracetic acid applications. We also use a surgical approach to wart removal called wide local excision.

Podophyllin and podofilox are two other effective topical agents applied to genital warts. Podofilox is still being tested clinically and has not yet been approved for use in women by the FDA. The compounds are painted on the small growths and then washed off. A few growths at a time are treated on a semiweekly or weekly basis, usually at a physician's office, until they are gone. Podophyllin should be applied under the supervision of a physician because, if it is absorbed through the vaginal mucous membrane or applied to the cervix, it can cause severe toxic effects. It should not be used during early pregnancy because absorption can harm the fetus.

Podofilox is less toxic, and when it becomes approved for use, patients should be able to self-apply this medication. A typical podofilox treatment cycle includes application of the topical cream twice a day for three days, followed by four days off the drug.

Other medications used in the treatment of warts are 5-fluorouracil, and, occasionally, interferon. Table 10-4 lists common drug therapy regimens for genital warts. Women for whom drug therapy is ineffective should have the warts removed with laser therapy.

The majority of women with genital warts can be treated satisfactorily, with the warts largely eradicated. It may not be possible to remove all the wart DNA (genetic material), and thus women should remain alert for recurrences.

Case Study

Melissa V, a 33-year-old paralegal, visited her obstetrician because she suspected she was pregnant. While giving her medical history, Melissa mentioned to the doctor that she had recurrent herpes, which she had contracted in college. The first few years she suffered from herpes, she had used topical acyclovir, but it hadn't seemed to help her. Her boyfriend with whom she shared an apartment was herpes-free, and they had been very careful to abstain from sex when Melissa had an outbreak. These had been decreasing and now seemed to occur only once every year or two.

The doctor examined Melissa and verified with tests that she was indeed two and one-half months pregnant. He also noticed that she had a small cluster of warts on her vulva. A Pap smear showed no abnormal cells, so he removed the warts with cryotherapy using liquid nitrogen. He also ran a series of tests on Melissa for gonorrhea, chlamydia, and HIV infection. Happily, all of those were negative.

As her pregnancy progressed, Melissa was cautioned to watch carefully for any outbreaks of herpes or warts and to notify the doctor immediately. Her plans and hopes were to have a successful vaginal delivery, but she knew that a cesarean section would be necessary if she had a herpes outbreak.

Key Points for Viral STDs

1. Sexually transmitted viral diseases are difficult to treat because there is no real cure for them. There are, however, therapeutic approaches, including drugs and lifestyle alterations that help women cope with these diseases.

2. Prevention is the most important thing a woman can do for herself and others, when it comes to sexually transmitted viral diseases. Male condoms plus diaphragm and spermicide and female condoms are the best ways to prevent sexually transmitted diseases.

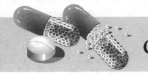

Chapter 10

3. AIDS is an ultimately fatal viral disease. If a woman is HIV-positive for the AIDS virus, a healthy lifestyle may fend off the full infection for a number of years. Drugs like AZT, DDI, and DDC slow the infection for a period of time, but eventually become ineffective.

4. Women with HIV positivity or AIDS should avoid pregnancy and breast-feeding, since the disease can be transmitted to an infant.

5. Women with herpes may lead a normal life, but should avoid all sexual contact until the recurring blisters have healed. Herpes may be with a person for a lifetime, but outbreaks tend to get milder and less frequent as years pass.

6. Topical or oral acyclovir, an anti-herpes drug, may be helpful in shortening the first outbreak of herpes. After that, oral acyclovir may help with recurring infections. Intravenous acyclovir is used to treat people with very severe herpes infections and lowered immunity.

7. Home remedies for herpes focus on keeping the blisters dry and as well aired as possible and relieving burning during urination. Cleanliness is very important to avoid a secondary bacterial infection.

8. Herpes can be dangerous to an unborn child at or near the time of delivery. If a woman has an outbreak of herpes just prior to delivery, she should undergo cesarean section.

9. Genital warts caused by human papillomavirus are said to be the most common of the sexually-transmitted viruses.

10. Although they may not be uncomfortable, warts should be removed because they occasionally lead to precancerous or cancerous lesions. Pap smears can indicate infection with HPV, even if no warts are visible.

11. Cryotherapy, topical medications, laser therapy, or wide surgical excision are all commonly used to remove warts.

12. Podophyllin, trichloracetic acid, and podofilox are topical drugs that are useful for removing warts. Because of its potential toxic effects, podophyllin should not be used during pregnancy.

Table 10-1

HIV/AIDS Infection Risk Assessment Questionnaire

1. Have you or your sexual partners used intravenous drugs since 1979?	yes	no
2. Have you had five or more sexual partners in any year since 1979?	yes	no
3. Have any of your sexual partners been sick with AIDS, AIDS-Related Complex (ARC), or a bleeding disorder (hemophilia)?	yes	no
4. Have any of your sexual partners had a positive HIV (AIDS) test?	yes	no
5. Have any of your partners' partners had a positive HIV (AIDS) test?	yes	no
6. Have you received any blood transfusions between 1979 and 1985?	yes	no
7. Have you had artificial insemination with donor semen since 1979?	yes	no
8. Have any of your male partners been bisexual or have they had sex with other men?	yes	no
9. Have any of your partners been sick with:		
genital warts	yes	no
herpes	yes	no
genital ulcers	yes	no
gonorrhea ("clap, " "drip")	yes	no
syphilis	yes	no
hepatitis (yellow jaundice)	yes	no
other STDs?	yes	no

Table 10-2

Topical Therapy for Genital Herpes

Agent	Comments
Burow's solution	Soothing for local relief only
Povidone iodine douche (Betadine)	2 teaspoons of Betadine per quart of warm water
Povidone iodine sitz bath (Betadine)	4 oz of Betadine solution in a warm tub two or three times per day
Acyclovir 5% (Zovirax)	Apply every 3 hours for 7 days

Table 10-3
Treatment of Herpes Genitalis with Acyclovir

Type	Acyclovir Dose
First genital episode	200 mg orally 5 times a day for 7-10 days
Recurrent episode	200 mg orally 5 times a day for 5-7 days
Suppressive therapy	200 mg orally 2-5 times a day for 1 year or 400 mg orally , twice daily for 1 year
Severe infection	5 mg/kg intravenous every 8 hours for 5-7 days

Table 10-4
Drug Treatment of Condyloma Acuminatum*

Agent	Comments
Podophyllin (10-25% in tincture of benzoin)	Wash lesion off first Do not apply to vagina or cervix Systemic side effects have been reported Contraindicated in the pregnant woman
Trichloroacetic acid (50-85%) Topical 5% 5-fluorouracil, (1.5 g intravaginally)	Protect surrounding tissues Use at bedtime once a week for 10 weeks If persistent disease, may repeat twice weekly for 10 weeks, if side effects minimal
Interferon α2b (Intron A, 0.1 m)	Inject 3-5 lesions at a time Increasing side effects with more lesions treated Treat 3 times week for 3 weeks

*Crythoerapy with liquid nitrogen or a cryoprobe is often recommended for patients with external genital, perianal, and vaginal warts.

Notes

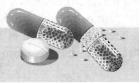

Chapter 11

Over-The-Counter Products for Women

by Kimberly A. Cantral, Pharm. D.

Consumers in the United States spend several billion dollars a year to purchase over-the-counter (OTC) feminine products. These include personal care items, vaginal contraceptives, antifungals, menstrual products, pregnancy and ovulation prediction kits, and preparations used by women who are breast-feeding. Misuse of these products can result in devastating economic and health consequences, i.e., unwanted pregnancy, delays in contacting a physician when prescription therapy is warranted, etc.

The 1990's have ushered in a new era in health care. Consumers are assuming a greater responsibility for their health than ever before. This chapter focuses on the appropriate use of nonprescription products and devices and the essential information that a woman should have for the safe and effective use of these products.

Vaginal Health Products

There are OTC products available for general cleansing of the skin surrounding the vagina and labia; for deodorizing; for relief of itching, burning, and dryness; and for the removal of vaginal discharge. The therapeutic value of many of these products is controversial; hence the term hygiene is seldom used in connection with them.

Vaginal secretions are part of the natural cleansing process of the body. In the absence of personal cleanliness and/or the presence of excessive discharge the secretions may accumulate on the external genitals where bacteria decompose, resulting in an unpleasant odor.

Douches

Douching is an ancient practice, that in its earliest years involved the use of wine and garlic for menstrual disorders as well as cassia oil for pelvic infections. Many women in the United States still douche for routine cleansing. A 1984 nationwide survey of women over 18 years of age reported that 32% of the nearly 7,000 women questioned had douched during the previous week. Despite its popularity, there are no good studies to demonstrate any advantage to regular douching, and its long-term effects on the vagina are unknown.

Douche products are available as premixed liquids, liquid concentrates, and two varieties of powders, one of which is diluted with water before use and the other is instilled as a powder.

An Advisory Review Panel on OTC contraceptive and other vaginal drug products evaluated data to determine the safety and efficacy of 38 active ingredients contained in various douche products. The panel's report was published by the Food and Drug Administration (FDA) in October 1983. As a result, currently there are only 20 active ingredients in douche preparations today. Antiirritants (e.g., eucalyptol, menthol, phenol, and sodium perborate) are included for their anesthetic and antipruritic (aids against itching and soreness) properties. Benzalkonium chloride, boric acid, and oxyquinolone citrate/sulfate are the usual preservatives found in these preparations. Povidone-iodine (Betadine) has antimicrobial activity and has been shown to be effective along with other drugs for fungal and trichomonal vaginitis. Astringents such as ammonium/potassium alum and thymol are included because they help reduce inflammation. Alkyl aryl sulfate, benzalkonium sulfate, cetylpyridinium chloride, citric acid, octoxynol 9, and sodium bicarbonate facilitate the spread of the douche over the vaginal folds. Ingredients that change the vaginal acidity or alkalinity of the vagina are also included (for example, acetic acid, citric acid, sodium bicarbonate, and sodium perborate).

Douching rarely causes problems, but it is very important to pay attention to the correct preparation and instillation of the product. Local irritation and allergic reactions can occur. The ingredients usually implicated in such problems are benzalkonium chloride, phenol, and povidone-iodine. New research indicates that, in some women, povidone-iodine (Betadine) douches encourage the overgrowth of infection-causing bacteria. When local irritation occurs, use of the douche product should be stopped immediately. If the reaction is severe, the short term use of oral steroids may be needed.

During pregnancy, the vagina has more blood circulation, which allows for increased absorption of many substances. When researchers studied the absorption of douche ingredients, it was found that, in most situations, no significant quantities were found in the bloodstream. On the other hand, evidence indicates significant absorption of povidone-iodine, following its use in the vagina. This is particularly dangerous to pregnant women. Iodine levels in the amniotic fluid surrounding the baby have been found to be elevated substantially following the use of douches that contain povidone-iodine. Until recently, doctors could only guess about the effects on the fetus. A recent study demonstrated that the use of a douche product containing povidone-iodine for 7 consecutive days resulted in too much iodine in the mother. This overload did not affect the mother's thyroid function; however, it did cause an increase in iodine levels in the fetuses' thyroid. Potentially, this could cause hypothyroidism (low thyroid function) in the fetus which, in turn, can lead to mental and physical retardation as well as breathing blockage and nervous disturbances. For this reason it is advisable to discontinue the routine use of any vaginal douche during pregnancy.

A great deal of controversy surrounds the question of vaginal douching as a risk factor for acute pelvic inflammatory disease (PID) *(See Chapter 9 for further discussion of PID)*. Until recently, there were no good studies on the topic. One study compared 100 women with documented PID who routinely douched with 762 randomly selected women without the disease. The study suggested that, for women who have a relatively small number of sexual contacts, douching may be a risk factor for PID, but for others who have a greater number of sexual partners this risk may be masked by a higher frequency of sexually transmitted diseases (STDs). Women who douche greater than three times per month seem to be at greater risk than women who douche less than once a month. Although this study did not prove a cause-effect relationship between douching and PID, it did suggest an association between these events.

Douche products do not contain sperm killing agents and are ineffective at removing seminal fluid (the material deposited after an ejaculation). Sperm migrate to the fallopian tube within 3-5 minutes following ejaculation so douching accomplishes nothing for contraception. Therefore they should not be used for contraceptive purposes. Some women like to douche after intercourse as a form of personal cleansing. However, if a vaginal contraceptive is used, douching should not be performed for 6 to 8 hours after its use since the douching process may remove the contraceptive substance.

Feminine Deodorant Sprays

Feminine deodorant sprays are aerosol products used to mask objectional odors. The FDA has classified them as "cosmetic" products and prohibits any reference to "hygiene" in connection with these products by the manufacturer. These products typically contain a germ-killing agent (similar chemicals to those in douche products) as a preservative, as well as perfumes, lubricating substances called emollients, and propellants (substances that "carry" the active ingredients out of the can). The emollients are included for their soothing effect on the skin. The emollients are often responsible for any sensitivity that may be experienced.

The most frequent problem associated with the use of these products is local irritation caused by holding the spray too close to the skin when applying it. The propellant evaporates once it is released from the canister, and if it has already reached the skin, its evaporation can result in "chilling" of the tissue. In some case reports this "chilling" and its resulting inflammation were significant enough to warrant the use of short-term oral anti-inflammatory drugs. Using feminine deodorant products has never been proved to be superior to routine bathing with soap. Nonetheless, these "feminine" products are aggressively marketed and widely used throughout the United States

Miscellaneous Products

A number of additional vaginal products are available as premoistened towelettes and anesthetic creams. Premoistened towelettes are used for deodorant purposes and contain the same ingredients found in feminine deodorant sprays, with the exception of the propellant. The towelettes may be an acceptable alternative to the use of an aerosol deodorant in women who are sensitive to the propellant.

Vaginal creams intended for the relief of pruritus (vaginal itching and sores) are also available. Vagisil, a product containing benzocaine (a local anesthetic) and resorcinol (an antimicrobial), is one example. Hydrocortisone products are also available for the relief of vaginal pruritus. The biggest concern with the use of these products is that their use may mask one of the most important symptoms of bacterial vaginitis, namely, pruritus, and result in a delay in seeking medical treatment.

A vaginal gel (Replens) has recently been marketed for the relief of vaginal dryness. After menopause the vaginal lining becomes thinner due to estrogen deficiency. This thinning can lead to discomfort during intercourse and pruritus. Unlike traditional vaginal lubricants that are applied just before intercourse, Replens should be applied three times per week on a routine basis. The active ingredient, polycarbophil, is 90% water. When applied to the vagina, it releases water to the underlying cells to provide continuous hydration. According to the manufacturer, two noteworthy side effects are sensitivity to the preservative and a white clumpy discharge occurring in approximately 8% of women who use this product. The discharge is due to cells coming off during the initial few weeks of use. The discharge typically disappears following approximately 3 weeks of continued use. Studies are currently in progress to determine the effectiveness of Replens in perimenopausal and postmenopausal women, in young oral contraceptive users, and in breast cancer patients who experience vaginal dryness as a result of medical therapy.

Contraceptive Products

Before oral contraceptives and intrauterine devices (IUDs), barrier methods were relied upon extensively for contraception. In the 1970s the use of barrier contraceptives fell into relative disfavor. As acceptance of oral contraceptives and the intrauterine device (IUD) increased, use of barrier contraceptives remained low until the 1980s, when fears of the adverse effects of the IUD and oral contraceptives as well as the spread of sexually transmitted diseases (especially AIDS) resulted in a dramatic shift back to the use of barrier methods. These products are now being used for protection against disease, as well as contraception. Many of the products in this category are available OTC.

Condoms

The earliest published reference to condom use was by an Italian anatomist who in the 16th century wrote of a linen sheath moistened with lotion for protection against venereal disease. Until the 1920s condoms were only available in places such as pool halls, gas stations, and barber shops. They were rarely sold in pharmacies, and even then they were stored in a drawer out of sight to the public. In the mid-1920s, Merle Youngs, a sundries salesman, started a condom manufacturing company and encouraged pharmacists to carry his product. His idea was to market a product of considerable quality and only available in pharmacies. Condoms subsequently became readily available in pharmacies throughout the country. Approximately 84% of the condom purchases today are made in pharmacies, with one third of those purchases being made by women.

Early condoms were made from the bladder of various animals or the intestines of sheep. Although this type of condom is still available today, they are no longer popular. Studies have shown that animal membrane condoms can be penetrated by smaller viruses (specifically those that cause AIDS and hepatitis) and may soon be off the market. The majority of condoms available today are made out of latex. Condoms are available in a variety of styles in an effort to make them more effective and aesthetically pleasing. First, they may have a plain or reservoir tip. The reservoir is designed to collect the semen following ejaculation, thus preventing its release into the vagina. If a plain-tipped condom is used, it is important that the man unroll his condom onto his erect penis and leave 1/2 to 3/4 inches of space at the end to accommodate the sperm containing material. Second, condoms may be lubricated or nonlubricated. If a lubricant is added, it is a water-based jelly that may or may not include a sperm-killing agent. The use of additional lubricant may also be desired by the consumer. Any lubricant used should be a water-based product. Petroleum jelly or other oils may cause the latex to deteriorate, thereby increasing the chance of rupture. For additional variation, condoms may be colored, scented, or contoured, or the outer surface may be roughened or ribbed. These later variations provide no additional therapeutic benefit but are present to satisfy the consumer's personal preferences.

Traditionally the condom is a contraceptive product utilized by the male partner. This may soon change with the marketing of the "female condom". This is a new form of barrier contraceptive being investigated for marketing in the United States. It consists of two diaphragm-like rings located at either end of a 15-cm soft, loose-fitting polyurethane sheath. The inner ring is placed high in the vagina, and the outer ring covers the labia and base of the penis. Following insertion of the device and before intercourse a vaginal spermicide is added.

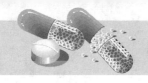

Unlike other barrier forms of contraception, this device is unique in that it covers the vaginal or labial opening where it is also possible to have the transmission of STD organisms.

Condoms are a very effective form of contraception (from 75% to 90% per 100 couple-years of use). In order to provide effective contraception, the male partner must place the condom on his erect penis before the penis comes into contact with his sexual partner, and it must be worn throughout the encounter. Following ejaculation, the penis should be withdrawn immediately. If the erection is allowed to subside before withdrawal, there is an increased risk of slippage and spilling of semen from the condom. To help prevent this from occurring, the ring of the condom should be held securely during withdrawal. Coating the condom with a vaginal spermicide provides an additional defense against spilling and provides lubrication for easier insertion. If a condom should tear, a vaginal spermicide should be inserted as soon as possible by the woman. Condoms should never be reused, and they should be stored in a cool dry place.

Vaginal Spermicides

Vaginal spermicides (sperm-killing substances) were introduced in the 1950s and are generally used with barrier-type contraceptives such as the diaphragm or condom. The FDA advisory panel in 1980 found both octoxynol 9 and nonoxynol 9 (N-9) to be safe and effective. N-9 is the only product available in the United States. Spermicides kill the sperm over a period of 4-6 hours. They may also offer protection against conception by forming a physical barrier against the entry of sperm to the uterus and fallopian tubes through the cervix. This is beneficial because fertilization typically occurs in the fallopian tubes. Effectiveness *positively corresponds to proper use* .

Vaginal spermicides intended for use with a barrier form of contraception provides less surface area coverage and a lower concentration of spermicide. In general, jelly formulations and products containing less than 2% N-9 should not be used alone (due to less surface area coverage). Product choice depends on personal preference. Creams provide a greater amount of lubrication, jellies afford easy removability due to their water solubility, and foams have the advantage of being nearly undetectable during use. Vaginal suppositories foam on contact with moisture. Therefore, women must wait 10 to 15 minutes between suppository insertion and intercourse. Recently the FDA officially approved VCF, a vaginal contraceptive film. This is a paper-thin 2 x 2-inch film that contains 72 mg (28%) of N-9. It is folded and inserted into the vagina close to the cervix no less than 5 minutes before intercourse. It has been suggested that the film may be placed on the penis and inserted at the time of intercourse. We do not recommend this, since placement over the cervix would not be guaranteed nor would the 5 minutes required for this product to dissolve and form a gel necessarily elapse.

All spermicides, *when used alone*, should be reapplied when intercourse is delayed beyond one hour after application . When these products are used in conjunction with a diaphragm, this period may be extended to 6 to 8 hours. If intercourse is repeated, reapplication of the spermicide is recommended in all situations and the diaphragm should not be removed for at least 6 hours after intercourse. Vaginal douching should be delayed for 6 to 8 hours following the use of a vaginal spermicide to avoid interfering with the spermicidal action of the preparation.

The most common complaint associated with the use of vaginal spermicide products is local irritation of the vaginal tissue. Studies done on the effects of spermicides on fetuses have concluded that there are no special dangers to unborn babies posed by these products.

Vaginal Sponge

In June 1983 the Today vaginal sponge was introduced in the United States. It is shaped like a mushroom with a loop attached to the back to aid removal. It is approximately 2 inches. in diameter and 1 1/4 inches thick. It is manufactured from a soft polyurethane material saturated with 1 gram of N-9. This is a sufficient amount of spermicide to maintain a concentration of 10% to 25% N-9 for 24 hours. The sponge is a unique contraceptive product with several actions. It serves as a barrier by covering the cervix, absorbing semen, and slowly releasing spermicide. One advantage to the sponge is that once it has been moistened with water to initiate the release of N-9, it will remain effective for up to 24 hours with no additional spermicide needed for multiple acts of intercourse. It should be left in place for 6-8 hours after intercourse for maximum effectiveness.

There has been considerable controversy regarding the efficacy of the Today sponge. A study conducted in the United States compared 723 sponge users (539 who had never had children and 184 who had) with 717 diaphragm/spermicide users (560 who had never had children and 157 who had). The investigators concluded that women using the sponge who had borne children were twice as likely to become pregnant as those who had never had a child. However, other studies conducted world-wide did not show this to be the case. The overall 1-year sponge effectiveness rate was calculated to be 13.3 pregnancies per 100 women.

Since its marketing, the contraceptive sponge has been associated with few problems. Typically, these are limited to local irritation caused by a sensitivity to the N-9. At the time of marketing the manufacturer included a warning about the possibility of toxic shock syndrome associated with use of the sponge. In addition the manufacturer recommends that the sponge not be used during menstruation, just after delivery or by women with a history of toxic shock syndrome and that it should not be left in place longer than 30 hours.

Chapter 11

Sexually Transmitted Disease

Information on the protective effects of vaginal contraceptives against sexually transmitted diseases is difficult to interpret. First, it is nearly impossible to determine the frequency with which a given individual is exposed to various diseases, and second, reliability of contraception is often poor, which may account for the high incidence of failure. Nonetheless, a National Institutes of Health study involving over 800 women addressed the protective effect of N-9 against the two most common sexually transmitted diseases, gonorrhea and chlamydial infections. They were able to demonstrate a significant reduction in the risk of disease caused by these two organisms. Another study was able to demonstrate a protective effect against trichomoniasis and bacterial vaginosis, with the risk of yeast infections increasing among their study subjects.

The contraceptive sponge has also been evaluated for its protective effects against sexually transmitted diseases. One study supported the protective ability of the sponge against chlamydial and gonorrheal infections. Women in this study, however, had an increased likelihood of vaginal infections with yeast associated with use of the sponge. To date there are no published studies assessing whether the sponge protects against the transmission of AIDS.

It is clear that barrier contraceptives are needed to control the rapid increase in rates of sexually transmitted disease, particularly by those individuals who have "high-risk" and/or multiple partners.

Topical Antifungal Products

Vulvovaginal candidiasis (yeast infections) is a gynecologic problem experienced by many women *(See Chapter 8)*. Recently, the FDA's Fertility and Maternal Health Drugs Advisory Committee unanimously voted in favor of the prescription-to-OTC switch for antifungal preparations used for this purpose, including clotrimazole, miconazole, and nystatin. The former two previously were available OTC for topical fungal infections only. Women who have had a short duration of symptoms, mild to moderate symptom severity, and four or fewer episodes in a 12-month period, as well as women who have had the diagnosis of vaginal candidiasis made by a physician in the past are the best candidates for use of these topical products. Use of these OTC products is contraindicated in pregnant women except with close physician supervision.

A homeopathic product (an extremely small dose of a pharmacologic agent) for treatment of vulvovaginal candidiasis also is available OTC, marketed under the trade names Yeast-Gard and Femicine. No research has been published on the effectiveness of these two products when used for this purpose.

Menstrual Discomfort Products

Several nonprescription products are available for the relief of symptoms associated with painful menstruation and PMS. Many of these products provide relief to women suffering from pain associated with menstruation. For women with "true" PMS, however, these products are usually ineffective *(See Chapter 2 for more information)*.

Analgesics

Selection of drug therapy for painful menstruation usually begins with the use of an OTC analgesic. Most of the nonprescription menstrual products contain aspirin or acetaminophen as analgesics. Since menstrual pain is largely caused by prostaglandins, aspirin theoretically would be effective because of its inhibition of prostaglandin formation. Interestingly, although acetaminophen does not inhibit the synthesis of prostaglandins, it has been shown to be effective for noninflammatory pain associated with painful menstruation. The recommended dosage for both aspirin and acetaminophen (Tylenol) is 500 mg every 4 hours, not to exceed 4 grams per day, and for not more than 10 days.

Research has shown that nonsteroidal anti-inflammatory drugs (NSAIDs), which are also prostaglandin inhibitors, provide significant relief to those suffering from painful menstruation. Currently, ibuprofen is the only drug from this category approved for OTC marketing by the FDA. Ibuprofen in a dose of 200 to 400 mg every 4 to 6 hours has been shown to be superior to aspirin and acetaminophen. Trials comparing aspirin with ibuprofen for the treatment of painful menstruation reported moderate to complete relief in 21% to 30% of patients receiving aspirin, with similar relief in 61% to 84% of women receiving ibuprofen. Dosages up to 1,200 mg/day of ibuprofen have been approved for OTC use, but the dosage often prescribed and the dosages used in many studies (400 mg every 4 hours) exceed the maximum recommended OTC dose.

Diuretics

Diuretics help with elimination of water accumulation and, consequently, the symptoms of weight gain and bloating during the menstrual and premenstrual periods. Ammonium chloride, caffeine, and pamabrom are all considered safe and effective when used for this purpose. Certain symptoms related to water retention such as breast tenderness and bloating do not seem to be affected by these drugs. Furthermore, there is often inconsistency between the amount of weight gain and the severity of PMS symptoms. These data suggest that the use of diuretic therapy for the treatment of PMS is unlikely to be successful all the time.

Antihistamines

Pyrilamine maleate is the only OTC antihistamine that has received the category I (safe and effective) rating by the FDA advisory panel. Its mechanism of action in PMS is unknown, but it is probably related to its side effect profile, namely sedation. Recommended doses are 25 to 30 mg every 3 to 4 hours or 60 mg every 12 hours, not to exceed 200 mg in a 24-hour period. Pyrilamine is only found in combination with an analgesic and/or a diuretic. This product is sold under the trade names, Maximum Strength Midol, Multi-Symptom Formula Caplets, Pamprin, and Multi-Symptom Relief Formula.

Miscellaneous

Phenylpropanolamine hydrochloride, ephedrine sulfate, and cinnamedrine hydrochloride, until recently, were contained in OTC premenstrual products for their theoretical ability to relax uterine smooth muscle. With no studies to support their use for this purpose, the FDA advisory panel recommended that they be removed from the PMS OTC market. Therefore, they are no longer available.

There are many products that contain extracts of botanical or vegetable herbs or contain vitamins (such as, pyridoxine) as a "natural" treatment for PMS. None of these ingredients are classified as either safe or effective for this purpose by the FDA advisory panel.

Feminine Napkins and Tampons

Toxic shock syndrome is associated with the use of tampons during menstruation in young, otherwise healthy women. The disease starts with the sudden onset of a high fever (102°F); a

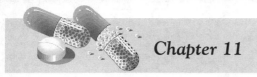

sunburnlike rash most prominent on the palms of the hands and the soles of the feet; and dizziness secondary to extremely low blood pressure. Toxic shock syndrome is thought to be caused by a specific strain of *Staphylococcus aureus* found to colonize the vagina.

Toxic shock syndrome has been reported with all brands of tampons marketed. The frequency with which they have been implicated in toxic shock syndrome is as follows; Playtex (used by 19% of women who developed the problem), Tampax (5%), Kotex (2%), and o.b. (2%). The Rely tampon, which was implicated in 71% of cases of toxic shock syndrome, has been removed from the market by the manufacturer.

The risk factors for toxic shock syndrome are controversial, but current recommendations include the following: (1) women who use tampons and have not had toxic shock syndrome are at very low risk of developing it (0.3% per year); (2) tampons should be changed four to six times each day; (3) alternating tampons and sanitary napkins is recommended; (4) any woman who develops a sudden onset of fever, sunburnlike rash, or low blood pressure should remove the tampon and seek medical attention immediately; and (5) women who have had toxic shock syndrome are at an increased risk of redeveloping the syndrome (45% in one study) and should wait for several menstrual cycles before using tampons again.

An alternative to the use of tampons for the absorption of menstrual flow is the feminine napkin or pad. They are available in various sizes and absorbencies. The "super" or "maxi" pads may be used during days 1 and 2 when the menstrual flow is usually the heaviest. During this time the pads may need to be changed as frequently as every 2 to 4 hours. "Mini," "light," "junior," or "teen" pads are designed to accommodate the lighter flow and smaller anatomy of adolescents or women using oral contraceptives. The "light" pads or the thin "shields" may also be used to protect undergarments from being stained by vaginal creams, suppository leakage, or normal vaginal discharge at times other than during menstruation.

Home Diagnostic Aids

It is projected that by the year 1995 consumers will spend approximately $2.2 billion annually on home diagnostic kits. When used properly, these tests provide relatively fast and accurate results.

Pregnancy Tests

The first home pregnancy test (e.p.t.) was marketed by Warner-Lambert in late 1977. Pregnancy tests, the fastest growing of the home testing products, account for one third of all home testing product sales.

The first hormone to be produced in appreciable amounts following conception and implantation of the fertilized ovum is human chorionic gonadotropin (hCG). Home pregnancy tests detect this hormone in the urine.

First-Generation Pregnancy Tests. These tests involve incubating a sample of the woman's first morning urine with the test reagent, which contains hCG-coated sheep red blood cells (RBCs) and rabbit anti-hCG serum. If hCG is present in the urine, it will bind to the rabbit antiserum after leaving the sheep RBCs and thus prevent them from sticking together. Rather than clumping, the RBCs settle to the bottom of the test tube in a doughnut-shaped ring, which is indicative of a positive test. If hCG is not present in the urine, a cluster of cells with no particular shape settles to the bottom of the tube.

There are several disadvantages to the use of these earlier tests. First, they are unable to detect small quantities of hCG in the urine and therefore are not considered reliable until approximately 9 days after a missed period. In addition, if testing is performed after the tenth week of pregnancy when hCG levels have declined, a false-negative test may result. These tests typically require a relatively long period of time to complete that ranges from 30 to 60 minutes. The slightest vibration of the test tube has been reported to produce a false-negative result due to disruption of the donut shaped ring formation. False-positive results (3%) occur more frequently than with the second-generation products because of their susceptibility to interference from sources of hCG production not associated with pregnancy. Many of these older kits are no longer marketed.

Second-Generation Pregnancy Kits. The newer second-generation test kits use highly sensitive methods and offer several advantages. These tests can be used as early as the day of the expected missed period; they are less susceptible to technical error and require less time to perform - from 3 to 30 minutes. As with the first-generation tests, performance of the second-generation test too early can cause false-negative results. Although the second-generation tests are less susceptible to interference from hCG not associated with pregnancy, false-positive results are possible when there is an ectopic pregnancy, when the test is performed in post-menopausal women, and when soap or detergent residues are present in the urine collection container.

Regardless of the type of pregnancy test selected, a first morning urine sample should be tested. Typically, this specimen contains the highest concentration of hCG, provided that the bladder has not been emptied within the last 6 to 8 hours. The urine should be collected in a clean, dry, detergent-free container. If the test cannot be performed immediately, the urine sample should be covered and stored in the refrigerator (not freezer) for no longer than 12 hours. Before testing, the sample should be allowed to return to room temperature. If a sediment has developed during refrigeration the specimen should not be shaken; rather the top portion should be removed and tested. If a negative result occurs, and no menstrual period starts, the test should be repeated in 1 week. If a positive result is obtained on the first or second test or a second negative result occurs, the woman should see her physician. Table 11-1 has a representative list of the currently marketed home pregnancy kits, the time required to perform the test, and the sign that indicates a positive result.

The manufacturers of home pregnancy testing products claim an accuracy of 98% to 99%. A recent study compared the accuracy of two of the newer second-generation testing kits (e.p.t. Plus, Advance) with two testing kits that are available for laboratory use only. In the hands of experienced laboratory personnel, the two "professional" brand pregnancy kits yielded identical results for all of the urine specimens tested. However, when lay people used the home test kits, 9.5% (e.p.t. Plus) and 12.5% (Advance) of the results showed a discrepancy with the results obtained by a trained technologist. To further test whether the discrepancies were due to the kits or to the individuals using them, the trained technologists repeated the tests by using the home test kits. Results showed an identical distribution of positive and negative results to that observed with the professional kits. The discrepancy between manufacturer stated and actual accuracy is thought to be due in part to the strict procedures that must be adhered to when conducting these tests.

Table 11 - 1
Pregnancy Tests

Product/Manufacturer	Time to Complete Test (min)	Indications of Positive Result
Advance®/Advanced Care Products	30	Color change from white to blue on tip of test stick
Answer 2®/Carter Products	60	Formation of red ring or button at the bottom of the test tube
Answer Plus®/Carter Products	30	Color change from yellow to blue on the lower color bead
Answer Quick and Simple®/ Carter Products	3	Color change from white to pink-purple on the lower area of color key
C & T/Healthcheck	5	Appearance of "+"
Clearblue®/Whitehall	30	Color change to blue on test stick tip
Clearblue Easy®/Whitehall	3	Blue line in large window
e.p.t. Stick®/Parke-Davis Consumer Products	30	Color change from white to pink on tip of stick
Fact Plus®/Advanced Care Products	5-8	Appearance of "+" on plus cube
First Response 5 - Minute Test for Pregnancy®/Tambrands	5	Appearance of pink color in test well
QTest for Pregnancy®/Becton Dickinson	9	Appearance of blue color on test pad area of test strip which is darker than "error control" pad

Ovulation Prediction Kits

The purpose of ovulation prediction is to determine the time period during which a woman is fertile in an effort to increase the chances of conception. This prediction is based primarily upon the detection of luteinizing hormone (LH), which is responsible for causing ovulation. Until recently, the only method available for in-home ovulation prediction was the measurement of basal body temperature. This method relies upon the changes in basal temperature that occur during the normal menstrual cycle. During the first 14 days of the cycle the basal temperature varies only slightly. Midcycle the temperature first drops 0.5°F to 1°F and then 24 hours later the temperature rises 0.5°F to 1°F above the normal temperature. The temperature remains elevated until menses occur. The rise in temperature indicates ovulation. The greatest drawback to measuring body temperature rise is that it does not allow one to predict ovulation but simply indicates that it has occurred within the previous 24 hours.

The in-home ovulation prediction test indicates an increased concentration of LH in the urine by a deepening color intensity of the sample. There are several products available that differ in the amount of time necessary to conduct the test, the number of tests provided in each package, and the specific procedure for determining when ovulation has occurred.

Before using the ovulation predictor test, the menstrual cycle length must be accurately calculated. If the woman has a fairly regular cycle, the average length of the previous three cycles can be determined. If, however, the woman's cycle varies by more than 3 days from month to month, the shortest of the last three cycles should be used to determine when testing should begin. Testing should begin 2 to 3 days before expected ovulation in order that the color change signaling ovulation can be observed. Since ovulation normally occurs 14 days before menses, a women with a 31-day cycle, for example, should begin testing on day 14 or 15. The test's accuracy can be increased by testing for a greater number of days. For example, if testing is done for 6 days in the middle of the cycle, ovulation can be successfully predicted in 66% of ovulating women. If the number of days of testing is increased to 10, ovulation will be predicted in 95% of fertile women using the test.

It is important that the urine sample be collected at the appropriate time of the month and at the same time each day. Some of the kits require a first morning urine while others require that the urine be collected between the hours of 10:00 a.m. and 8:00 p.m. If the sample collected is not a first morning specimen, fluid intake must be restricted during the 1 to 2 hours preceding the collection. This will avoid possible dilution of the sample. As for the pregnancy test kits, the urine can be refrigerated for up to 12 hours if the test cannot be performed immediately, provided that it is allowed to return to room temperature before testing. If a sediment develops during refrigeration, the liquid on top should be used for testing.

Ovulation test kits are indicated only to facilitate conception. *They are not a reliable means of contraception.* Sperm can survive for up to 72 hours following ejaculation. in the female reproductive tract. Consequently, it is possible for fertilization of an ovum to take place even though intercourse occurred before the LH surge and ovulation.

Urine should be collected in the containers provided with the testing products and those containers discarded with each use because soap or detergent residue can alter the test results. False-negatives have not been reported with the use of these kits. It is possible, however, to miss the LH surge by beginning testing too late. Since ovulation can occur at different times each month, the tests must be performed during each cycle. Because LH is similar to follicle-stimulating hormone (FSH) and thyroid-stimulating hormone (TSH), medical disorders involving these hormones may cause false-positive results. These include menopause (elevated levels of FSH) and hyperthyroidism (elevated TSH levels). Drugs used to stimulate ovulation (i.e., menotropins) in infertile patients can stimulate FSH and LH and thereby cause false-positive results. Danazol, a drug used for the treatment of endometriosis, inhibits the release of FSH and LH from the pituitary, thus inhibiting ovulation. The use of an ovulation prediction kit by a women receiving danazol therapy would therefore not be a good idea. Table 11-3 contains a list of representative ovulation prediction kits currently available as OTC products.

Breast Care Products

The practice of breast feeding among women has been increasing over the past decade. Most women who breast feed will experience some degree of nipple pain during the first few weeks. This often contributes to the early abandonment of breast-feeding.

Home remedies for nipple pain have been suggested over the years, including the application of egg whites, salad oil, cocoa butter, and a variety of creams and lotions. It has also been suggested that breast milk and colostrum have lubricating and bacteriostatic properties and therefore should be left on the nipple and allowed to dry following each feeding as a "natural" means of treating nipple pain. The pharmacologic "protectant" receiving the most publicity over the years has been lanolin, and it is the principal ingredient found in Masse Breast Cream. The effectiveness of lanolin was compared with the application of expressed breast milk to the nipple after breast-feeding for the prevention and reduction of nipple pain. The amount of nipple pain and trauma experienced by these women was similar between the two groups.

Reports of pesticide residue in lanolin have recently been published. Although the level of pesticide is low and not thought to present any immediate toxic hazard, the potential effects on the nursing infant are unknown. For this reason and in light of the fact that products containing lanolin have not been shown to be superior to non-drug techniques, it would seem prudent to avoid the use of products that contain this ingredient.

Case Study

Sybil F. was married, with three children ranging in ages from 7-12. She and her husband were happy with the size of their family and enjoying their lives, with the children being older and less dependent upon them.

Sybil was in good health, although she smoked a pack of cigarettes a day, in part to control her tendency to gain weight. Now 40, because of her smoking and extra pounds, Sybil had been advised not to take oral contraceptives. She had always been afraid to try an IUD because some of her friends had bad experiences with them. Her periods had always been very regular, so she used the rhythm method and Delfen foam for contraception. Sybil also like to use Massengill Disposable Douche as a deodorant and cleanser..

When she missed her usually regular period, she was taken by surprise. She purchased an e.p.t. kit at the drugstore, and to her and her husband's shock, the test turned positive for pregnancy.

Sybil contacted her gynecologist immediately. After close questioning the doctor learned that Sybil had douched only an hour after intercourse at a date midway through her menstrual cycle. The doctor reminded her that a woman should wait at least 8 hours before douching after intercourse, when protecting herself with a barrier method such as foam, jelly, or cream.

Although taken aback by the unplanned pregnancy, Sybil and her husband decided they were willing to welcome another child into the family. They scheduled a genetic amniocentesis to be done at the end of her fourth month of pregnancy.

Key Points for Over-The-Counter Drugs

1. Despite its popularity, regular douching has not been proven to offer women any advantages in vaginal health or hygiene. Douching with povidone-iodine may be harmful to the fetus during pregnancy and may even increase the chance for vaginal infections. Women should wait 8 hours or more before douching after intercourse if vaginal spermicides have been used.

2. Other products such as feminine deodorant sprays and premoistened towelettes occasionally produce irritation. Vaginal premoistened towelettes occasionally produce irritation. Vaginal creams for the use of itching and soreness can relieve symptoms but may mask more serious problems.

3. Latex condoms are an effective form of contraception and help prevent some sexually transmitted diseases. Female condoms may soon be marketed in the U.S. for further protection.

4. Vaginal spermicides come in a variety of forms - cream, foam, jelly and in sponges. It is important to apply jellies, creams and foams *each time* intercourse is repeated. Nonoxynol-9, the main ingredient, has been proven effective in preventing transmission of chlamydia and gonorrhea.

5. Several nonprescription products aid with menstrual discomfort and symptoms of PMS. These include aspirin, acetominophen, and ibuprofen for pain; ammonium chloride, caffeine, and pamabrom for water retention; and pyrilamine maleate for anxiety.

6. Tampon usage occasionally causes toxic shock syndrome. To minimize chances of getting the disease, change tampons frequently, alternate tampon usage with pad usage, see a doctor immediately if high fever, dizziness or rash develop, and do not use tampons if you have had toxic shock syndrome.

7. Home pregnancy tests are useful and accurate. However, directions must be followed very carefully, in order to get accurate results. If a period does not occur within a week after results, another test should be made or a doctor's visit scheduled.

8. Ovulation prediction kits are effective in predicting ovulation to help schedule conception. They are not recommended as a form of contraception.

9. Lanolin-containing breast creams have not been proven superior to home remedies for sore nipples, such as salad oil or cocoa butter. Breast milk and colostrum are believed to have healing properties, also.

Table 11- 2 Ovulation Prediction Kits			
Product	Manufacturer	Number of Tests	Time to Complete Test (min)
Answer	Carter	6	30
Clearplan	Whitehall	10	30
First Response	Tambrands	6	20
Fortel	NMS Pharmaceuticals	9	30-40
OvuKIT	Monoclonal Antibodies	9	60
OvuQUICK	Monoclonal Antibodies	6 or 9	5
Q-Test	Becton-Dickinson	5	35

Chapter 12

Birth Control Pills and Other Hormonal Contraceptives

In 1960 the first form of nearly 100% reliable contraception was marketed - Enovid 5 a high-dose estrogen birth control pill. This drug changed the course of social history because it gave women nearly complete control over their reproductive lives. At long last women could have children when they wanted to or never have them, if that was their choice. It's no coincidence that the so-called sexual revolution and the availability of birth control pills started at the same time; and that the women's liberation movement followed soon after.

Oral contraceptives and physicians and women's attitudes about them have changed a lot in 30 years, but one thing remains the same: "the pill" is still the most popular and reliable form of reversible contraception in the world (Table 12-1). (Sterilization is the number one method, but it is seldom reversible.) In developed countries such as the United States, Canada, The Netherlands, New Zealand, West Germany, and Australia, almost 20% of women of reproductive age are taking the pill. In the U.S. alone this represents about 10 million women. An estimated 5-10% of women in third world countries use oral contraceptives and their use is increasing.

In spite of their popularity, however, after 12-24 months of usage, many women discontinue the use of birth control pills with its ultra-reliable contraception. Since most of these discontinuances do not have to do with side effects from the pill, physicians have concluded that women have been frightened by media reports questioning oral contraceptive safety or that they simply do not like to take pills. Thus, the search for a more perfect contraceptive continues as the world population reaches the 2.5 billion mark.

How Does the Pill Work?

What exactly are the millions of women who swallow their contraceptive pill every day taking? Oral contraceptives are small tablets containing steroidal female sex hormones, either combinations of a synthetic estrogen and a synthetic progesterone (called a progestin) or a progestin alone. They work by preventing ovulation (egg formation) and, at the same time, thickening cervical mucus so sperm have difficulty getting through the cervix. The synthetic estrogen has two forms, ethinyl estradiol and mestranol. Combination pills can deliver the same concoction of hormones each day, or they can deliver proportionately different dosages over a 21 or 28 day cycle.

During a normal menstrual cycle, two naturally-produced hormones are in charge of regulating egg production and menstruation - estrogen and progesterone. In the approximately 14-day-long portion of the monthly cycle before ovulation (production of the egg) the estrogen hormone is in charge. After the egg has been released from the ovary into the fallopian tube, it finds its way down into the uterus and progesterone takes over. The secretion of progesterone for the next 14 days causes the lining of the uterus to become thicker. and more receptive to implantation of an egg.

During this time the ratio of estrogen and progesterone changes each day, with progesterone levels mounting as the day approaches when menstruation begins. The lining sloughs off at the end of the cycle as progesterone secretion stops. The resulting menstrual period lasts for about 5 days, and then the entire process starts over again with estrogen secretion. Fig. 1 on page 3 illustrates the anatomy of the uterus, cervix, and vagina, where the menstrual cycle takes place.

Oral contraceptives attempt to match much of the normal menstrual cycle, but prevent conception by holding back the normal production of estrogen and progesterone by the ovaries and thus prevent ovulation. Under natural conditions estrogen and progesterone are secreted by the ovary and pass directly into the general blood circulation of the body. The hormones contained in oral contraceptives must be absorbed by the intestines, pass through the circulation of the liver, and then enter the general circulation of the body where they can do their work. For the synthetic hormones to work on the reproductive organs, the amount swallowed in the pills must be at least three times higher than what the body would normally produce. This is because most of the synthetic hormones in the pills are broken down by the liver and are not used by the reproductive organs.

Differences between the natural hormone secretion cycle and the synthetic hormone cycle of the pill are as follows: *(1)* The synthetic hormones enter the body through the intestines and then the liver, whereas natural hormones go into the general circulation directly from the ovary. *(2)* The ratio of estrogen to progestin is constant within the pill, unless the triphasic oral contraceptives are used; the ratio of natural hormones varies constantly. *(3)* With the pill estrogen and progestin are administered together. Natural hormones are still secreted more or less separately by the ovary but at a lower level since the estrogen-progestin pill suppresses stimulating hormones from the pituitary gland. If no stimulation from the pituitary occurs, ovulation is not possible. That is the major effect of the pill.

Effects on the Reproductive Organs

Oral contraceptives affect the reproductive process in many ways. The pill suppresses the stimulating hormones released from the brain reproductive centers known as the hypothalamus and the pituitary gland. This suppression causes the ovaries in women taking oral contraceptives to become small and inactive. The uterus changes also, becoming firmer and smaller. The lining of the uterus called the endometrium, is affected to the point where menstrual flow becomes scanty. As long as she has regular monthly spotting, pill use is satisfactory. If a woman feels that she would like to have more bleeding during her period, the pill can be changed to one with less progestin in it. If her period stops altogether, a woman is usually advised to refrain from taking the pill to let her uterus and lining regain their normal capacities or to change pills.

The cervix, the opening of the uterus, is very sensitive to the effects of synthetic estrogen and progestin. It too sometimes becomes firm, and cervical mucus changes to a consistency that is nearly impenetrable to sperm. The opening of the cervix sometimes becomes irregular in shape when oral contraceptives are used, but no definitive evidence has been found to show that the incidence of cancer of the cervix is any higher in women who have taken the pill. Other risk factors such as becoming sexually active at an early age, a history of sexually transmitted diseases, and multiple sexual partners are much more important in cervical cancer risk.

A woman may notice that her vagina is drier when she is taking the pill, and she may be more susceptible to certain kinds of fungal infections such as those caused by *Candida albicans*. The condition of a woman's vagina while she is taking the pill is affected by the particular pill she takes, the amount of sexual activity she engages in, the number of partners she has, and her personal hygiene. If she runs into a problem with chronic vaginal infection, any one of these items might be the cause.

Both when she is pregnant and when she is using birth control pills, a woman's breasts may increase in size and be more tender than they normally are Nursing mothers who take oral contraceptives, particularly before 4 weeks post partum, may find that their milk flow

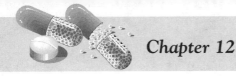

decreases. Some studies have shown that the composition of milk changes during pill use. For the most part these problems do not occur when the mother is taking low-dose estrogen pills.

Interestingly, there is a significantly lower incidence of fibrocystic breast disease in pill users, anywhere from 25% to 80% lower, than in women who don't take the pill. This common disorder, characterized by small, benign tumors that form in the breasts, seems to be associated with a slightly higher incidence of breast cancer.

The association between breast cancer and pill usage is still controversial, and research continues on large numbers of women to try and determine the level of risk of breast cancer for pill users. Some researchers have seen a very slight increased risk of breast cancer in young women (under age 45) who used oral contraceptives for a long time, but most experts don't agree with this. Evidence to support a pill-breast cancer connection surfaced in a large Swedish study where women were taking a different type of estrogen than that found in contraceptive pills prescribed in the United States. Use of oral contraceptives is not associated with an increase in the chance of developing ovarian cancer.

Many studies are now in progress to determine the effects of accidental use of oral contraceptives early in pregnancy. Some researchers in the past have suggested that the number of miscarriages due to genetic abnormalities is higher in women who were taking oral contraceptives than in nonusers.

The weight of evidence today seems to be shifting to indicate that use of contraceptive hormones early in pregnancy is not very harmful. No information exists to date indicating that either congenital diseases or genetic defects are higher in babies whose mothers used oral contraceptives early in pregnancy. We would certainly not recommend an abortion just because a mother had been using oral contraceptives at the time of conception.

On balance we feel that there are more positive effects from the pill on the reproductive system than negative ones. Table 12-1a summarizes these positive features.

Table 12-1	
Comparative Effectiveness of Contraceptives	
Method	*Percent Pregnant within First Year*
No contraception	85%
Norplant system	0.2-0.3%
Female sterilization	0.2-0.4%
Oral contraceptives	0.1-0.5%
Intrauterine device	1-2%
Condom without spermicide	2-12%
Cervical cap	6-18%
Diaphragm with spermicide	6-18%
Vaginal sponge	6-20%
Spermicide alone	3-20%

Table 12-1a
Advantages and Benefits of Oral Contraceptive Usage

- One of the most carefully studied drugs in modern medicine

- May be used by healthy non-smokers all the way to menopause

- Decreased blood loss from period, helps prevent anemia

- Decreased number of accidental pregnancies (less than 1% per year of pill-users)

- Decreased number of ectopic pregnancies

- Decreased incidence of fibrocystic breast disease

- Decreased incidence of ovarian cysts and ovarian cancer

- Decreased incidence of endometrial cancer

- Decreased incidence of PMS

- Decreased incidence of endometriosis

- Decreased incidence of pelvic inflammatory disease

Table 12-2

Warning Signs of Potentially Serious Problems for Oral Contraceptive Users

Symptoms	Potential problem
Abdominal pain (severe)	Gallbladder disease, liver tumor, blood clot, pancreatitis
Chest pain (severe); shortness of breath coughing up blood	Blood clot in lungs or heart attack
Headaches (severe)	Stroke, hypertensive episode, or migraine headache
Eye problems: blurred vision, flashing lights, blindness	Stroke, hypertensive episide temporary vascular problem at many possible sites
Severe leg pain (calf or thigh)	Blood clot in legs

Effects on Other Organs of the Body

Since the pill was first marketed many discoveries have been made about how it affects the body. In fact, oral contraceptives are the most extensively studied drugs ever used in medical practice. Table 12-2 lists symptoms of possible problems for oral contraceptive users.

The Liver

As mentioned, the liver is strongly impacted by the synthetic hormones in the pill. Particularly in cases when a woman already has an underlying liver disorder, jaundice (yellowing of the skin) may appear when she begins taking the pill since the liver isn't circulating bile properly. This can be conducive to gallstone formation, if other factors are present too. Again we wish to emphasize that most of these complications were reported before the introduction of low dose estrogen or mini-pills. When a woman is taking a pill that has the correct ratio of estrogen to progestin for her system, these problems seldom occur.

High Blood Pressure

High-dose estrogen birth control pills correlate with increased blood pressure. In one carefully monitored study, blood pressure increased by an average of 13.5 mm Hg systolic and 6.2 mm Hg diastolic in all pill users. For women with preexisting hypertension, oral contraceptives are probably not advisable regardless of the dosage. If there are no other workable choices, a woman with high blood pressure should use a combination pill with a low dose of estrogen (0.35 mg or less). She should also plan to check her blood pressure at home at least weekly and report any upswings to her physician immediately.

Blood Clots

The most serious problem we see in pill users is blood clots. The vulnerable areas in a woman's body are the same as those associated with late pregnancy and delivery: the lower legs, the pelvis, and the lungs *(See Chapter 17, Managing Medical Problems During Pregnancy)*.

Other factors that increase the risk of blood clots for contraceptive users are overweight, smoking, heredity (clots are three times as common in mothers and daughters or sisters), major surgery, chronic diseases such as diabetes, varicose veins, and being very sedentary or confined to a bed. Deep vein thrombosis is 5 1/2 times more common in women who take the pill. This risk, once again is greatly reduced with the use of low-dose estrogen pills. *However, if a woman has or has ever had a blood clot. she should not take oral contraceptives.* Women with varicose veins or superficial thrombophlebitis are best advised not to use oral contraceptives either. Note: A currently popular form of therapy to prevent blood clots and other vascular problems is to take one baby aspirin a day. Talk to your physician about this if you are concerned about blood clots.

Heart and Blood Vessel Disease

Contraceptive use has been studied intensively in the United Kingdom, where they have found that the chance of having a stroke (a clot or bleeding in a specific part of the brain) when using oral contraceptives is four times higher than normal although, overall, the risk is still very low. Once again estrogen seems to be the culprit, and the risks are lessened if a low-dose pill is being used. If there is a history of stroke in the family, or if a woman has headaches or notices a tendency to muscle weakness on one side of her body, she should not use the pill. These all indicate a possible predisposition to stroke.

The risk of a heart attack is significantly higher in women taking oral contraceptives who also have high blood pressure and high levels of fatty substances in their bloodstream. If these women smoke, the risks increase even more and they continue to increase with age. Table 12-3

(Page 126) shows the risks of heart attack for smoking and non-smoking women who take oral contraceptives in various age groups.

Mitral valve prolapse (a weakness in the leaflets of a heart valve) is very common in women. In the great majority of cases it causes no symptoms or problems, nor, is it, by itself, a contraindication to the use of the pill. One subgroup that seems to be at special risk, however, are women with mitral valve prolapse combined with symptoms of vascular disease. If your doctor has told you that you have a prolapsed mitral valve and you also have headaches and associated vascular or cardiac disease you should avoid oral contraceptives.

In every age group pregnancy is riskier than any contraceptive method except in women over the age of 40 who smoke. In this group, using the pill is more dangerous than being pregnant. Smoking evidently outweighs all other risk factors in women over age 40 who take oral contraceptives. Smoking and the pill just don't go together.

Who Should Not Use the Pill

From the preceding discussion we can develop a profile of the woman who should not use oral contraceptives. She is 35 or older, is and has been a heavy smoker (1 1/2 to 2 packs or more of cigarettes per day) for several years. (Her risk drops precipitously if she quits smoking!) She is 20 pounds or more over the recommended weight for her height and body build. She has one or more of the following medical disorders: high blood pressure, blood clots or a family history of blood clots, high fat and cholesterol levels in her bloodstream, heart disease of any kind, epilepsy, diabetes, gallstones, or liver disorders. If two or more of these characteristics apply to you we recommend that you find an alternative to birth control pills. Table 12-4 (Page 126) lists a number of medical problems that make oral contraceptives relatively inadvisable or absolutely contraindicated.

Years ago we hesitated to prescribe oral contraceptives to women over 40, regardless of the state of their health. Studies have shown us that, if a woman over 40 does not smoke or carry any of the other major risk factors, she can safely take low-dose oral contraceptives until her menopause. Since the progestin-containing pills are known to help with problems like fibroid tumors (a common cause of bleeding in women approaching the menopause), they may even help avert perimenopausal difficulties. Combination birth control pills have been shown to reduce a woman's risk for both ovarian cancer and endometrial cancer.

Who May Use the Pill

Healthy women who do not smoke and who maintain a suitable weight for their height and body build should feel confident that birth control pills are a safe and reliable form of contraception provided that they have not had menstrual problems or other difficulties with their reproductive organs. This is true for all ages up to the menopause. The pill is an ideal form of contraception for women who want children but plan to postpone their arrival for anywhere from 1 to 5 years. Particularly for those women who feel they would not be able to accommodate a pregnancy for economic, psychological, professional or any other reason, we recommend the pill because it has one of the highest effectiveness rates of all methods available today. As a bonus it lowers your risks of fibrocystic breast disease and ovarian cancer and cyst formation. Certain menstrual problem such as irregular periods and cramps often improve greatly during and after pill use.

A drawback to oral contraceptives (if there are no associated medical problems) is cost. They normally range in price from $17.20-$28.26 for one month's supply, a cost that may over-stretch some women's budgets. Planned Parenthood does offer reduced rates on contraceptive materials. Women who are economically strained should visit their local Planned Parenthood chapters for assistance in purchasing low-cost contraceptives. The 17 year patents on several pills recently expired. These pills are now manufactured with fewer restrictions and can be obtained for $2-4 less per month at some places.

Which Pill is Right?

Choosing the right pill is not always easy. It may be necessary to try different kinds before settling on one that can be tolerated for a number of years. Right now several pharmaceutical houses market at least 35 different compounds that are prescribed to an estimated 10 million users in North America alone.

The major difference among the preparations is the amount of synthetic estrogen or progestin that they contain. The range is from 20 to 150 mcg of synthetic estrogen and from 0.9 to nearly 10 mg of progestin. Table 12-5 (Page 127) lists some of the popular, currently available brands of oral contraceptives with their dosages of synthetic estrogen and progestin.

Each active tablet contains a specific concentration of estrogen and progestin to be taken daily for 21 or 28 days each month. The tablets are packaged in containers that have some sort of calendar to help count the days of use. Some packages contain 28 pills; the last seven pills are inactive, but they are helpful to the user as she counts the days. When taken properly, the pills are nearly 100% effective. Even the lowest dose pills, which contain only 35 mcg of synthetic estrogen, have a pregnancy rate of only 0.2% per 100 women years of use. We advocate using the low dose compounds because they have fewer side effects with only a slight difference in the occurrence of unwanted pregnancies.

Table 12-6 (Page 128) describes different oral contraceptive formulations and their respective advantages and disadvantages.

Getting Started on the Pill

Oral contraceptives are prescribed not because a woman is ill, but because she needs a family planning method. Therefore contraceptives should not *(1)* initiate any medical problems, *(2)* aggravate any existing medical condition, *(3)* allow an unwanted pregnancy to occur, or *(4)* be associated with future dangers to pregnancies or a woman's health. Because caution is necessary to be sure that none of these things happen, we recommend starting with a low dose pill. (less than 35 mcg of synthetic estrogen and less than 1 mg of progestin) Higher doses may be necessary if side effects such as no period or breakthrough bleeding in between periods occur.

Women routinely begin a contraceptive pill regimen on the fifth day of their normal period; the pill should be effective within 2 or 3 days. If periods have been irregular or if the pill wasn't started on the fifth day, a backup method such as a diaphragm should be used with the pill for a full month. Following pregnancy, women should wait at least a month or until they have their first period before going back on the pill. Nursing mothers should wait at least 3 or 4 months before resuming pill usage. If a woman has had a miscarriage or an abortion, she may begin taking the pill within a week if there are no other complications.

If you miss taking your pill, here is what you should do:

If you miss one pill:

• Take the missing pill as soon as you discover that you forgot it and continue to take the rest of the pills on their correct days (*This means you may take your "makeup" pill and your regularly scheduled pill on the same day*).

If you miss 2 pills:

• Take one of the two missed pills on each of the next two days along with your regularly scheduled pill so you end your pill pac at the usual time.

If you miss 3 or more pills:

• Take an extra pill each night along with your regularly scheduled pill until you catch up. *In addition,* you must use additional contraceptive protection, such as the condom, diaphragm. or sponge for at least 7 days in a row.

Side Effects

Side effects can occur when you are taking oral contraceptives and will be most noticeable during the first 3 months of pill usage. That is why we recommend a 3-month trial before rejecting any particular pill. Women should schedule a visit to the doctor after using the pill for 3 months to make sure there have been no adverse side effects. A yearly office visit is wise even if there are no apparent problems. During this visit a woman should have a breast examination, a pelvic examination, a blood pressure reading, an analysis of any physical changes such as weight gain, and laboratory blood tests to check the levels of fat and cholesterol.

The thought of using a drug as potent as the contraceptive pill is upsetting to some women, who may need reassurance and emotional support during their first months of pill usage. Some of the symptoms these women experience may be due merely to nervousness or worry about the consequences of taking the drug. In other cases symptoms may indicate that the proportion of estrogen or progestin should be adjusted by switching to a different pill. Symptoms that resemble PMS such as nausea, nervousness, irritability, weepiness, water retention, and headaches probably result from these excess hormones. Symptoms similar to those of pregnancy such as fatigue, sluggishness, depression, increased appetite, and weight gain may be attributed to too much progestin.

As is true for most drugs, oral contraceptives may interact with other drugs to produce unanticipated side effects (Table 12-7). The desired effect from either the contraceptive or the other drug may not be fully achieved, or undesirable symptoms may occur in the body. Antibiotics have been the most important drug class found to interact with oral contraceptives. Tetracycline and ampicillin, which are commonly prescribed for respiratory and other types of infections appear to decrease the effectiveness of oral contraceptives. Rifampicin (an antituberculosis drug) and penicillin V are also thought to do so. Drugs whose own effectiveness appears to be changed by oral contraceptives are the sedative and hypnotic benzodiazepines and barbiturates; all blood-thinning drugs; insulin and the oral antidiabetes drugs; guanethidine and occasionally methyldopa (Aldomet); drugs that control high blood pressure; and all the phenothiazines including reserpine and the tricyclic antidepressants. In some situations it is possible to modify pill usage to overcome the drug interaction problem; in others it may be necessary to discontinue the pill and find an alternate method of contraception.

Alternatives to the Pill

The Norplant Contraceptive System

Introduced to the U.S. public in 1990, but already tested in other countries for almost 20 years, the Norplant system represents a major innovation in contraceptive technology. Norplant levonorgestrol implants deliver a sustained-release contraceptive hormone through 6 small Silastic tubes about the size of a matchstick that are placed just under the skin of the upper arm. Implanted through a simple surgical procedure done in the doctor's office, the Norplant tubes will provide continuous contraceptive protection for as long as five years.

Norplant is a progestin-only system, but it differs from the progestin-only pill in that it maintains constant low-level hormone delivery rather than the "peak and trough" effect that pills produce. This means that contraception can be maintained predictably with very low levels of synthetic hormones.

Sustained-release contraception is attractive for women who don't want to be bothered with swallowing a pill every day, but who still wish reliable long-term contraception. It is also a good choice for those who may be considering sterilization, but aren't sure. Finally, it is a good alternative for those who wish to avoid taking estrogen.

Injectable Hormones

Injectable hormones are an important contraceptive method outside the United States and have been approved and used in more than 90 countries, including The United Kingdom, Sweden, and West Germany. The most commonly used injectable contraceptive is depo-medroxyprogesterone acetate (Depo-Provera). This synthetic progestin is given by injection every 3 months. Depo-Provera has been approved by the FDA for use for contraception in the United States. The Upjohn Company markets an injectable Depo-Provera contraceptive for widespread use, also. Menstrual irregularities similar to Norplant have occurred with Depo-Provera injections.

Contraception Following Intercourse (Morning-After Pills)

While not to be recommended as a regular form of contraception, hormones given after intercourse are effective in preventing pregnancy. These post-intercourse treatments, which actually have been on the market for about 20 years, most often provide a form of high-dose estrogen (ethinyl estradiol, 200 mg) in combination with a progestin (dl-norgestrel, 2 mg) in tablet form. Two of these are given as soon as possible after intercourse, followed by two more tablets 12 hours later. Previously these drugs have been prescribed for as long as 4 days, but because of ensuing nausea and discomfort, this is not commonly done anymore. Only slightly more than 1% of women became pregnant after taking these high-estrogen hormone pills within 12 hours of sexual contact. About 4.5% became pregnant when they started therapy 48 hours or more after intercourse.

A drug called RU 486, which is classified as an antiprogesterone, has had good results for post-intercourse contraception. A single dose taken on Day 27 of the menstrual cycle (i.e. the day before a period was expected) by 62 women yielded only one pregnancy. RU 486, which is also used to induce abortions is not available in the United States, but has been studied and used extensively in France.

Male Contraceptives

Steroid hormones given to men to suppress sex hormones and sperm production were developed several years ago. Unfortunately, these have sometimes had the effect of reducing sexual desire and performance as well. Currently, combinations of a drug called DMPA and androgens (important male sex hormones) have been effective in reducing and immobilizing sperm without reducing sexual desire. However, the jury is still out on other side effects such as the risk of vascular disease and liver cancer.

Pulsatile GnRH *(See Chapter 14, Fertility Drugs)* has been used in men to *promote* fertility. The drug is currently used for the treatment of prostatic cancer, as well. Now, the intriguing possibility of a role for GnRH in male contraception has also arisen. Research on the male contraceptive application of this drug is going on right now.

Non-hormonal Contraception

Among the best non-hormonal alternatives to birth control pills are the intrauterine device (IUD) and the diaphragm or condoms used in conjunction with contraceptive cream or jelly. The IUD is highly effective in guarding against pregnancy the first year it is in position, with no more than a 1% to 2% pregnancy rate. Complications such as excessive bleeding cramps and discomfort can occur but do so in fewer than 10% of users. The IUD may have to be removed if complications create too many difficulties.

The optimal time for inserting an IUD is during the first menstrual period after delivery of a baby, when the uterus is still somewhat enlarged. An IUD may be inserted immediately after a first-trimester abortion or miscarriage or 2 weeks after a second trimester abortion or miscarriage. It can also be inserted at any time during the menstrual cycle.

Diaphragms produce virtually no side effects but are associated with a higher rate of pregnancy (estimates range from 6-18% per year). Most physicians feel this is the result of failure of the user to conform to the requirements of diaphragm usage rather than with specific defects of the device. Diaphragms must always be used with a spermicidal jelly or cream like Ortho-Gynol, which must be reapplied every time intercourse is repeated. The diaphragm is inserted no more than 6 hours before intercourse and must stay in place at least 8 hours after intercourse has taken place. The diaphragm must be checked periodically for perforations or wear, and it should be refitted if a woman has undergone a weight change of 10 or more pounds or had a baby. During the first month of using either the IUD or the diaphragm, a backup contraceptive method such as foam and condom is advisable.

What's on the Horizon?

Researchers predict that even better types of contraception will be marketed in the U.S. within the next five to ten years. These fall into categories of:

1. Contraceptives with new synthetic progestins: norgestimate, desogestrel, and gestodene. The potency of these progestins is high, so they can be given in small doses. When combined with estrogen, they offer the advantage of not having an adverse effect on lipids (for women concerned with cardiovascular disease) or carbohydrate metabolism (for women concerned with diabetes). They also have fewer masculinizing effects like acne or facial hair growth.

2. New and different IUDs that contain more copper (the active contraceptive agent) but are smaller with fewer side effects such as bleeding or cramps. Other new IUDs, will release progesterone or progestins into the uterus, with their effectiveness lasting, in some cases, up to seven years.

3. Modified implants, similar to Norplant, but with two solid rods instead of the six capsules, will be more easily inserted under the skin.

4. The vaginal ring, a small ring, inserted into the vagina, which releases either progestin alone or estrogen and progestin in a time release fashion. Since women themselves can insert the ring, dependency on a health care professional is lowered. After 3 weeks, the ring is removed, and the woman menstruates. Subdermal implants and skin patches are being tested for future marketing. The implants will release progestin into the system slowly over a year; the skin patch will be in place for 3 weeks and off for one week to allow bleeding.

Case Study

Linda G. became sexually active in high school and when she entered college she decided to take birth control pills. Some of her friends warned that the pills had dangerous side effects and that she was doing bad things to her body by taking them. Nevertheless Linda was healthy and wanted to be completely free of worry about pregnancy The contraceptive that offered her that type of freedom was the pill. She started on Ortho Novum 1/35 without difficulty and stayed with it about 9 months. At that time she began to spot between her periods and then she missed a period. Panic-stricken, she went to the doctor but he explained to her that it was not pregnancy causing her to miss the period, but rather the effects of the birth control pills. Her friends said, "I told you so."

The doctor, however, thought that Linda's problem was that she was not using a pill with a high enough estrogen dosage. He suggested that they give a higher dosage pill a chance so Linda agreed to go with pills one more time. She began taking Ortho Novum 1/50. After 9 months she was once again established on a normal menstrual cycle with no spotting and with periods from 3 to 5 days in length. Her blood pressure was normal, but she did put on 5 pounds which may have been due to fluid retention. Linda decided that 5 extra pounds were worth the freedom from worry she enjoyed by using the pill.

Key Points for Contraceptives

1. In the 30 years since the birth control pills were marketed, we have made great progress. We now understand more about the dosages of hormones necessary to inhibit ovulation. The amounts of estrogen and progestin are about 5 times lower than they were in the early oral contraceptives. We have also determined contraindications for usage, and those medical disorders where the pill should not be used.

2. Oral contraceptives are a safe, highly effective form of birth control when used correctly by healthy women with no contraindicative medical problems. If she has no risk factors a woman may take the pill until her menopause.

3. With use of birth control pills, women are less likely to have fibrocystic breast disease, endometrial cancer, ovarian cancer, menstrual discomfort or anemia.

4. Oral contraceptives do have strong effects on both the reproductive system and on other organs of the body. Sometimes women will experience nagging symptoms, especially during the first 3 months of pill usage. If a pill does not work out after a 3-month trial a woman should visit her doctor to request a different pill or an alternative method of birth control.

5. Usually, the lower the dose of estrogen in the pill, the fewer the noticeable side effects. For practical purposes lower dose estrogen pills are just as effective as high-dose estrogen compounds.

6. The pill is risky for women with certain medical problems, such as high blood pressure, blood clots, diabetes, heart or blood vessel disease, epilepsy, liver disorders, or gallbladder problems. Smoking increases the hazards from pill usage, especially for women over age 35.

7. It is important to see your doctor regularly when you are taking the pill. You will need a routine examination after the first 9 months of pill usage and annually from then on.

8. Oral contraceptives interact with certain other drugs. Sometimes the effectiveness of the contraceptives will be reduced; at other times the effectiveness of the other drugs will be diminished when the two are taken simultaneously. Always tell the doctor who prescribes your birth control pills about any other medications you are taking.

9. The "morning after" pill is a high-dose estrogen birth control pill given for 3 to 5 days to prevent implantation of the fertilized egg. It is not to be taken routinely for birth control but is helpful in cases involving rape, incest, or possible failure of a condom, diaphragm, or IUD.

10. The newest birth control method on the American market is Norplant (6 small tubes of levonorgestrol) which are implanted in the forearm or upper arm of a woman. They are effective for five years. Occasionally Norplant causes light vaginal bleeding.

11. The alternatives to pill usage, such as a diaphragm or an IUD, should be carefully considered before the pill is discontinued. The copper-containing IUD is effective for four years.

Table 12-3

Risk of Death from Myocardial Infarction (Heart Attack) in Smoking and Non-smoking Women Using Oral Contraceptives

Age	Death rate (non-smokers)	Death rate (smokers)
25-34	1/59,000	1/10,000
35-44	1/6600	1/2100
Over 45	1/2500	1/500

Table 12-4

Contraindications and Relative Contraindications to the Use of Combination Estrogen-Progestin Oral Contraceptives

U.S. FDA-listed contraindications
  Thromboembolic disorders, present or past
  Cerebral vascular or coronary artery disease
  Carcinoma of the breast
  Estrogen-dependent neoplasm
  Undiagnosed abnormal genital bleeding
  Pregnancy
  Liver tumors, benign or malignant

Other commonly accepted contraindications
  Blood dyscrasias (leukemia, polycythemia)
  Sickle cell disease
  Active liver disease (hepatitis, porphyria, cirrhosis, history of
    cholestatic jaundice of pregnancy)
  Hypertension
  Hyperlipidimia

Relative contraindications-evaluation and close care needed
  Diabetes mellitus
  Amenorrhea (evaluate first)
  Lactation
  Migraine headache
  Mitral valve prolapse, symptomatic
  Varicose veins, severe
  Gallstones
  Recurrent monilial vaginitis

Table 12-5
Composition of Oral Contraceptives in Current Use in the United States, 1990

Trade Name*	Progestin	Estrogen
Progestin-only		
Micronor (NorQD)	NE,† 0.35 mg	None
Ovrette	*d,l*-NG,† 0.075 mg	None
Combination-monophasic		
Norlestrin	NEA,† 2.5 mg	EE, † 0.050 mg
Norlestrin -1	NEA, 1.0 mg	EE, 0.050 mg
Loestrin 1-5/30	NEA, 1.5 mg	EE, 0.030 mg
Loestrin 1/20	NEA, 1.0 mg	EE, 0.020 mg
Ovral	*d,l*-NG, 0.5 mg	EE, 0.050 mg
10/Ovral	*d,l*-NG, 0.3 mg	EE, 0.030 mg
Nordette (Levlen)	levo-NG, 0.15 mg	EE, 0.030 mg
Ortho-Novum 1/50 (Norinyl 1/50)	NE, 1.0 mg	ME, † 0.050 mg
Ovcon 50	NE 1.0 mg	EE, 0.050 mg
Ortho-Novum 1/35 (Norinyl 1/35)	NE, 1.0 mg	EE, 0.035 mg
Modicon (Brevicon)	NE, 0.5 mg	EE, 0.035 mg
Ovcon 35	NE, 0.4 mg	EE, 0.035 mg
Demulen	ED,† 1.0 mg	EE, 0.050 mg
Demulen 1/35	ED, 1.0 mg	EE, 0.035 mg
Multiphasic		
Ortho-Novum 10/11	NE, 0.5 mg, and EE, 0.35 mg (first 10 days)	
	NE 1.0 mg, and EE, 0.035 mg (next 11 days)	
Ortho-Novum 7/7/7	NE, 0.5 mg, and EE, 0.035 mg (next 7 days)	
	NE, 0.75 mg, and EE, 0.035 mg (next 7 days)	
	NE, 1.0 mg, and EE, 0.035 mg (last 7 days)	
Triphasil (Tri-Levlen)	levoNG, 0.050 mg, and EE, 0.030 mg (first 6 days)	
	levoNG, 0.075 mg, and EE, 0.040 mg (next 5 days)	
	levoNG, 0.125 mg, and EE, 0.030 mg (last 10 days)	
Tri-Norinyl	NE, 0.5 mg, and EE, 0.035 mg (first 7 days)	
	NE, 1.0 mg, and EE, 0.035 mg (next 9 days)	
	NE, 0.5 mg, and EE 0.035 mg (next 5 days)	

*Trade names are used for ease of identification. A second, identical formulation by a different manufacturer is identified in parentheses.

†EE = ethinyl estradiol; ME = mestranol; NE = norethindrone; NEA= norethindrone acetate;

ED = ethynodiol diacetate; D,L-NG = *d.l*-norgestrel; levo-NG = levonorgestrel.

Table 12-6

Different Types of Oral Contraceptives and Their Potential Advantages and Disadvantages

Formulation	Advantages	Disadvantages
Monophasic	Ease of patient usage (only one "active" pill formulation per pack)	Higher total hormonal content than other pill formulations
Biphasic	Less total hormonal content than monophasic pills More closely mimics hormonal changes in normal menstrual cycle	Greater incidence of midcycle breakthrough bleeding
Triphasic	Significantly less hormone content than monophasic pills (25-39% less). Comparable breakthrough bleeding rate to monophasics	Up to four different doses are taken per cycle. May be difficult to determine where woman is in cycle should problem occur.
Progestin-only	Estrogen-related side effects or complications such as nausea, headache, hypertension may be avoided.	Less predictable menstrual patterns. Irregular bleeding problems. Reduced effectiveness.

Table 12-7

Summary of Drug Interactions With Oral contraceptives*

Drugs that interfere with oral contraceptive effectiveness

Drugs that reduce effectiveness
  Anticonvulsants
    Phenytoin, phenobarbital, methylphenobarbital,
    primidone, carbamazepine, ethosuximide
  Antibiotics
    Rifampin (proven)
    Ampicillin, tetracycline, other broad-spectrum antibiotics (possibly)
    Griseofulvin (possibly)

Oral contraceptives increase plasma levels of the following drugs:
  Benzodiazepines
  Theophylline and caffeine
  Cyclosporine
  Metaprolol
  Phenazone
  Prednisolone
  Alcohol (possibly)

Oral contraceptives decrease plasma levels of the following drugs:
  Aspirin
  Clofibric acid
  Morphine
  Pracetamol
  Temazepam

Perspectives on Obstetrics

If like Rip van Winkle, we had slept for the past 20 years (instead of practicing medicine and writing about it), it would be difficult to appreciate or understand the changes in modern-day obstetrics that have been made during this time. Obstetricians and researchers have committed themselves to identifying the causes of maternal death and succeeded. Excellent programs have been established to eliminate these causes. For example, hypertension (high blood pressure), for many years the number one cause of death in pregnant women, now rarely causes a maternal death. Research and clinical programs to identify early disease, such as diabetes, and treat it have resulted in a decline in the death of mothers. During the next decade even further strides will be made in this area.

All indicators point to place of delivery as a determinant of safe and healthy deliveries. Home deliveries now constitute less than 1% of deliveries in this country. We believe that people are convinced that even a normal, healthy pregnant woman can run into trouble during labor. About 15% of the babies whose mothers develop risks during labor will require special nursery observation and care.

Since childbirth is important for both the mother and her offspring, it is important that she talk to her doctor prior to conception. We call this *preconceptual counseling,* and its purpose is to correct the mother's health problems ahead of time, to provide the baby with the best possible environment for growth and protection in the uterus. Such health problems include control of diabetes and high blood pressure, correction of anemia, elimination of infection, especially of the cervix or vagina, checking immunity against such diseases as rubella (German measles), elimination of sexually transmitted diseases, and withdrawal from nicotine and recreational drugs. To say it simply, we work to develop the optimum environment for the growth and development of the fetus.

A major knowledge explosion has occurred in obstetrics, especially in the development of instruments which help provide a safer environment for the baby during pregnancy and during labor and delivery. The first wave of these new tools resulted from studies on the uterus and how it works. We found out how it is stimulated and how it can be stopped.

We have made progress in safe deliveries, but we have a long way to go. Preterm delivery is the greatest single problem in the world today, comprising 8%-16% of all deliveries, and a solution to it is still being sought.

The next phase of study centered around the heart rate of the baby - a difficult task, since the electrical current of the baby's heart is more than 100 times less than the mother's heart current. We developed monitoring methods with recommendations that any mother who is at risk should have electronic fetal monitoring during labor. These studies were later translated into evaluating the fetus prior to labor to assess its health.

Some of the things we came up with have been abandoned, for instance, chemical tests on the mother to try to determine fetal health. One diagnostic procedure has stood the test of time - amniocentesis. This drawing off of fluid from around the baby teaches us many things. Special importance is being able to tell if there is any infection or if the fetal lungs are mature enough for the outside world.

The obstetrician's quest to know and understand the fetus *in utero* was greatly enhanced by the development of real-time ultrasound, some 25 years ago. The tools have evolved into sophisticated instruments that make diagnoses of problems *in utero* possible as early as 6 to 10 weeks of pregnancy. It is used for detecting birth defects and to reassure the mother and the obstetrician that growth and development are on target. Once, more than 50% of multiple births came as a complete surprise at delivery. Now, thanks to modern diagnostic tools, we usually detect multiple fetuses well in advance of delivery. Ultrasound instrumentation also allows us to measure flow through blood vessels, especially of the placenta, when high risk pregnancies need special evaluation.

Many women who now have babies would never have been able to conceive 25 years ago. Reproductive technologies allowed us to produce the first "test tube" babies. Major advances have taken place in reproductive endocrinology and infertility. These have led to a better understanding of fertilization and development of the fertilized egg, how implantation takes place, and further refinement of in vitro fertilization (union of the sperm and egg outside the body). Not that such techniques have been problem free. Drugs like Pergonal and Clomid can overstimulate the ovary, resulting in multiple gestations that present new problems to the obstetrician. Even so, reproductive endocrinology has produced many happy parents who appreciate all it has done.

Consumerism has had a vital influence on scientific obstetrics. The voices of consumers have been heard, resulting in more positive delivery environments, allowing for very positive bonding of both father and mother to the baby, and more hospitable labor and delivery areas. Women now play a more active role in delivering their babies, with a resulting decrease in the need for excessive drugs during labor, expansion of relaxation and self-help techniques, and the increase of epidural anesthesia.

Cesarean section rates have risen from 10% to 20% of all deliveries, as our assessment of the indications for cesarean section have changed. The focus of attention continues to be on the mother and fetus, but new attention is now paid to the fetus and newborn.

We now have the ability to diagnose Down's syndrome and other chromosomal abnormalities by *chorionic villi sampling*, done at 9 to 11 weeks of gestation. The cells are grown in tissue culture and results become available from 1 to 3 weeks after the procedure. Certain tests can be done on the parents to determine the transmission of specific diseases and permit genetic counseling prior to or after conception.

Before the newborn baby goes home, tests are done to assure the newborn's health, such as bilirubin levels for jaundice; tests for phenylketonuria, hypothyroidism, bleeding tendencies, and major birth defects. The mother, after the first week of the baby's life when the tests are done, can leave reassured that her baby is off to a healthy start.

Finally, in the rare but still possible event that the baby or mother is ill or has a serious defect, a large number of new drugs have come on the market, which can treat these problems very effectively. *The Women's Health & Drug Reference* details those drugs, their applications, and their limitations for all those interested in the latest information on drug therapy. Scientific obstetrics is a balance of assets with a few liabilities.

The development of neonatal intensive care units (NICU) during the past 25 years has allowed smaller and smaller newborns to survive, some of whom will never be completely

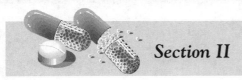

normal. Seventy-five percent of all newborn problems are seen in those who weighed less than two pounds in a preterm delivery. Thankfully, 90% of these babies are perfectly normal, but how can obstetricians tell who they will be and prevent the 10% who are not normal?

A major liability is an escalation in health care costs. Does everyone need state-of-the-art sophistication in care and testing? The answer is a resounding, NO! Which patients and which obstetricians vote to omit this sophistication in their care and testing? The answer is, we can't tell, because it is impossible to identify everyone who does or does not need it. Hence, in spite of the objections of the insurance industry, we will continue to overtest and overmonitor the fetus and its mother, to assure a positive birth outcome.

Another major issue of the last decade has been malpractice, which has led to further escalation of health care costs. Many obstetricians retire long before they used to, often by the time they reach age 50 because of the emotional trauma of lurking malpractice suits. The anxiety caused by this process is truly overwhelming, since a lawsuit may be initiated against the obstetrician or the estate as long as 20 years after the event in question took place. Major reform is needed in this area to help reduce the escalation of health care costs.

It is a privilege to be part of these advances in health care delivery. Things have improved greatly and the consumer is part of these advances, from laboratory to bedside. In writing this book, we show our continued support for educated consumers and the valuable contribution they make to health care advances.

Notes

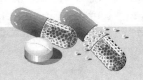

Chapter 13

Preparing for Pregnancy

More and more women are learning (or relearning their grandmothers would probably say) the value of an ounce of prevention when it comes to health matters. Nowhere is this more relevant than during pregnancy. Prenatal care is one of the best examples of preventive medicine. One of the best ways to do this is through preconception counseling.

Preconception Counseling

Preconception counseling starts with a visit to the gynecologist, scheduled before a woman takes any steps to become pregnant. When this visit is arranged, she should ask for some extra time to discuss plans for pregnancy. This will be her preconception counseling session. To prepare for that interview a women must gather any information the doctor may need about her health history, especially if she ever had any problems.

Important details include whether or not she has conceived in the past and the outcome of that pregnancy, that is, a birth, a miscarriage, an abortion. The doctor will want to know how she felt during that pregnancy and if anything abnormal happened.

If she suffers from a chronic disease such as hypertension, epilepsy, or diabetes, she should remember to bring a medical history from her regular doctor or the specialist who cares for her and, especially important, a list of medications taken. If there is a hereditary disease in her family, for example, sickle cell anemia, muscular dystrophy, Tay-Sachs syndrome, or cystic fibrosis, she should plan to discuss with the doctor if and how this could affect her child.

Also important are any sexually transmitted diseases she has had or been exposed to, such as chlamydia, herpes, gonorrhea, or AIDS. If she or her sexual partner are at risk from any of these problems, it is necessary to inform the doctor so that appropriate preconception testing can be undertaken.

If she smokes, drinks alcohol, uses drugs, drinks coffee, or works in a place with environmental hazards, such as a plant, a farm, or a hospital, she should be sure to mention these to the doctor. It is in her own best interest and that of her future child to be completely honest with her physician. The doctor is there to help her carry out a successful pregnancy and can only do so if given accurate and detailed information.

Women with nutritional deficiencies may need dietary and adjustments to help them prior to pregnancy. Supplements like folic acid may be advisable before conception, especially for women who have had a previous child with spina bifida or a neural tube defect or for women taking anti-seizure medications like Dilantin.

Finally, physicians are starting to consider factors that affect the health of the male as well as the female partner in a pregnancy. Recent studies have linked the use of tobacco, street drugs (cocaine in particular), alcohol, and toxins in the workplace to sperm damage, birth defects, and a variety of childhood diseases. Some studies have indicated that lack of adequate Vitamin C in the diet results in abnormal sperm. Reproductive health has become a two-way street, and men, too should consider lifestyle changes several months prior to conception if they want to maximize their chances of creating a healthy baby.

People who are trying to give up smoking should be aware of a new smoking cessation tool that reached the market in 1992. Manufactured under names such as Nicoderm and Habitrol, it is comprised of a skin patch that delivers nicotine to the system in timed released doses, thus relieving nicotine craving while the individual works to overcome other aspects of her dependency on cigarettes. The nicotine skin patch is meant to be used with a comprehensive smoking cessation program that includes behavior modification and motivational techniques. If possible, smoking cessation programs and use of aids like Habitrol should occur before conception, but stopping smoking is always advisable no matter when you start. Women should talk to their doctors about smoking cessation methods, especially if they are already pregnant. Patches for smoking cessation are not recommended for use during pregnancy by the manufacturer.

After the doctor has assessed a woman's medical history to decide if there are any apparent risks to a pregnancy, he or she will want to do a physical examination and take some tests. Table 13-1 shows a number of problems that can be identified during preconception counseling and what can be done to alleviate them before a baby is actually on the way.

Preconception counseling also allows women to take a realistic look at what pregnancy may be like for them so that they can prepare psychologically as well as medically for the big event, should it be undertaken. We encourage all women who wish to become pregnant to use preconception counseling as an important first step to insuring a healthy pregnancy.

Immunization Before and During Pregnancy

In addition to tests and an examination, the doctor may want to bring a woman's immunizations up to date. The preconception period is an ideal time to handle immunization because giving shots that protect against diseases to pregnant women is not always advisable. In North America, women of childbearing age should be routinely vaccinated against measles, mumps, rubella (German measles), polio, diphtheria, and tetanus. Some women may need additional immunizations if they have special risk factors. Table 13-2 lists the diseases women need to be vaccinated against and the advisability of being vaccinated prior to becoming pregnant.

Some vaccines - also known as immunobiologic agents - could have an effect on the fetus because they contain live, attenuated (greatly weakened) viruses or bacteria. Others contain killed biological agents that do not pose any threat that we know of to a fetus. Still others, called immune globulins, are proteins taken from the blood of people who have already been immunized. These proteins, when injected into another person, offer short-term immunity to particular diseases. Immune globulins are safely given during pregnancy and are often used as a temporary replacement for vaccinations. Immune globulins are taken from human blood, but because of the special processing they undergo, we consider them to be very safe and free from viruses such as hepatitis or AIDS.

Once again, it is important that the doctor get complete information about lifestyle, work, places travelled to, and diseases to which which a woman may have been exposed so that he or she can decide if immunizations are needed either before or during pregnancy.

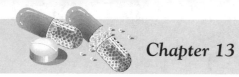
Table 13-1
Problems Identified During Preconception Counseling

Problem	What May Be Identified and Prevented
Lack of immunity to rubella (German measles)	Outbreak of a disease that is dangerous to the fetus. Rubella vaccination given 3 months prior to conception. (A preconception blood test can confirm whether or not you have immunity to rubella).
Previous miscarriage	Malformations of the uterus, possibly caused by hormones ("DES") given to woman's mother.
Previous premature labor	Defects of the uterus or infections of the cervix or vagina.
Hypertension (high blood pressure)	Presence of hypertension and condition of kidneys, eyes, and heart. Best drugs to control hypertension during pregnancy chosen. Woman taught to monitor her own blood pressure.
Chronic kidney disease	Serum creatinine tested to see if favorable pregnancy outcome is likely. Check for infection, lupus, and other side effects of chronic kidney disease so these may be treated.
Organ transplant	Women with liver transplants who are without symptoms for 18 months may be able to undertake pregnancy successfully. Women with kidney transplants must be watched very closely because of their high incidence of preeclampsia. At this time we do not have enough experience with heart and lung transplants to make recommendations.
Diabetes mellitus	Evaluation of insulin dosage. Woman taught to monitor her own blood sugar. Hemoglobin A1C test evaluates likelihood of favorable pregnancy outcome. Eyes and kidneys evaluated for effects of diabetes.
Nutritional deficiencies; Weight problems	Anemias, underweight, overweight, identified and try to correct before pregnancy occurs. Prenatal vitamins may be needed in some cases.

Table 13-1 (continued)

Hereditary diseases	Blood tests, chromosome tests to identify, especially if woman comes from high-risk background. Genetic counseling offered to assess chances of a successful pregnancy.
Age over 35 years	Undergo counseling to understand statistical risk of problems. Explain various tests (amniocentesis, chorionic villi sampling) woman should take during pregnancy.
Substance abuse	Dangers of various substances to fetus explained. Chemical dependency treatment undertaken prior to conception.
Sexually transmitted diseases and other infections	Many of these can be treated with drugs and cured prior to conception. Others, such as HIV infection (AIDS) and hepatitis B pose strong dangers to the fetus and mother during pregnancy and pregnancy may not be appropriate. This is particularly true with AIDS.

Table 13-2

Immunization Before or During Pregnancy

Disease	When to vaccinate?	Risk of disease to mother or fetus
Measles	Prior to pregnancy	Significant illness for mother; can cause miscarriage, malformation in fetus
Mumps	Prior to pregnancy	Increased risk of early miscarriage
Polio	Prior to pregnancy unless actually exposed	Increased risk of fetus getting disease with 50% mortality; disease may be more severe during pregnancy for mother
Rubella	Prior to pregnancy	High rate of miscarriage and problems

Table 13-2 (continued)		
Influenza	Prior to or during pregnancy, if mother is at risk	May be serious for mother; may increase miscarriage rate
Rabies	Prior to or during pregnancy, but only if exposed	Nearly 100% fatal
Hepatitis B	Prior to or during pregnancy, if mother is at risk	May be more severe during pregnancy; may increase miscarriage and premature delivery; newborn may be a carrier
Pneumococcus	Prior to or during pregnancy, depending on risk to mother	Mothers at high risk may be very ill
Tetanus-diphtheria	Prior to or during pregnancy, if mother has not had boosters on schedule or not had original series	Severe illness for mother w/30% chance of death from tetanus 10% death from diphtheria; 60% death from tetanus for newborns

Immunization data provided courtesy of American College of Obstetrics and Gynecology (ACOG)

Case Study

Carrie J and her husband had been married for a year and wanted a child very much, but both had concerns about their previous health history, so they scheduled a counseling session with Carrie's gynecologist.

Carrie, 25, was about 20 pounds overweight. She smoked a pack of cigarettes daily, had several coffees and cokes each day, and occasionally smoked marijuana at parties. She also had mild high blood pressure (145/95). Her husband smoked as well, and, prior to their marriage, had been sexually active with several partners. Both Carrie and her husband were completely honest with the doctor about their habits and medical history. First the doctor tested both of them for sexually transmitted diseases, including AIDS. The tests revealed that they both carried the infectious chlamydia organism. The doctor put them on a 15 day course of tetracycline, which eradicated the infection. Next he gave Cathy a complete physical and explained the risks of high blood pressure during pregnancy. While he did not prescribe medication at that time, he told Carrie that she might have to take anti-hypertensive medication during pregnancy. He also warned her that she might have to rest in bed a great deal towards the end of her pregnancy.

The couple was strongly encouraged to quit smoking, and they enrolled in a smoke-stoppers clinic at the hospital. They also decided to stop using recreational drugs. Carrie cut back on caffeine-containing beverages, by choosing decaffeinated colas, coffees, and teas. After two months, the couple felt healthier, and much more comfortable with starting a pregnancy.

Key Points for Preconceptual Counseling

1. Preconceptual counseling is recommended for all couples contemplating pregnancy. Many problems can be cleared up or avoided by seeing a doctor before getting pregnant.

2. Records of a woman's previous health history and medication schedule should be brought to the preconceptual counseling session.

3. A woman should be completely open with her physician about any problems or habits she has that might impact on a pregnancy. He or she is there to help her do everything possible to bring a healthy child into the world.

4. Necessary immunizations are best given before a woman gets pregnant. Along with her medical history, she should bring a record of previous immunizations to her preconception counseling sessions.

Chapter 14

Fertility Drugs

Some couples cannot conceive a child no matter how hard they try. *Infertility* affects from 10-15% of all couples who want to become parents. More commonly, these men and women are in their mid-thirties or older and have put off childbearing for several years. While worrying about unwanted pregnancies - and having them - is certainly no fun, the pain of wanting a child and being unable to conceive may go even deeper. Besides the frustration of failure with many and different means, repeated unsuccessful attempts to achieve a pregnancy can put emotional, sexual, and financial strain on couples.

Happily, research and scientific work within the past 20 years, especially in the past five years, have made great strides in reversing infertility. This is particularly true with respect to inducing ovulation. We estimate that, through various means, almost half of all infertile couples can create a pregnancy, and the majority of these will result in a healthy, normal infant.

New technologies now allow fertilization of an egg to occur outside the uterus, with the fertilized egg implanted either back into the biological mother or a surrogate mother (a woman not biologically related to the child who lets the embryo develop inside her body and who gives birth to it).

Causes of Infertility

The medical definition of infertility is the inability to conceive after a year of frequent intercourse without using contraceptive protection of any sort. If a couple continues for this length of time without a pregnancy occurring, they may wish to consult an obstetrician-gynecologist who specializes in infertility problems.

It is very important that both the man and the woman be part of the solution to reversing infertility. Regardless of the source of the problem, both partners will have to cooperate closely with the physician when the diagnostic tests are performed and when the actual program for conception begins.

Only half of the infertility cases brought to the attention of physicians are related exclusively to the woman's reproductive system; at least 40% are due to problems with the man's reproductive system, and about 10% are due either to a combined problem or to causes that simply cannot be determined. Of the 50% that represents the female proportion of infertility, about 5% concern a problem with cervical mucus; about 60% are due to an obstruction of the fallopian tubes or a problem with the ovaries, the cervix or the uterus; and about 35% are due to lack of ovulation (egg production).

Cervical mucus problems may be treated with antibiotics if there is an infection or with estrogen if the mucus is too thick. Surgery will sometimes help a blocked fallopian tube, but often the infertility continues after the unblocking because related problems still exist. There are procedures available to help with problems such as a cervix that is not tight enough to hold a developing fetus. If conception takes place, the cervix can be tightened with stitches for the duration of the pregnancy, a technique called *cerclage*. Problems such as endometriosis can be treated by laser surgery or hormone-suppressing drugs *(See Chapter 3)*.

The most common cause of infertility in men, and one that is easily correctable, is a condition called a *varicocele,* an enlarged vein in the spermatic cord leading from the testicle, much like the varicose veins people have in their legs. Pressure from the swollen vein blocks sperm passage and also elevates the temperature in the region, which has a negative effect on sperm production. One study established that these varicoceles were the cause of about 40% of all male infertility. Varicoceles can be corrected by a simple, surgical procedure that is sometimes done on an outpatient basis. The doctor simply ties off the enlarged vein and reroutes the blood through another vessel. Depending on how low the sperm counts were before operation, the operation is from 30% to 70% effective. Hormone supplements following the operation can improve these statistics greatly.

Good progress is being made currently on the other causes of male infertility, such as glandular disorders and congenital defects of the reproductive organs. New research is beginning to point to tobacco, crack cocaine, and alcohol use as possible contributors to a low sperm count in men and to formation of defective sperm. Most substances concentrate in the seminal vesicles and this can affect the movement of sperm.

Pregnancy Loss

Pregnancy loss, often called miscarriage or spontaneous abortion, especially if repeated, may result from hormonal imbalances in the mother, such as a luteal phase defect, the lack of progesterone secreted by the organ that forms after the egg is released, the corpus luteum . Repeated pregnancy loss may also result from physical defects such as a loose cervix. Such problems can be treated by a gynecologist specializing in infertility.

However, there are other causes of miscarriage, as well, including incompatibility between the mother's and father's immune systems or injury. Very often, we simply don't know why a miscarriage occurs. While a pregnancy loss, especially in the later months can be a sad and difficult experience, after many years of trying to prevent them, physicians have come to realize that neither drugs nor bedrest will stop a miscarriage that is destined to happen. A miscarriage is Nature's way of correcting a problem pregnancy that never would have resulted in a healthy child.

Treatment for the mother following miscarriage varies, depending upon when in the pregnancy the miscarriage occurred:

One to eight weeks: Often, little or no treatment will be needed for these very early miscarriages, but if bleeding is heavy or if it continues for more than a few days, 0.2 mg of ergotrate or Methergine can be prescribed. These drugs cause the uterus and the blood vessels to contract and thus stop the flow of blood.

Eight to 14 weeks: Spontaneous abortion during this phase of pregnancy will leave a membrane attached to the inside of the uterus called Nitabuch's layer. This layer must be removed with a D&C (dilation & curettage), a gentle scraping of the inside of the uterus. Either ergotrate or Methergine may be given in conjunction with the D&C.

More than 14 weeks: Treatment of a woman experiencing pregnancy loss at this phase would be similar to that given after a birth. Pitocin, a strong uterine-contracting drug, might be given within the first couple of hours of delivery. Ergotrate or methergine might be given following that for heavy bleeding, if needed.

What Happens at the First Infertility Appointment

Much of a couple's first visit to a gynecologist who specializes in infertility will involve a discussion session with questions on many aspects of the couple's lives. The doctor will need to know both medical histories, including any problems with their reproductive systems, their occupations, sports and recreational activities, and their sexual habits and techniques. The physcian will attempt to explain the various causes of infertility and to dispel any fears and misinformation the couple may have. The doctor will then schedule a complete physical examination for both the man and the woman. After that a series of tests will be given to determine the cause of infertility.

Testing

The major tests given at the beginning of the infertility consultation are described below. After the tests have been completed, the doctor will make recommendations on the treatment of the infertility problem. These recommendations may include a surgical procedure for either the man or the woman, medical treatment for the woman, a change of certain sexual or other habits, or a fertility drug if it is clear that no egg is being produced.

Semen analysis. The man will have to provide a fresh semen specimen so that the sperm can be counted, their structure and movement analyzed, and the volume of the ejaculate (material containing the sperm) measured. A normal sperm count is more than 40 million sperm per cubic centimeter. Fertility can usually be attained with counts as low as 20 million sperm per cubic centimeter. The motility of sperm, that is, their activeness and ability to swim, is also a key to successful conception.

Determination of egg production. The woman's basal body temperature will have to be measured several times during the monthly menstrual cycle. At the time of egg production, the temperature goes up 0.5 to 1 degree. Ovulation usually occurs just prior to this temperature rise, and at this point production of an egg can be verified. A window of about 24 hours exists for the egg to be fertilized. Sperm, on the other hand, have a longer life and can sustain fertility for at least 48 hours.

X-ray examination of uterus and fallopian tubes. A special x-ray examination, called a hysterosalpingogram, will be made. This consists of inserting radiopaque dye into the uterus through the cervix. Using the x-ray apparatus the doctor will watch the dye, checking primarily to see if there are any deformities of the uterine cavity and if the dye passes through the fallopian tubes and spills out. If it does not, fallopian tube blockage is indicated, and measures must be taken before a pregnancy will occur. The chance of conception usually increases during the first 4-6 months after the hysterosalpingogram. This is because the test itself may open up the tubes by breaking up tiny scar tissue fibers.

Postcoital cervical mucus test. This test must be performed around the time of ovulation, which usually occurs two weeks before the onset of menstruation. The couple will be asked to have intercourse 2 to 4 hours before the test is made. The doctor will then examine the mucus that surrounds the cervix. Normal cervical mucus at the time of ovulation should be stringy, thin, and clear (a phenomenon known as *spinnbarkheit* mucus). Under a microscope the action of the sperm and their number in the mucus are examined.

Drugs That Stimulate Egg Production

The most popular fertility drugs are clomiphene citrate (Clomid), human menopausal gonadotropin (Pergonal), gonadotropin-releasing hormone (GnRH, Factrel), and bromocriptine (Parlodel). Since each of these drugs acts in a different way, we shall discuss them separately.

Clomid

Ovulation can be induced with Clomid in more than 80% of women who don't ovulate, but who still have normal estrogen levels. Of these, the pregnancy rate is between 50-80%. Clomid acts on two important brain centers - the pituitary gland and the hypothalamus - to stimulate production of the hormones that cause ovulation. Clomid counteracts the production of estrogen and thus induces the hypothalamus to produce luteinizing hormone and follicle-stimulating hormone. These are the hormones that actually cause the egg to ripen and be released. If the lack of egg release is caused by severe pituitary gland or hypothalamus dysfunction, Clomid will probably not work.

Dosage schedule. In the Clomid treatment cycle, 5 days after the start of menstruation (which is often artificially induced) the woman receives 50 mg of Clomid in tablet form daily for 5 days. When she stops the Clomid, ovulation should occur from 5 to 11 days later. Ovulation must be monitored closely, and intercourse will have to be carefully timed to correspond with its occurrence. If the Clomid cycle does not work, the daily dosage can be increased 50 mg each time it is tried (up to 250 mg per day). The treatment is sometimes lengthened two more days. However, both prolonged treatment and higher dosages can result in overstimulation of the ovary and the production of more than one egg.

Usually, fertilization will take place within the first three ovulation cycles. If it has not occurred after three to six treatment cycles with Clomid, retesting for other problems must begin. Sperm counts, fallopian tube opening, conditions of the uterus, and quality of the cervical mucus should all be examined. If, after six more cycles, pregnancy has not yet occurred, the likelihood of it happening, at least by using Clomid, is small, and there is no point in continuing the drug.

At this point the doctor might consider laparoscopy (looking into the pelvis with a special telescope mounted on a long, thin, flexible tube). During this procedure, which will require hospitalization and a general anesthetic, a blue dye is injected into the fallopian tubes to verify that they are open. The doctor will also check to see if there are signs of endometriosis or some other fallopian tube disease.

Adverse effects. The most highly publicized problem with fertility drugs is multiple births, a real concern, but not as great a one as it used to be. Sometimes the media give the impression that taking fertility pills guarantees quintuplets. However, the incidence of women taking Clomid and producing more than two children is less than 1%. The incidence of twins is 4-9%, almost all of these being fraternal (nonidentical) twins. Multiple births result from excessive stimulation (hyperstimulation) of the ovaries. Hyperstimulation of the ovaries can also lead to temporary ovarian enlargement. Ovarian enlargement probably occurs in fewer than 10% of women taking Clomid, although some studies have reported this figure to be as high as 19%. When ovarian enlargement does occur, Clomid treatments should be suspended until the problem can be resolved.

The other major problem for women taking fertility drugs is the increased rate of spontaneous abortion, that is, miscarriage. For women who have taken Clomid, the rate of miscarriage is 20%, whereas in normal conceptions it is 10-12%. While miscarriage can be a harsh blow, once it has been established that a woman can conceive using Clomid, she should try again, if her physician sees no contraindications to her making another attempt. Remember, the odds are 80% in your favor!

The number of birth defects reported for women who take Clomid is no higher than those found in women who were treated for infertility in other ways. A slightly higher incidence of birth defects has been reported when women accidentally took Clomid after becoming pregnant (5.1% versus 2% to 4% in the normal population).

Pergonal

Whereas Clomid stimulates the production of the hormones necessary to induce ovulation, Pergonal actually replaces them with hormones called gonadotropins extracted from human menopausal urine. Use of Pergonal is indicated when treatment with Clomid has not worked, probably because the pituitary gland or other structures that stimulate the ovary are functioning poorly. In some places, especially outside the United States, treatment regimens combining Clomid and Pergonal have become popular.

Pergonal is composed of two hormones crucial to ovulation (luteinizing hormone and follicle-stimulating hormone). Although the idea of merely supplying the needed hormones seems simpler than trying to make the body produce them, it is actually more difficult. Pergonal is more expensive than Clomid, it must be given by needle injections, it requires close laboratory monitoring by the doctor, and it has more severe side effects. Therefore we recommend that Pergonal be used only after Clomid or other appropriate measures have failed to solve the infertility problem. Pergonal treatment is usually administered only by infertility specialists.

Dosage schedule. In a typical Pergonal treatment cycle the woman receives a daily injection of Pergonal for 3 or 4 days. At the same time, she must keep a daily temperature chart, her cervical mucus and ovaries must be examined daily, and she must have a daily blood test to determine estrogen levels. If the estrogen in her blood serum goes up, the same dosage of Pergonal should be continued. If it does not, the dosage should be increased for 9 more days. Twenty-four to 96 hours after the estrogen has reached a satisfactory level, an injection of another hormone, HCG (human chorionic gonadotropin), is given to maintain conception if it has taken place. If the estrogen levels have gone too high, the doctor will withhold the HCG shot, since high estrogen levels may indicate multiple egg production or ovarian enlargement. Four to 8 days later this hormone is reinjected to support the pregnancy if it has occurred. The incidence of pregnancy using this method is about 50%.

Adverse effects. Multiple births average about 25% when this method of conquering fertility is used. Most of these will be no more than twins if the physician has been very cautious in monitoring the estrogen levels during the treatment cycle.

Ovarian hyperstimulation does occur in this program, but again careful monitoring of estrogen levels and withholding the HCG injection if estrogen is too high should help to prevent the problem. A woman may have to be hospitalized if ovarian hyperstimulation occurs because she may have symptoms of abdominal discomfort, dehydration, and abnormal blood clotting. In rare cases surgery will be necessary, for example, if an ectopic pregnancy (pregnancy outside the uterus) has occurred or the ovary is bleeding.

Miscarriage rates using Pergonal range from 20% to 25%; a significant portion of these miscarriages are two or more conceptions.

Gonadotropin-releasing Hormone

One of the newest methods for treating infertility is the use of gonadotropin-releasing hormone (GnRH) to induce ovulation. This substance is normally secreted by the pituitary gland after stimulation from a portion of the brain called the hypothalamus, and it will act on the ovaries to produce eggs.

The secret to success with GnRH is a technique called *pulsatile administration.* The drug must be given intravenously or subcutaneously (a needle injection just under the skin) by a portable, battery operated machine that pumps it into the bloodstream in closely timed cycles of 60, 90, or 120 minutes. This action mimics the normal pituitary GnRH-release, which also occurs over a 60-120 minute cycle. A woman does not necessarily have to be hospitalized during this treatment because the pump is small and portable and can be carried in a case attached to a belt. The doctor will check estrogen levels in the bloodstream approximately every 3 days. When they are high enough or the ovaries are ready to produce an egg, he will administer a shot of HCG, the same as is done with Pergonal. Alternatives to that are progesterone suppositories or continuation of the pulsatile GnRH pump until pregnancy is confirmed.

Adverse reactions. We have less information about the results of this form of infertility therapy because it has been in use for a shorter time than Pergonal and Clomid. Some mild ovarian hyperstimulation has occurred, and some multiple births have occurred, although the incidence seems to be lower than that when Pergonal is used.

We feel this is a promising new method of combating infertility, especially for women with amenorrhea (lack of menstruation) caused by pituitary insufficiencies.

Bromocriptine

In a few cases of infertility the lack of ovulation is associated with the body's excessive production of prolactin, the hormone that stimulates the production of breast milk. Nursing mothers have high blood prolactin levels and are usually less fertile than women who are not breast-feeding. In fact, many women never ovulate while they are nursing. Perhaps this is nature's way of helping women to space the births of their children. (But, never count on breast-feeding to provide reliable birth control. Many women do ovulate and get pregnant while nursing).

For some unknown reason, the mechanism of prolactin production occasionally goes awry, and, even though no baby has been born, the body produces prolactin. The cause of the excessive prolactin production must be sought before bromocriptine is prescribed because tumors of the pituitary gland may be responsible. Since these tumors sometimes grow very rapidly during pregnancy, inducing conception may be dangerous when they are present.

Bromocriptine, a drug that suppresses lactation is taken in tablet form. We advise that you swallow it at bedtime because it may lower the blood pressure. The drug is taken every day for 5 weeks; if, at the end of 4 weeks, pregnancy has not resulted, the dosage is increased. Once again, ovulation must be monitored by temperature charts and, if it is thought to occur, the drug should be stopped until menstruation begins.

The conception rate with bromocriptine used under these circumstances is at least 60%, and the number of miscarriages and birth defects associated with the use of this drug is thought to be the same as in women who have conceived normally. When bromocriptine is first begun, women often experience nausea, headaches, high blood pressure (as well as an initial episode of low blood pressure), dizziness, and vomiting. However, these symptoms seem to clear up with dosage adjustments and time.

Test Tube Babies

Test tube babies - babies produced by in vitro fertilization - have fascinated the public. The first "test tube baby," a girl born on July 25, 1978, in England, now has thousands of counterparts that have been conceived in many other parts of the world.

How is a test tube baby created? The mother receives a drug like Clomid or Pergonal to make her produce eggs and preferably more than one egg at a predictable time. At just the right moment, a long needle is inserted through the vagina to the ovary where the eggs are suctioned out under ultrasound guidance. Next, the eggs are incubated in a warm, moist chamber with a known concentration of carbon dioxide, like the interior of the human body, for 6 to 8 hours. The father then contributes some of his sperm, and the eggs and sperm are mixed carefully in a clear plastic dish.

For the next two days the doctors observe the contents of the dish, and when a four- to six-cell conception has been achieved, it is removed and inserted through the vagina into the mother's womb. If more than one conception has occurred, up to 3 embryos are inserted, and the rest are kept as frozen embryos.

The most difficult hurdle comes next - that is, actual implantation in the wall of the uterus. As in nature, only about one in every four conceptions will successfully implant and go on to develop into a baby.

Chances are high that the entire process will have to be repeated, which is not only discouraging but also expensive, as much as $5000 to $6000 per attempt. Nevertheless, many couples go on to try again because the accomplishment of a pregnancy is the uppermost priority in their lives.

Another procedure called gamete intrafollicular transfer (GIFT) was first done successfully in 1984. This technique requires at least one normal fallopian tube. The procedure is similar to in vitro fertilization with respect to ovulation induction and retrieval of eggs, either with a laparoscope or under ultrasound monitoring. No more than 2 eggs are mixed with sperm in a tube and this mixture is transferred to each fallopian tube, where fertilization may occur. The ectopic pregnancy rate is reported to be 3-8% with GIFT conceptions. Recent figures report that GIFT pregnancy rates of 27% compare favorably with the 27% pregnancy rate achieved with transfer of embryos fertilized in the laboratory (a procedure known as ZIFT or zygote intrafallopian tube transfer) and 19% for in vitro fertilization and embryo transfer. GIFT is less costly because there is no laboratory culture or delicate early embryos to deal with.

Case Study

Brian and Cindy H. had been married for 5 years, and during that time they had developed successful careers as a metallurgical engineer and an accountant. Cindy was nearing 40 when she and Brian decided to start a family. After over a year of regular, unprotected sexual activity and no sign of pregnancy, Cindy consulted her gynecologist, who examined both Brian and Cindy. They were in good physical condition, with no obvious anatomical defects. Brian's sperm count was a healthy 60 million per milliliter and his sperm were vigorous and active.

Cindy then began to take her temperature daily for a month. A clue appeared when her temperature never fluctuated more than two tenths of a degree, even when she should have been ovulating. After obtaining the same temperature pattern for 3 consecutive months, Cindy's doctor decided that she was not ovulating.

He prescribed Clomid, which she began to take each day, from day 5 to 10, following her menstrual period. At the same time she and Brian were told to plan intercourse for every other night from the 14th to the 18th day of Cindy's menstrual cycle.

Three months went by and Cindy had still not become pregnant. The couple felt slightly discouraged and unhappy about scheduling their sex life so tightly while using the fertility drug. Cindy's doctor told them to try one more month of Clomid, and if nothing happened he would prescribe another drug. At the end of the fourth month Cindy's menstrual period did not appear and she noticed some breast tenderness. A sensitive blood test showed up positive for pregnancy. Her doctor examined her by ultrasound 3 weeks later. The ultrasound image depicted a gestational sac and fetus about 8 weeks size.

After an uncomplicated prenatal course, Cindi went into labor near her estimated due date. Because the baby was in a breech position, the doctors decided to perform a cesarean. At that time they noted that Cindi's uterus, ovaries, and fallopian tubes appeared to be perfectly normal. She gave birth to a tiny but healthy 5-pound 8-ounce girl to the delight of her husband and the new grandparents.

Key Points for Infertility

1. Infertility is a concern for about 10% of couples who wish to be parents. In roughly half of them, infertility is due to a defect or deficiency of the female reproductive system, 40% are due to a male reproductive problem, and the remainder either a combination of the two or unknown.

2. Overcoming infertility takes a strong commitment to doing exactly what is necessary in the treatment cycle. Both partners must be committed to treatment plan, regardless of the source of the problem.

3. A careful history and physical examination of both the man and the woman must be obtained and a special regimen of tests conducted before a doctor can consider treating the infertility problem.

4. Clomid and Pergonal are the two major drugs used to treat infertility caused by the lack of egg production occurring in approximately one third of women found to be infertile. Clomid is less expensive and has fewer side effects, so it is the first choice when the treatment cycle begins.

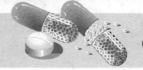

5. In special cases where lack of egg production is caused by excessive prolactin production, the drug bromocriptine has proved to be quite effective.

6. Very careful surveillance by both the patient and doctor are necessary to determine when ovulation occurs. The use of fertility drugs requires strict timing and patience if treatment fails.

7. The risk of miscarriage or multiple births with the use of fertility drugs is lower than it used to be but still higher than for normally conceived pregnancies.

8. Laparoscopy, viewing the pelvic contents with a medical telescope inserted just below the navel, is an important tool in the diagnosis and treatment of infertility.

9. If 3-month to 1-year trial of these medications is unsuccessful, reevaluation for other causes of infertility is indicated. This may required diagnostic surgery. Ultimately, couples may have to consider adoption or a similar alternative, if fertility cannot be induced by any means.

Notes

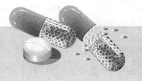

Vitamins, Diet Supplements, and Nausea Control During Pregnancy

The informed and aware pregnant woman knows the importance of eating well during those very special 9 months. Some will find food even more attractive than when they weren't pregnant, with fantasies zeroed in on ice cream sundaes or pizza. Others develop bizarre eating habits and cravings. Still others, an unfortunate but substantial minority of prospective moms, find that food isn't appealing at all. Each meal is force-fed because they know that the baby needs the nutrition that only its mother can supply.

Diet and Nutrition

Every obstetrician emphasizes a good diet during pregnancy. Whatever the mother's cravings, her menu must contain plenty of protein-rich foods, such as meat, fish, eggs, dairy products, nuts, tofu, or beans. She should consume a variety of fresh fruits and vegetables, and she needs whole grains and fiber from wheat, oats, rice or corn which can be found in breads, cereals, pancakes and other grain-product foods.

Pregnancy is not the time for a reducing diet, even when a woman is not at her ideal weight. Overweight pregnant women should not fall below their beginning weight at the time of conception and may even safely gain up to 30 pounds. We prefer to see all of our pregnant patients gain at least 25 pounds. Weight loss programs can be undertaken after the baby is born. Medications which cause the body to lose fluids should be avoided, as well. Salt intake does not need to be restricted during pregnancy, unless a woman has hypertension.

All pregnant women should avoid the well-known "junk" foods, like diet pop, candy bars, and salt and fat-laden foods. Four or five small but nutritious meals spread throughout the course of the day work well for those with a good appetite but less space for food.

A sensible, regular exercise program should be maintained along with a good diet. Activities like walking, swimming, and biking are all very beneficial to a healthy pregnant woman, provided that she does not strain herself or become too breathless. The best advice is do what you did before pregnancy - in moderation - but don't take up tennis or high-impact aerobics for the first time while pregnant.

Expectant mothers should be good to themselves and can enjoy a few indulgences like milk and graham crackers at midnight or lazy weekend mornings in bed with the newspaper. On the other hand, spoiling yourself must be done in a way that's good for the baby too. *The single best thing you can do for both you and the baby is to take a 1 to 2 hour nap or rest, lying on your side, each day.*

Habits like smoking, drinking, or consuming lots of caffeinated beverages (i.e., coffee, tea, chocolate, and cola drinks), and using drugs of any kind (unless prescribed by a doctor) should be curtailed. We now know that excessive use of alcohol can cause major birth defects. Tobacco and marijuana smoking are associated with low birth weight. Several other drugs, like crack cocaine and heroin also may have bad and sometimes permanent developmental effects on the baby.

A prospective mother has more control over her diet and lifestyle than any other aspect of pregnancy. Good nutrition, a sensible exercise program, rest, and avoidance of dangerous habits cannot be overemphasized. She will achieve great satisfaction knowing that she helped in every way you could to make her baby beautiful and healthy.

Multi-vitamins and Minerals

The value of extra vitamins and minerals for pregnant women (as well as others) is the subject of ongoing debate. Nutrition programs insisting that pregnant women take enormous quantities of food supplements to produce a healthy child have never been scientifically proven. On the other hand, many women eat a substandard diet, and supplementation may be necessary. Most obstetricians feel that some supplementation is advantageous (especially calcium, iron, and folic acid), but excessive vitamin usage is both unnecessary and undesirable. Recent information suggests that prenatal vitamins, especially those with folic acid, may decrease the incidence of neural tube defects in the baby (for example, spina bifida), if taken prior to conception. Folic acid is also crucial to the formation of healthy red blood cells.

Table 15-1 lists several prenatal and over-the-counter vitamin preparations with their iron and folic acid content. Note the differences between pills in amounts of both substances. Many over-the-counter vitamin pills contain no iron or folic acid and are not suitable for pregnant women. If you question the value of a particular food supplement, consult a physician or nutritionist.

Iron

Pregnant women need significant amounts of iron in their diet to make red blood cells. Without it, anemia causing fatigue or weakness in late pregnancy and after delivery can occur. A normal woman has about 4 liters (5 quarts) of blood in her body. During pregnancy blood volume expands to nearly 6 liters, almost a 40% increase. The fetus, the placenta, and the umbilical cord all demand quantities of iron-rich blood.

Iron deficiency anemia is the most common medical problem found during pregnancy. It occurs in 60% of pregnant women not taking supplementary iron and accounts for 97% of the anemias diagnosed in pregnancy. Even if she eats iron-rich foods or takes iron supplements, a woman will benefit from only about 10% of the iron she swallows, since not all of it is elemental iron, which can be easily absorbed by the digestive system.

One of the first things an obstetrician will recommend to a pregnant patient is a blood count to determine the adequacy of her present iron levels. If a woman starts her pregnancy in a nonanemic state, she will probably not need iron supplements until her fourth month. However, if she is anemic, she will need to take at least 30 mg of extra elemental iron per day, beginning immediately. *Important*: by the fourth month of pregnancy all women should be taking at least 20 mg of supplementary iron per day. Despite recent studies showing a link between iron and heart disease, we still believe it plays an important role in the health of pregnant women.

Unfortunately not all people tolerate iron pills well. They can cause nausea, gas, diarrhea, or constipation. Occasionally, they will give bowel movements the color and consistency of tar, which could be mistaken for blood. Taking iron pills after meals may help prevent some of these side effects, but less iron is absorbed at this time. Some iron pills contain a stool softener that counteracts their constipating effects. Certain preparations of vitamin C taken along with iron improve its absorption. Antacids should not be taken at the same time as iron pills because they hinder absorption of the iron.

Physicians sometimes find that their pregnant patients remain anemic even if they have prescribed iron.

The main reasons for pregnancy related anemias after iron supplementation are:

1. Women did not take the pills in the manner prescribed.

2. Women could not tolerate or absorb the iron.

3. The particular iron preparation used could not be absorbed well by the body.

4. Undetected bleeding had occurred somewhere in the body.

5. Antacids were being taken along with iron pills.

6. Women had an intestinal infection, inflammation, or growth that hindered the body's absorption of iron.

7. Women had another type of anemia that was unrelated to iron deficiency.

Women who have uncomfortable side effects from iron pills or who don't properly absorb oral iron can receive iron injections or even intravenous iron, if they cannot tolerate injections. Oral liquid iron capsules are now available too.

Iron preparations must be regarded as dangerous drugs in homes with small children and kept out of their reach. An overdose of iron can be fatal; every year in the United States many children die from eating iron pills. They look like candy, with their often colorful, mildly sweet coating. As few as four or five high-dose iron pills have killed a small child.

Folic Acid

Pregnant women must get adequate folic acid in their diets to aid red blood cell production. Folic acid deficiency is another leading cause of anemia during pregnancy. Several of the vitamins recommended in Table 15-1 have adequate amounts of folic acid and, combined with a balanced diet with plenty of green and leafy vegetables, should supply a pregnant woman with her necessary folic acid. About twice as much folic acid is needed during pregnancy as is normally required (0.8 mg vs 0.4 mg). Women who must take medications to prevent epileptic seizures or women who have previously given birth to a child with a neural tube defect (spina bifida or anencephaly) will need extra folic acid (1 mg per day at conception and during pregnancy).

Calcium

Calcium is also important during pregnancy. Most mothers-to-be should be able to get their needed calcium in a diet containing milk, cheese, yogurt, or ice cream. Unfortunately, milk and other dairy products do not agree with all adults, including pregnant ones. Bloating, excess gas, and abdominal cramps can occur after eating dairy products, due to a condition called lactase deficiency.

Lactase, an enzyme found in the intestinal tract is necessary to break down lactose, the natural sugar in milk, and lactase production tends to decline as people get older. Seventy percent of people of African-American, Asian, Mediterranean, Jewish, southern and central European, and native American origin have a lactase deficiency. In fact, it is the normal condition of the vast majority of the world's adult population. The exception: Most people of northern European extraction seem able to continue drinking milk successfully into adulthood.

Lactose intolerance is sometimes a matter of degree, that is, a woman may be able to drink 2 cups of milk a day (more than 60% of the daily calcium requirement) with no ill effects, but will feel ill after drinking 3 or 4 cups.

Many non-dairy foods contain substantial calcium. These include sardines; canned mackerel and salmon; broccoli; collard, turnip, mustard, and especially dandelion greens; sesame seeds; and torula yeast.

We do not routinely recommend calcium supplements during pregnancy if milk or other calcium-rich foods are consumed along with prenatal vitamins. The body makes adjustments during pregnancy that allow it to better absorb calcium; unlike iron, the calcium taken into the body is used rather efficiently. The old myth of "one tooth per child," can be laid to rest because the fetus takes only about 2.5% of the calcium circulating in the mother to make its bones and teeth.

Some doctors think that calcium supplementation (2 g/day) may decrease the incidence of pre-eclampsia high blood pressure in pregnancy. This concept is currently under study.

A few women with digestive tract diseases that do not permit them to absorb food nutrients may need calcium supplements. If a woman has undersized parathyroid glands, she may also need extra calcium, for it is the enlargement of the parathyroid glands during a normal pregnancy that allows the increased calcium absorption.

Other Nutritional Supplements

Prenatal fluoride supplements have been recommended recently for pregnant women. Preliminary evidence suggests that the enamel of prenatal fluoride-exposed teeth during fetal development, may carry a resistance to caries later in childhood.

Whether an additional daily 1 mg dose of elemental fluoride during the second and third trimesters is truly more beneficial than the fluorides commonly found in the water remains to be seen.

Greater quantities of vitamin A and several of the B vitamins may be necessary during pregnancy. The Food and Drug Administration's (FDA) recommended daily allowances of vitamins for pregnant and nonpregnant individuals are reported in Table 15-2.

No one should take Vitamin A in excessive amounts. It is toxic in dosages over 100,000 units daily. This is more than 10 times the dosage found in a typical prenatal vitamin pill, so there is no need for concern about them. Vitamin D is toxic in excess of 50,000 units per day, but again, prenatal vitamins normally contain no more than 400 units of Vitamin D. Mineral oil taken as a laxative may prevent the absorption of Vitamins A, D, and E, so we recommend choosing a different laxative, such as bisacodyl (Dulcolax) if constipation is a major problem during pregnancy.

Women who are strict vegetarians should be certain that they supplement their diets with vitamin B12. Lack of this vitamin can lead to certain anemias and nervous system disorders in the mother.

Gastrointestinal Upsets During Pregnancy

Nothing can spoil the excitement of pregnancy like "morning sickness," the nausea, vomiting, and indigestion that at least 50% of pregnant women experience during the early months.

It may be comforting to know that this nausea is actually a good sign, indicating the rising hormone levels of a healthy pregnancy. The nausea of pregnancy can occur at any time of day, and will usually last no longer than 4 months. If it does, you should speak with your doctor.

Dietary adjustments are the first route to controlling pregnancy-induced nausea. Obstetricians now recommend alternating dry foods and liquids in small quantities a couple of hours apart. The old standby, soda crackers, can be part of this regimen, but more nutritious foods, particularly those containing protein, should be included too. Upset stomachs will tolerate rice, pasta, white meat poultry, mild-tasting fish, and mild cheeses better than red meats, beans, or nuts. Bananas are easily digested, but citrus fruits, tomatoes, and other highly acidic foods will probably not stay down. Cooked green vegetables in place of raw ones may be preferable during bouts of nausea. Ginger ale and decaffeinated colas are also helpful.

Drugs to Control Nausea

Just as the first edition of this book went to press in 1983, the Merrell-Dow Pharmaceutical Company decided to cease production of Bendectin, a drug that had been popularly prescribed for very difficult cases of morning sickness. Adverse publicity based on unscientific evidence presented in a lawsuit influenced this decision. To date, there has been no scientific evidence presented that Bendectin causes birth defects. However, it is unavailable to pregnant women in this country. The therapeutic gap caused by the loss of this widely used drug causes us to reflect on the effects litigation has on health care.

A category of drugs known as the phenothiazines (promethazine, trade name Phenergan); prochlorperazine, trade name Compazine) can also be used in resistant cases of nausea, but these drugs are not approved by the FDA* for use during pregnancy, although no birth defects have been shown to be associated with their use. They may be familiar to you because they are commonly prescribed to control motion sickness, for which they are FDA approved.

Common side effects of antinausea drugs include drowsiness and relaxation. Painkillers, sedatives, and alcohol should not be used along with these drugs because the combination may create even further sleepiness. You should not drive or undertake any action requiring close attention and coordination when you take these antinausea drugs, either alone or with other substances.

Again, these drugs are dangerous to small children. If a child swallows Compazine or Phenergan, call for help immediately. Make the child vomit, using syrup of Ipecac as directed, and then give him activated charcoal to absorb the poisonous material. Vomiting should be induced very carefully because there is a chance the child will lose motor control and breathe the vomited material into the lungs. In any case a fast trip to the Emergency Room is indicated.

A drug delivery system, pioneered by the ALZA Corporation, where medication is absorbed through the skin, is on the market. The drug is called Trans Derm V and is a small, plastic patch applied behind the ear, usually for control of motion sickness. It contains a drug called scopolamine, which has been used during labor and delivery for many years with no harmful effect on babies. Only a few physicians have used it to date, but it may be appropriate for controlling nausea and vomiting during pregnancy. You will need to discuss with your physician whether he or she is comfortable prescribing it to you.

Currently the only drug of this type with FDA approval for use in pregnancy is ritodrine for prevention of premature labor.

One study has indicated that taking vitamin B6 helps control the nausea of pregnancy. More information is needed with regard to Vitamin B6, although a 10 mg daily dose is probably harmless.

Antacids

Heartburn, indigestion, and gas are frequent companions of pregnancy, especially in the last few months as the baby grows larger and the mother's internal space is more crowded. Avoiding spicy and acidic foods and eating small, frequent meals will help with the problems of heartburn and indigestion. Many physicians recommend sleeping with the head, neck, and shoulders slightly elevated to the right side to prevent acid from coming back up the esophagus. Bland foods like crackers or toast near bedtime may also assist in controlling the symptoms.

Antacids may not seem like medicine, and you may be tempted to swallow or chew them every time a little discomfort occurs. The truth is, they should be reserved for cases of strong heartburn or indigestion and used only after dietary adjustments have failed. Many antacids contain aluminum or bismuth, both of which can be absorbed through the placenta in small amounts. Doctors don't know much about the effects of these substances accumulating in the fetus, but generally we would prefer to avoid having it happen. Some antacids contain bicarbonate of soda, which if used excessively, may cause fluid accumulation in pregnant women.

Antacids also can cause side effects such as constipation or diarrhea, which add to the misery of pregnancy-related digestive upsets, as well as creating the need for more, possibly inadvisable, medications.

We recommend antacid liquids such as Gelusil, Maalox, Riopan, Digel, Kolantyl, or Phillip's Milk of Magnesia, although chewable tablets are more convenient. All of the tablets contain sodium, with the difference between the low-dose and higher-dose preparations being insignificant. In excess they would not be advisable for pregnant women.

Case Study

Barbara G., 26, worked part time as a secretary and cared for her husband and 3 year old son at home the rest of the time. When she was pregnant with her first child, she felt well with very few discomforts and no medical problems. With her second pregnancy she had considerably more demands on her time and energy and soon began to notice she was tired and did not feel as well. Almost immediately she had bouts of nausea and indigestion. Her morning cup of coffee and afternoon chocolate bar were replaced by saltines, toast, and noodle soup.

Before trying medication, she attempted to manage her nausea and vomiting with frequent small meals, alternating between dry and wet foods. Her doctors persuaded her to change from Alka-Seltzer and Bromo-Seltzer to Mylanta to help with heartburn.

Barbara's digestive symptoms went away after her fourth month, but she found herself coping with colds, sinus infections, and a chronic runny nose throughout the windy and damp winter of her second trimester. Her doctors reminded her at each visit that she needed plenty of fresh fruits and vegetables in her diet. She took Sudafed as a decongestant and an occasional dose of Tylenol to relieve general discomforts and headaches.

In her eighth month, the entire family came down with a violent gastrointestinal flu. Barbara was very ill and was almost hospitalized for dehydration. She took Kaopectate for diarrhea and stayed in bed for more than a week. Her appetite gradually came back, and she drank all the liquids she could manage to consume.

Barbara eventually recovered but worried that the health problems and drugs she had during pregnancy would adversely affect her baby. Her doctor told her that the baby would gain a large proportion of its weight during her last month, as much as two pounds. He encouraged Barbara to eat well at that time and be particularly conscientious about getting enough protein.

Two weeks after her recovery from the flu, after a short but intense labor, Barbara gave birth to a healthy baby girl weighing 6 pounds 10 ounces. She requested sterilization after delivery, the decision being related to her difficult pregnancy. Because of her young age, her doctors counseled her to reconsider and she was persuaded to use a low-dose estrogen birth control pill as a contraceptive method.

Key Points for Nutrition and Lifestyle

1. Proper diet is a highly important part of pregnancy, one over which a woman can exert a great deal of personal control.

2. The most important dietary supplement is iron and every pregnant woman should be taking it by the start of her fourth month of pregnancy.

3. Other vitamins may be helpful, particularly if a woman eats an inadequate diet. Prenatal multivitamins should never be regarded as a substitute for nutritious food.

4. Nausea in the first 4 months of pregnancy is quite common and should disappear by the beginning of the fifth month. To manage nausea dietary adjustments should be tried first. If they do not work, a physician may be able to prescribe medication.

5. Over-the-counter antacids, anti-nausea drugs, laxatives, and anti-diarrhea drugs should be used sparingly. Consult your doctor about the safest ones for use during pregnancy.

6. Hospitalization may be necessary if nausea and diarrhea persist, causing dehydration. Don't put up with symptoms if they are unbearable. Your physician can provide you with relief.

Table 15-1
Common Prenatal and Over-the-Counter (OTC) Vitamins

Trade name	Elemental Iron Content (mg)*	Folic Acid Content (mg)+
Prenatal vitamins		
Filibon#	18	0.4
Filbon F.A.	45	1
Filibon Forte	45	1
Materna 1.60	60	1
Natalins#	30	0.5
Natalins Rx	60	1
Pramilet FA	60	1
Stuart Prenatal#	60	0.8
Stuartnatal 1 + 1	65	1
Over-the-counter vitamins for general use		
Dayalets Plus Iron	18	0.4
Mi-Cebrin	15	0
One-A-Day	0	0.4
One-A-Day Plus Iron	18	0.4
Stresstabs 600 with Iron	27	0.4
Theragran-M	12	0
Theragran Hematinic	67	0.33

* Minimum daily requirement of absorbed elemental iron during pregnancy and lactation is 4 mg. However, approximately 10% of elemental iron is absorbed.

+Minimum daily requirement of absorbed folic acid during pregnancy and lactation is 0.8 mg.

#OTC prenatal vitamins

Table 15-2

United States Recommended Daily Nutritional Allowances (USRDA)

Nutritional needs	Nonpregnant	Pregnant or lactating
Calories (kcal)	2100	2400
Protein (gm)	50	80
A (IU)	5000	8000
D (IU)	400	400
E (IU)	30	30
C (mg)	60	60
Folic acid (mg)	0.4	0.8
Niacin (mg)	20	20
B1 (mg)	1.5	1.7
B2 (mg)	1.7	2.0
B6 (mg)	2.0	2.5
B12 (mg)	0.006	0.008
Iron (mg)	18	30
Calcium (mg)	800 to 1200	1200

*IU, International units

Notes

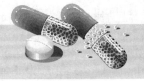

Chapter 16

Drug Effects on the Unborn Baby

Women have worried for a long time that the use of drugs and medications during pregnancy could affect their unborn child - and not without reason. The "thalidomide babies" of the 1960s were a particularly sad example of what happens when the wrong substance reaches a fetus. These unfortunate people, some with no arms or legs, still remind us of the damage that can be done by a drug that wasn't fully understood before it was prescribed. Another case in point: The "DES daughters" of the 1970s, girls who were born with reproductive tract disorders because their mothers took diethylstilbestrol to prevent miscarriage.

These days, doctors and drug manufacturers know much more about the effects of drugs on fetuses, and it is rare that a prescription drug produces widespread birth defects. Unfortunately, many women are using street drugs like crack cocaine during pregnancy, and we are just beginning to see the results. Children who are hyperactive, unable to learn and who cannot control their behavior are reaching school age, and we are beginning to realize that some of these effects may be permanent. *Indiscriminate use of drugs is definitely out of place during pregnancy!*

At the other extreme, some women believe that no drug can be safely taken during pregnancy. They will suffer for months with nausea or respiratory and urinary tract infections, refusing all medications for fear of damaging their unborn child. Prospective mothers can be reassured that there is a middle ground. They do not necessarily have to endure illness or discomfort to protect their babies from harm.

Two facts can be stated: (1) drugs taken by a mother-to-be generally do reach the fetus; (2) the majority of pregnant women take drugs, both prescribed and nonprescribed. Women need to be aware of the large variety of substances that fall under the category of drugs and of what their own drug consumption habits are. They need up-to-date knowledge on which drugs can be taken with relative safety, and then, with the advice of their physicians, can decide the benefits of a given drug versus its hazards. Armed with this knowledge, they can minimize drug use while remaining healthy and happy expectant mothers.

How Drugs Affect the Fetus

To understand the effects of drugs on the fetus growing in the uterus, it is necessary to understand what happens to the mother's body, then the placenta, and then the fetus. In studies of pregnant animals, researchers have found that drugs concentrate in the umbilical cord and blood of the newborn at levels close to those in the mother's blood. In other words, what the mother gets, the fetus gets too. This is especially true if she has been taking the drug for a long time. The placenta acts like a big sponge, sucking up as many of the substances in the mother's bloodstream as it can. What she swallows, smokes or injects, be it good or bad, usually reaches the unborn baby through the placenta, which has many areas where exchange of substances takes place. (This fascinating temporary organ is quite large and would equal a rug laid out in a room 16 feet by 16 feet if it were flattened out to one layer!)

Some drugs can reach the fetus very quickly. These include ampicillin, penicillin G, cephalothin, kanamycin, tetracycline, streptomycin, diazepam (Valium), phenytoin (Dilantin), phenobarbital, alcohol, aspirin, and propranolol (Inderal), a popular heart medication. Alcohol and recreational drugs such as heroin and cocaine get to the fetus in a matter of minutes. A few substances will attain *higher* levels in the fetus than in the mother - Valium being a prime example. Therefore it is especially important to avoid drugs like these or use them only if absolutely necessary.

The dosage received is definitely a factor in determining how much a particular drug will affect the unborn child. Because its organ systems are not fully developed, a fetus breaks down and clears drugs more slowly than an adult. Thus, drug concentrations can build up, even if the mother never took a high dosage. The total exposure of the fetus to a drug over the long range is probably more important than a single high dose of drug at any given time.

How a drug will affect a fetus partially depends on its prenatal age at the time it is exposed to the drug. Exposure to a substance that causes defects in very early pregnancy (the first 5 weeks following the last menstrual period) results in miscarriage infrequently. During the fifth through the twelfth weeks after the last period, major organs are formed, and a drug that causes defects may have an effect on their development. Beyond 12 weeks, delay in the unborn baby's growth and brain development is a major concern.

The majority of defects caused by drugs are difficult if not impossible to diagnose before the baby is born. A procedure for getting fluid from around the baby called amniocentesis can be performed from the 12th through the 18th weeks of pregnancy. However, this is useful for detecting hereditary diseases like Down syndrome rather than for drug-associated problems.

Drug interaction, the interplay between two or more drugs, can be hazardous to the fetus' health. For instance, drug A may be dangerous only in the presence or absence of drug B. Adding drug C may create an entirely new situation. After birth the newborn remains susceptible to drugs that have crossed the placenta during labor and may have symptoms caused by them for hours or even days. The newborn's kidneys and liver are still not mature enough to break down drugs efficiently, so this may delay their passing from the newborn's system.

Almost any drug circulating within the mother can be transferred into her breast milk and thus reach the baby. Generally speaking, however, we encourage mothers to continue breast-feeding, even if they must take a drug for a while when nursing. Newborns do not necessarily absorb the drugs acquired in breast milk through their immature gastrointestinal tracts, and for the most part the benefits of breast-feeding outweigh the drawbacks of drug transfer. If you question the safety of a drug while breastfeeding, always get your doctor's advice.

Drug-Taking Habits of Pregnant Women

Studies show that women do take drugs during pregnancy; in fact, the average woman consumes two or three different drugs while pregnant. Not counting vitamin and iron preparations, 82% of all pregnant women take a prescription drug while they are expecting their babies, and 65% take drugs that have not been prescribed by a physician. Caffeine, alcohol, tobacco, and vitamins are used so routinely that sometimes people lose sight of the fact that they are drugs. One study of several hundred pregnant women showed that marijuana, diet pills, and birth control pills were the three drugs most commonly being taken at the time of conception. For women overall, pregnant or nonpregnant, tranquilizers and other mood-altering drugs are among the most frequently prescribed substances. For years, before physicians began to appreciate its addictiveness, the drug most commonly prescribed to women was diazepam (Valium), a tranquilizer.

All drugs should be used with caution during pregnancy. This includes over-the-counter drugs like aspirin and habitual drugs like alcohol, tobacco, and caffeine. Drugs should be taken only for a specific reason, in the lowest possible dosage, for the shortest amount of time needed to get results. Pregnant women should let their doctors know of any drugs they are taking or are likely to take, including those purchased over the counter.

A small number of drugs are clearly harmful to the unborn baby, but these account for no more than 5% of all recorded birth defects. Hereditary and environmental factors cause another 30%, and for the remaining 65% the cause remains unknown. Several drugs have aroused suspicion, and we recommend caution in their use. An even larger number of drugs have at one time or another been associated with a particular disease. In this latter category there is too little information for us to make specific recommendations. With pregnancy, it is always better to err on the side of being too careful, however. Thus, when the effects are unknown or suspect, a drug should be avoided.

The tables in this chapter give a detailed list of well-known drugs, with the findings to date regarding their effects during pregnancy. Readers, along with their physicians, can evaluate them for their own purposes.

Fetal Drug Effects
Known Harmful Effects

That small number of drugs definitely known to produce a specific birth defect are listed, along with the problems they create, in Table 16-1. If at all possible, use of these drugs should be avoided during pregnancy, except for phenytoin (Dilantin), which is used for the treatment of epilepsy. When women have serious medical conditions like epilepsy, blood clots, or cancer, the use of agents known to produce birth defects must be carefully considered along with the seriousness of the mother's need for the drug. The final decision lies with the woman and her doctor.

Suspected Harmful Effects

Certain drugs, again not a large group, have raised enough suspicion that doctors recommend avoiding them during pregnancy. Table 16-2 lists these drugs and their effects. When more extensive and detailed studies have been completed, these drugs may move up into the proven-to-be harmful category. Right now we recommend that these drugs be avoided if at all possible, but we do not recommend that you automatically terminate a pregnancy because you have been using them. Chances are still in your favor that your baby will not have a birth defect or other problem. It might be possible to find a safer substitute, as in the case of the sulfonylureas for treatment of diabetes. Or, a woman can consciously choose to discontinue use of a drug, as in the case of nicotine.

No Proven Harmful Effects

This category is rather sweeping in that it covers the majority of drugs on the market today. Some of them have been studied in animals, with occasional problems noted along the way. We know that the results of research in animals clearly do not always apply to humans: What may harm an animal may do nothing whatsoever to a human (or vice versa). Thalidomide was studied extensively in animals, and no harmful effect was ever noted. Researchers could never have realized that only in humans was a particular by-product of thalidomide formed, and it was this by-product that would cause the malformations.

Single reports of birth defects that could be associated with drug-taking abound in the medical literature, but the evidence is too scanty for physicians to draw definite conclusions. At this time we can say that, if a pregnant woman needs to take these drugs, the benefits to her health will probably outweigh the remote chance that the drug will cause a problem for the baby.

These apparently safe drugs, as well as many others, and their reported effects from isolated case reports in human infants appear in Table 16-3. Only the generic (chemical) names of the drugs are listed. Often several manufacturers will market the same drug under different trade names. *The Physician's Desk Reference* provides information about trade name and generic drugs and their effects. Updated yearly, this useful guide is available at most major book dealers.

Recommendations for Drugs Commonly Used During Pregnancy

Several of the drugs most commonly used during pregnancy are discussed, along with our recommendation for their use.

Pain Relief Medications

Aspirin, acetaminophen (Tylenol, Datril), and ibuprofen (Motrin, Nuprin, Advil), when used in moderation, have not caused problems that we know of in the early stages of fetal development. There is some evidence that prolonged aspirin use in large doses in the last 3 months of pregnancy causes bleeding problems, prolonged onset and duration of labor, and premature closure of a major heart-to-lung artery in the fetus before birth. However, physicians are now studying the possible *beneficial* effects of low-dosage aspirin (baby aspirin in 80 mg tablets) as a means of decreasing the incidence of high blood pressure throughout pregnancy.

We recommend that aspirin be avoided in the last third of a pregnancy and that acetaminophen be substituted if a painkilling remedy is needed - unless your physician prescribes aspirin for a specific reason. Heavy doses of acetaminophen must be avoided also. While acetaminophen is often recommended as a substitute for aspirin, more time is needed to study it before definitive conclusions can be drawn about its safety. Acetaminophen is toxic to the liver if taken in very large doses.

Ibuprofen has become widely used for menstrual discomfort, toothache, and arthritis pain over the last few years. Its side effects are thought to be similar to those of aspirin, so we would issue the same kinds of warnings regarding its usage in later pregnancy.

Decongestants and Antihistamines

Pregnant women often suffer from nasal congestion and upper airway infections, which can last for the full 9 months. Decongestants containing pseudoephedrine (Sudafed) have been studied and appear to be safe for use during pregnancy. Brompheniramine, chlorpheniramine, and meclizine are antihistamine-decongestants found in many over-the-counter cold and allergy-relief medications. They have been studied in pregnant women, and no increase in birth defects has been noted with their usage. They also appear to be relatively safe when used during nursing. Despite these favorable reports, we recommend that such drugs be used in the lowest possible dosages. Nasal sprays may be a safer alternative to oral decongestants, but, if overused, can lead to a rebound effect (meaning, after the drug wears off, the original problem gets worse) and an undesirable dependency on the product.

Antacids

Heartburn and indigestion can plague a woman during pregnancy, worsening in the later months because of increased pressure on her insides. Antacids are safe when taken in normal dosages, but keep this in mind:

1. Some antacids, such as Alka-Seltzer and Bromo-Seltzer, contain sodium (salt). Those few pregnant women with salt limitations should read the labels carefully and avoid antacids with a high sodium content.

2. Antacids can also cause constipation, making an already common side effect of pregnancy even worse.

3. Antacids can cause decreased or delayed absorption of food and certain drugs.

You should discuss the use of antacids with your doctor if you are taking them in combination with any other drug, particularly antibiotics. We believe the liquid antacids such as Gelusil, Maalox, Mylanta, and Riopan are more effective than the chewable tablets, although the tablets have the advantage of being easy to carry, so you can have them with you at all times.

Penicillins

The two most common infections encountered during pregnancy are urinary tract infections and upper respiratory tract infections. Penicillin type drugs are commonly used to treat respiratory problems, and amoxicillin is sometimes used for urinary tract infections.

As far as we've been able to determine, penicillin does not have any adverse effect on the developing fetus. In most of its forms, it should be safe for pregnant women who are not allergic to it. On the other hand, the penicillins will appear in breast milk and may cause diarrhea and candidiasis, a type of oral fungus infection, in the nursing infant with long-term exposure. Penicillin is found in a variety of different forms, the more common of which are ampicillin, amoxicillin, penicillin G, benzathine penicillin, methicillin, nafcillin, carbenicillin, dicloxacillin, and ticarcillin.

Penicillin drugs, along with almost all antibiotics, destroy the normal organisms in the vagina, often resulting in an imbalanced growth of yeast. Itchy yeast infections, which add to the discomfort of pregnancy, can be avoided if you insert an anti-yeast vaginal suppository when taking antibiotic drugs. These suppositories are now available over-the-counter.

Anti-nausea Drugs

Anti-nausea drugs help reduce the discomforts of nausea and vomiting, which can be very intense during the first few months of pregnancy. Promethazine (Phenergan) and prochlorperazine (Compazine) are used for "morning sickness;" although they appear to be safe, they can create unwanted side effects such as drowsiness, disorientation, low blood pressure, and difficulty in walking or sitting properly. Note that these two drugs have not been approved by the U.S. Food and Drug Administration for use during pregnancy, although they are approved for use in motion sickness. Chapter 14 discusses nausea control during pregnancy in more detail.

Diet Pills

Some women take diet pills before they know they are pregnant, perhaps even as a result of the weight gain and fluid retention of pregnancy, which can begin very early. These pills sometimes contain amphetamines, powerful stimulants that make a person very jumpy and jittery at the same time that they kill the appetite. No one has shown any clear relationship between the use of amphetamines and birth defects, but the drugs are still suspect by many physicians. Other substances commonly used in diet pills, such as phenylpropanolamine, caffeine, and methylcellulose, have not been proved to cause birth defects, but we still believe their use should be minimized during pregnancy.

Safety considerations aside, diet pills should be immediately discontinued once you discover you are pregnant because of the need for good nutrition.

Caffeine

This much used and sometimes invisible drug is found not only in coffee, but also in tea, chocolate, cola and other soft drinks, headache tablets, diet pills, and cold and allergy capsules. Caffeine crosses the placenta without difficulty and has been detected in the blood and urine of newborns. It also appears in breast milk, and even moderate doses can produce irritability in infants.

In September 1980 the Food and Drug Administration suggested that pregnant women limit their consumption of caffeine severely, primarily as a precautionary measure. Since then more than 15,000 pregnant women have been studied by researchers at Harvard and other universities and no link between caffeine consumption and birth defects in humans has been found. In fact, although it has been implicated many times, caffeine has never been proven to cause any known medical disease. Currently, we believe that, while caffeine is a relatively safe drug to use during pregnancy, its use should be kept to a minimum.

Pregnant women should try to limit themselves to no more than 300 mg of caffeine per day, the equivalent of about 2 cups of coffee or 2 cola drinks. We would encourage substitution of decaffeinated products whenever possible.

Birth Control Pills

Once a woman discovers she is pregnant, she will want to discontinue the use of birth control pills. Studies done in the early eighties associated birth control pills with certain birth defects during early pregnancy, but these have never been substantiated.

One of these is a defect involving the spine, anus (rectal opening), esophagus (food pipe), trachea (windpipe), and the arms and legs. It is known as the VACTERL syndrome. New information acquired since then indicates that the danger of VACTERL syndrome was overestimated in these early studies. Women should be reassured that the incidence of these defects is probably less than 1% among those who have taken contraceptives while pregnant. The odds are still overwhelmingly in their favor that they will bear a normal child if the pregnancy continues.

Cigarette Smoking

There is no longer any doubt that smoking can have a negative effect on an unborn infant. Low birth weight, problems with the placenta that result in hemorrhage, premature rupture of the membranes surrounding the fetus, and newborn death have all been documented.

Four thousand separate compounds have been identified in cigarette smoke, but the two most studied are nicotine and carbon monoxide. Nicotine causes changes in the mother's circulation and heart rate and seems to lower the baby's oxygen consumption. It can appear in noticeable amounts in the breast milk of heavy smokers. Carbon monoxide, a truly dangerous substance also crosses the placental barrier easily. It competes with oxygen for a place in the blood of the fetus and can lead to insufficient weight gain and retarded growth. More studies need to be done on the effects of smoking in terms of actual birth defects, miscarriage, and slower mental development, but physicians already know enough to strongly recommend that their pregnant patients stop smoking altogether.

New evidence is emerging about the effects of *passive smoke inhalation,* that is, breathing in other people's smoke. Babies and young children living with adults who smoke suffer more respiratory diseases than children living in smoke-free households. The same is true for non-smoking adults with chronic respiratory problems such as asthma. While evidence on the effects of passive smoke inhalation on pregnant women is still being gathered, we suspect that it will show a negative impact on both the mother and the fetus. Therefore, if a pregnant woman lives with a smoker, she should encourage them to quit or to smoke in a place where she will not be exposed.

More and more public places such as restaurants, airports, stores, and theaters are creating smoke-free environments for their patrons. Many medical centers no longer allow smoking anywhere on their indoor premises. It is in the best interest of pregnant women to frequent places like these rather than "smoke-filled rooms." If you are exposed to smoke on the job, contact the National Institute for Occupational Safety and Health (NIOSH) to learn about your right to protection from environmental smoke at your workplace.

Alcohol

For decades doctors have suspected that drinking was responsible for some birth defects, and in 1973 a landmark study described a group of associated abnormalities that came to be known as *fetal alcohol syndrome.* These include nervous system disorders, growth deficiencies, and facial abnormalities. Mental retardation is also common. Undersized heads (microcephaly), the so-called water heads (hydrocephaly), and incomplete development of the brain occur also in conjunction with alcohol overuse.

How much alcohol does it take to produce these results? Recent studies indicate that a daily intake of six or more "hard" drinks (whiskey, vodka, gin) or an equivalent 12 bottles of beer or 12 glasses of wine significantly increases the chance of these abnormalities developing in the fetus. The effects of "light" or "moderate" drinking are not as clear cut. No absolutely safe level of consumption has been determined, so all pregnant women are cautioned to reduce alcohol drinking to the barest minimum, or to none at all, and to concentrate on eating well.

The DES Story

In the early 1950s and 1960s, a sizable number of women received the hormone, diethyl-stilbestrol (DES), a form of high-dose estrogen, to prevent threatened miscarriage. About 15 years later a small percentage of the girls who were born to these women were found to have diseases of the reproductive tract. Our two principal concerns about these "DES daughters" have been whether they have cellular changes in the upper vagina or cervix or structural deformities of the uterus and cervix.

Cells not normally found on the vaginal surface may be glandlike and resemble cells normally found on the inner lining of the cervix. This finding, known as adenosis, is very common among women exposed to DES during their mother's first 9 months of pregnancy, but it does not cause any symptoms. The extent of the cellular abnormality can be determined in the doctor's office by inspection of the upper part of the vagina and cervix through a magnifying lens called a colposcope, using special, washable stains.

Because of the different chemical changes that take place in the vagina, once in a great while these abnormal cells undergo further changes, which are cancerous. This serious disease is known as adenocarcinoma or clear cell carcinoma. Fortunately, these changes occur only once in about every 10,000 women who have adenosis. We tell this to our DES-exposed patients to reassure them, and we do not treat their adenosis, other than to have the women come in annually for a pelvic examination and Pap smear. In those rare cases of adenocarcinoma, surgery and radiation treatment are usually very successful, especially if the cancer is detected early.

A second and perhaps more worrisome condition is the DES-exposed woman who is pregnant or who has had repeated miscarriages. Certain defects can occur in the female reproductive organs of DES-exposed women that make it difficult to carry through with a pregnancy.

These defects and their locations are listed below:

1. Upper vagina: vaginal septum

2. Cervix: cervical hood, cockscomb cervix, incompetent cervix

3. Uterus: T-shaped uterus

4. Fallopian tubes: distortion as the tube enters the uterus

Even though these defects are more typically found in DES-exposed women than other woman, they are not at all common in either group.

Many women come to us greatly concerned because they are uncertain about whether they were exposed to DES. We do not take any sort of action for these women until they reach their childbearing years. If, after a pelvic examination, there is no evidence of adenosis or abnormalities, we offer reassurance that they are unlikely to have problems. When an abnormal Pap smear or if staining of the vaginal cells suggests adenosis, we will continue to watch the woman and certainly treat her if that is necessary. If she has any of the deformities just listed or if she has had several miscarriages or premature deliveries, we will perform an x-ray examination of her reproductive tract (the X-ray technique known as the hysterosalpingogram). Under most circumstances, we cannot correct these deformities surgically, but at least we can be aware of the deformities and watch very closely for signs of miscarriage or premature delivery during pregnancy. Sometimes, especially in women with a T-shaped uterus, a cerclage (tightening with stitches) of the cervix will prolong the pregnancy.

Case Study

Sarah J was 17 and a senior in high school. Her mother took her to the doctor immediately when she suspected that the plump teenager might be pregnant. Her fears were confirmed when the doctor announced that Sarah's pregnancy test was positive. He estimated that Sarah was in her tenth week. Sarah took the news in stride, although she seemed uncertain about her plans for marriage or taking care of the baby. Her mother was very upset and deeply concerned about a number of substances Sarah and her boyfriend had been using at the time she became pregnant. She smoked both cigarettes and marijuana and drank beer at parties. Her boyfriend had been using cocaine for the past 2 years. Like so many of her friends, Sarah used Dietac from time to time to try to lose weight. She had already gained five pounds with her pregnancy, so she had started taking the drug four weeks prior to her doctor's appointment.

The doctor's interview revealed that Sarah had also taken birth control pills sporadically. Frightened when she missed her period, Sarah had gone back on the pill, even though she was already pregnant.

Even though they were very worried about the impact of the lifestyle of both Sarah and her boyfriend on her pregnancy, the family was opposed to an abortion. So, Sarah's doctor referred her to a high-risk pregnancy clinic at the state university medical center 65 miles away. In a conference with one of the obstetricians there, Sarah and her mother were told that, in spite of all the drugs Sarah had taken, the risk of birth defects caused by any one of them was less than 5%. The doctor did qualify her remarks by stating that she did not know if the particular combination of drugs might be more dangerous for the unborn infant's development.

The family resigned itself to the fact that 17-year-old Sarah was going to have a baby. She quit smoking and refrained from other drug use throughout her pregnancy. Her diet consisted of too much junk food, but she took her prenatal vitamins regularly. A community agency offered childbirth preparation classes for teenage mothers, and she was able to attend some high school courses so that she could graduate before the baby arrived. Sarah delivered a healthy 8 pound boy at term. She remains at home to care for him, and is being supported by her parents.

Key Points for Drug Effects on the Fetus

1. An unborn baby will be affected not only by any type of drug taken, but by:
   The amount of drug actually reaching the fetus.
   The individual genetic differences of the mother and child.
   The age of the fetus at the time it is exposed.
   The length of time over which a fetus is exposed to the drug.
   The presence and interaction with drugs.

2. Once a pregnancy is confirmed any of drugs used near the time of conception should be reported to the doctor.

3. Only a few drugs definitely or probably cause birth defects (see Tables 16-1 and 16-2), although taking them does not always result in birth defects. Those should be avoided unless the medical benefit to the mother outweighs the danger to the unborn child.

4. The effects of most drugs have never been thoroughly investigated, although many appear to be safe.

5. Consult with a doctor before taking *any* drug, even those which were used habitually before pregnancy or purchased without a prescription.

6. If there is a definite medical problem and the physician has prescribed a drug, it should be taken. Drugs that improve a mother's health will often benefit a fetus much more than they will harm it.

7. Use of a questionable drug at or before conception should not solely determine seeking an abortion. This should be carefully considered for other personal reasons. Discuss the problem with informed people and find out what the odds are of producing a defective infant.

8. We do not advise the use of either amniocentesis or ultrasound to test for drug effects on the fetus, since in most cases it neither proves or disproves anything. Occasionally, these tests may be given to provide reassurance and comfort to the mother and to date the pregnancy more accurately.

Table 16-1
Drugs Known to Cause Birth Defects

Drug	Birth Defect
Anticonvulsants Trimethadione Phenytoin	Facial dysmorphogenesis (characteristic facial expression), mild mental retardation, growth retardation
Anticoagulants Coumadin and related drugs	Nasal hypoplasia (underdeveloped nose bridge), stripping of bones, optic atrophy
Alcohol	Fetal alcohol syndrome: growth retardation, mild mental retardation, increase in anomalies
Antihypertensives ACE Inhibitors (captopril, fosinopril, benazapril, ramipril, lisonopril, enalapril, quinapril)	Reduced urine output in fetus; kidney damage; hypotension; fetal death
Dermatologics Isotretinoin (Accutane)	Hydrocephalus, microcephalus, ear abnormalities, cardiovascular abnormalities, facial abnormalities
Folic acid antagonists Methotrexate, Aminopterin	Abortion, multiple malformations
Hormones Diethylstilbestrol and related drugs Androgens	Vaginal adenosis, carcinogenesis, uterine anomalies, epididymal anomalies Masculinization of female fetus
Methyl mercury	Central nervous system damage, growth retardation
Thalidomide	Phocomelia (short limbs)

Table 16-2
Drugs Suspected of Causing Birth Defects

Drug	Birth Defect
Alkylating agents Aminopterin	Abortion, anomalies

Hormones
  Oral contraceptives
  Progestins
	Limb and heart defects (?)

Lithium carbonate(?)	Ebstein's anomaly (heart defect)(?)
Nicotine	Growth retardation
Sulfonylureas	Anomalies(?)
Tranquilizers Benzodiazepines	Facial clefts(?)

Table 16-3
Drugs and Reported Effects on the Fetus

Drugs	1st Trimester Effects	2nd and 3rd Trimester Effects
Acetaminophen	None known	Hepatotoxiciy and Nephrotoxicity (?)
Narcotics	None known	Depression, withdrawal,
Salicylates	Frequent reports none proven	Prolonged pregnancy and labor, hemorrhage, altered hemostasis, intracranial hemorrhage
Anesthetics		
General	Anomalies (?), abortion(?)	Depression
Local	None known	Bradycardia, seizures
Appetite Suppressants		
Phenylpropanolamine	Eye(?), ear (?), hypospadias (?)	None known
Amphetamines	Cardiac defects (?), hemorrhagic brain infarction	Irritable, poor feeding, growth retardation
Phenmetrazine	None known	None known
Meclizine	Oral cleft (?) Eye (?) Ear (?)	None known
Antiasthmatics		
Theophylline	None known	Jitteriness, tachycardia
Terbutaline	None known	Tachycardia, hypothermia, hypocalcemia, hypoglycemia, and hyperglycemia
Metaproterenol	None known	None known

Table 16-3 (continued)
Drugs and Reported Effects on the Fetus

Drugs	1st Trimester Effects	2nd and 3rd Trimester Effects
Anticoagulants		
Heparin	None known	Hemorrhage (?), stillbirth (?)
Anticonvulsants		
Barbiturates	Malformations (?)	Bleeding withdrawal
Carbamazepine	Craniofacial, neural tube (?)	Bleeding, withdrawal, Growth retardation
Clonazepam	None known	Withdrawal, depression
Ethosuximide	None known	None known
Primidone	Orofacial clefts	Hemorrhage, depletion of vitamin K-dependent clotting factors
Valproic acid	Spina bifida, facial dysmorphogenesis	Perinatal distress, behavioral abnormalities
Anti-infection agents		
Aminoglycosides	None known	Nephrotoxic (?), ototoxic(?)
Azalone-quinolones	None known	None known
Cephalosporins	None known	None known
Chloramphenicol	None known	Vascular collapse
Clindamycin	Unknown	Unknown
Erythromycin	None known	None known
Isoniazid	Malformations	Behavioral abnormality
Metronidazole	None known	None known
Nitrofurantoin	None known	Hemolysis (?)
Penicillins	None known	None known
Rifampin	Malformations (?)	None known
Sulfonamides	None known	Hyperbilirubinemia (?)
Trimethoprim	Unknown	Unknown
Tetracyclines	None known	Stained deciduous teeth (enamel hypoplasia)
Cancer chemotherapy		
Alkylating agents	Abortion, anomalies	Hypoplastic gonads, growth retardation and delay

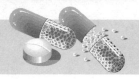

Table 16-3 *(continued)*

Drugs	1st Trimester Effects	2nd and 3rd Trimester Effects
Antimetabolites		
Pyrimidine analogues (Cytosine arabinoside)	Same as above	Same as above
Purine analogues (Thioguanine, Mercaptopurine)	Same as above	Same as above, transient anemia
Antibiotics (actinomycin)	Same as above	Same as above
Vinca alkyloids (Vincristine)	Same as above	Same as above
Cardiovascular drugs		
Antihypertensives		
Methyldopa	None known	Hemolytic anemia, tremor hypotension,
Hydralazine	Skeletal defects (?)	Tachycardia, thrombocytopenia
Propranolol	None known	Bradycardia, growth retardation, hypoglycemia, respiratory distress
Reserpine	None known	Lethargy, respiratory distress
β-Sympathomimetics	None known	Tachycardia
Digitalis	None known	Bradycardia
Colds and cough preparations		
Antihistamines	None known	None known
Cough suppressants	None known	None known
Decongestants	None known	None known
Expectorants	Fetal goiter (?)	None known
Dextromethorphan	None known	None known
Diuretics		
Furosemide	None known	Death from sudden hypoperfusion, electrolyte imbalance
Thiazides	None known	Thrombocytopenia, hypokalemia hyperbilirubinemia, hyponatremia
Fertility drugs		
Clomiphene	Meiotic nondisjunction (?) Neural tube defects(?)	Unknown
Hormones		
Androgens	Masculinization of female fetus	Adrenal suppression (?)
Corticosteroids	Orofacial cleft in animals, not in humans	Growth retardation (?)
Estrogens	Cardiovascular anomalies (?)	None known

Table 16-3 (continued)

Drugs	1st Trimester Effects	2nd and 3rd Trimester Effects
Progestins	Limb and CV anomalies (?) "VACTERL" syndrome, masculization of female fetus(?)	None known
Danazol	Virilization of female fetus (?)	None known
Hypoglycemics		
Insulin	None known	None known
Sulfonylureas	Anomalies (?)	Suppressed insulin secretion
Laxatives		
Bisacodyl	Unknown	Unknown
Docusate	None known	None known
Mineral oil	Decreased maternal vitamin absorption	Decreased maternal vitamin absorption
Milk of magnesia	None known	None known
Psychoactive drugs		
Antidepressants (tricyclics)	None known	None known
Benzodiazepines	Facial dysmorphism (?)	Depression, floppy infant, hypothermia,withdrawal
Hydroxyzine	None known	None known, behavioral abnormalities
Meprobamate	Cardiac anomalies (?), major malformations (?)	None known
Phenothiazines	None known	TcMuscle rigidity, hypothermia, tremor
Sedatives	None known	Depression, slow learning
Lithium	Facial clefts; Cardiovascular anomaly (?)	Lithium toxicity (neurologic and hepatic dysfunction)
Radiolabeled diagnostic drugs		
Albumin	Does not cross	None known
Technetium	Does not cross	None known
13 (diagnostic)	None known	None known
Thyroid drugs		
Antithyroid (therapeutic)	Goiter, abortion, anomalies	Goiter, airway obstruction, hypothyroid, mental retardation
Propylthiouracil	Goiter	Same
Methimazole	Aplasia cutis (?), goiter	Same, aplasia cutis (?)
Thyroid USP	None known	None known
Thyroxine	None known	None known

173

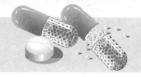
Table 16-3 (continued)

Drugs	1st Trimester Effects	2nd and 3rd Trimester Effects
Magnesium sulfate	None known	Hypermagnesemia, respiratory depression
β-sympathomimetics	None known	Tachycardia, hypothermia, hypocalcemia, hypo- and hyperglycemia
Vaginal preparations		
Antifungal agents	None known	None known
Podophyllin	Metagenesis (?)	CNS effects (?)
Vitamins (high dose)		
A	Urogenital and craniofacial anomalies (?)	None known
C	None known	Scurvy after delivery (if deficient)
D	Supravalvular aortic stenosis (?)	None known
E	Unknown	None known
K	Unknown	Hemorrhage, if deficiency
Street drugs		
LSD	None known	Withdrawal, behavioral effects
Marijuana	Fetal alcohol syndrome	Behavioral effects, growth retardation
Methaqualone	None known	Withdrawal
Heroin	None known	Depression, withdrawal
Methadone	None known	Withdrawal, growth retardation
Pentazocine	None known	Withdrawal , growth retardation
Phencyclidine	None known	Withdrawal, neurobehavioral, growth retardation
Cocaine	Placental abruption, vascular disruption, urinary tract anomalies	Withdrawal, placental, abruption, vascular disruption, growth retardation, behavioral difficulties
Other		
Cimetidine	Unknown	Liver impairment (?)
Caffeine	Anomalies (?) in high doses, abortion (?)	Jitteriness
Azathioprine	Abortion	Anemia,. thrombocytopenia, lymphopenia, growth retardation
Bromocriptine	None known	None known
Spermicides	None known	None known
Lead	Abortion, CNS disorders	Stillbirth, mental retardation

*Proven teratogen.

Unknown = no studies to investigate fetal effects; None known = no malformations reported in human studies or no consistent malformations in animal studies (when no human studies reported); (?) = conflicting information to question any increase risk of a previously reported anomaly.

Notes

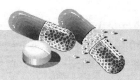

Managing Medical Problems During Pregnancy

While every woman thinks about her personal health during pregnancy, Nature has made it possible for most to adjust to the situation with a minimum of problems. In fact, many women feel better during pregnancy than at any other time in their lives. But, although pregnancy is a normal physical event and not a disease, it creates big changes in the body and makes strong demands on it as well. And, for the substantial number of women who go into pregnancy with an underlying health problem, stress and even danger can occur. Sometimes these medical problems remain undiscovered until pregnancy; sometimes the mother is well aware of them before she conceives. In either case, very careful attention must be paid to the mother's health problem and the treatment needed to control it.

About one in every five pregnant women has an underlying medical disorder, but medicine has made great strides in managing diseases that used to make completing a pregnancy impossible. We are treating a higher proportion of women with medical complications all the time. The list of diseases that can complicate pregnancy is very long, but the most common are anemia, including both iron and folic acid deficiency; high blood pressure (hypertension); heart problems other than hypertension; diabetes; thyroid disease, both overactive (hyperthyroid) and underactive (hypothyroid); epilepsy; phlebitis, that is, blood clots in the legs, pelvic region, or lungs; asthma; morbid obesity (100 or more pounds overweight); organ transplantation; and sexually transmitted diseases.

Besides worrying about her own well-being, the mother-to-be with health problems will be concerned about the effects of her disease on her baby plus the effects of the medication or therapy that must be used to control it. All of the problems just mentioned require the use of drugs in their medical management. Many of them are discussed in the following sections in more detail.

Hypertension

Hypertension or high blood pressure is caused by constriction or tightening of the blood vessels of the body. To pump the blood through the body at the necessary rate, the pressure in the vessels must be higher than normal because their diameter is smaller. Some cases of hypertension are related to underlying heart disease or "hardening" of the arteries, but other cases seem to exist by themselves. Hypertension is often symptom-free and for this reason is especially dangerous. People sometimes don't even realize they are hypertensive until it is too late and they suffer a stroke or other blood vessel damage.

There are four different types of hypertension found during pregnancy: (1) acute hypertension, also known as preeclampsia-eclampsia, pregnancy-induced hypertension, or toxemia (this develops only during the last 3 months of pregnancy); (2) chronic hypertension; (3) chronic hypertension with additional acute hypertension; and (4) transient hypertension, which occurs during labor or immediately after delivery and then subsides.

Acute Hypertension

Acute hypertension or preeclampsia is not preventable, but it is treatable. It is seen more commonly with first pregnancies and is a disorder doctors will watch for closely in first pregnancies, which is why your doctor will take your blood pressure at each prenatal visit. When it is discovered in its mild stage, its most dangerous complications can be avoided almost completely. If not treated in time, both mother and infant may suffer the consequences. The first symptoms are usually noticed after the 20th week of pregnancy. They include swelling of the face and hands, blood pressure greater than 140/90 (or big jumps over previous readings), and the presence of significant protein in the urine. One of the things the doctor looks for in the urine sample you leave at each visit is protein, which may indicate signs of preeclampsia.

A diagnosis of mild preeclampsia means you will have to check into the hospital for awhile. A woman with preeclampsia must have complete bed rest, preferably lying on her side. She will need a nutritious diet. If all goes well, within a couple of days she should have a noticeable loss of water, and her other symptoms should begin to subside. If she is at or near term, the doctor may consider inducing labor.

With severe preeclampsia, blood pressure rises even higher (to 160/100 or more), protein in the urine increases, urination may be inadequate, visual or mental disturbances may arise, abdominal pain can occur, and there may be difficulty in breathing. With such symptoms, the expectant mother will need her blood pressure monitored several times a day. She should be given intravenous magnesium sulfate, a drug that prevents the convulsions sometimes resulting from preeclampsia. Nearly all obstetricians use this drug around delivery time when it becomes necessary to treat any worsening hypertensive complications. The drug does not actually lower blood pressure a great deal. Rather, it seems to prevent severe fluctuations in blood pressure, which are damaging to the fetus. Most studies have shown that it does not have severe toxic side effects for the mother and fetus when given in proper dosages. Excessive magnesium can cause a slowing down of muscular responses and ultimately breathing and heart rate for both mother and child. Calcium chloride counteracts the effects of excessive magnesium and can be given if such symptoms are noticed.

If a woman with severe preeclampsia does have a convulsion, she now has eclampsia. We believe that, once the doctor has treated these symptoms adequately, labor should be induced and the baby delivered, for this is the only true cure for preeclampsia/eclampsia.

Remember, preeclampsia is most common in first pregnancies in young women under age 25. (It occurs in 8% of them.) To prevent it, see your doctor early in pregnancy and at frequent intervals. Lay on your left side in bed for at least 60 minutes per day, starting at the 14th week of pregnancy, and eat a nutritious diet high in protein. Promising new research indicates that taking a low dose of aspirin (50-80 mg/day or 1 baby aspirin/per day) and extra calcium (2000 milligrams per day) may prevent preeclampsia.

Chronic Hypertension

Chronic hypertension usually exists in the mother prior to pregnancy, whether or not she is aware of it. Pregnancy tends to provoke chronic hypertension, which, unlike preeclampsia, is more common in women who have had two or more children or who are over age 35. Even in its milder forms, it is dangerous for the fetus: the fetal death rate goes as high as 15% when the disease is left untreated.

With chronic hypertension, your doctor will prescribe a chest x-ray examination, electrocardiogram, and laboratory studies and then a medication to control the hypertension. Once you discover you are pregnant, we recommend that you stop taking any diuretics (fluid pills).

If her blood pressure changes are not too great, the pregnant woman can monitor blood pressure herself at home twice a day, three times a week. She should see her doctor more often, since it may even be possible to discontinue the high blood pressure medication, at least for a period of time. But if blood pressure continues to rise, hospitalization and bed rest combined with appropriate medications are the only alternatives.

Note: The three most important things a woman with chronic hypertension can do for herself are monitor her blood pressure conscientiously, rest in bed on her side at least 2 hours per day, and eat a nutritious, high-protein diet.

Drugs used to Treat Hypertension

The doctor's challenge in treating hypertension is to be able to find the right combination of therapy and drugs that will do a minimal amount of harm to the unborn child while adequately treating medical problems.

Obstetricians avoid diuretics (fluid pills) during pregnancy because they suspect these drugs create undesirable side effects in both mother and child. The thiazide diuretic drugs (Diuril, Hydrodiuril, Dyazide) are often prescribed to nonpregnant women but have been associated with jaundice (a blood disorder causing yellowish skin), low sodium, and low platelet count (cells necessary for blood clotting) in the infant. Other diuretics, such as furosemide (Lasix), ethacrynic acid (Edacrin), spironolactone, and chlorthalidone, have been studied less, and their use is recommended only in severe cases of water retention.

Alpha-methyldopa (Aldomet) is widely used for blood pressure control. More studies of this antihypertension medication have been made than of any other drug used for the same purpose. To date it appears to be safe for both mother and child, and it is the primary drug that we recommend for control of chronic hypertension in pregnancy.

Propranolol (Inderal) is also used in the management of hypertension. Right now, we feel its effects on the fetus are likely minimal, despite a few early reports noting growth delay and slowed respiration and heart beat in newborns. Other drugs being used to control hypertension during pregnancy are labetalol (Trandate, Normodyne) and nifedipine (Procardia).

Recently, several drug companies have issued new warnings about the use of ACE inhibitors in the second and third trimesters of pregnancy. These drugs can cause injury and even death to the developing fetus, and should be discontinued as quickly as possible after pregnancy is discovered. ACE inhibitors are a new class of drugs used in the control of hypertension. They come under the names of captopril, fosinopril, benazapril, ramipril, lisinopril, enalapril, and quinapril. Most other antihypertension drugs are relatively safe during pregnancy, provided a physician supervises their use carefully.

Hydralazine (Apresoline) helps to dilate constricted blood vessels. Wide experience with this medication has convinced us that it is not harmful during pregnancy. Given in combination with methyldopa, it appears to be a relatively safe form of hypertension control. In cases of acute hypertension it will have to be given intravenously, although in less serious situations it is effective when taken orally.

Heart Disease

With the improvements in the treatment of heart birth defects and other heart diseases, many women are alive today who would never have survived twenty or more years ago. As a result, obstetricians frequently see pregnant women with histories of cardiac disease. We estimate that anywhere between .1.0% and 3.7% of pregnant women have some kind of heart disease. It is the fourth leading cause of death in pregnant women in the United States.

Pregnancy puts a lot of demand on the heart. The volume of blood in the arteries, the heart rate, and the amount of blood pumped by each heartbeat rises to a peak in the second to early third trimesters. The heart must do a great deal of work during and after labor and this can cause great stress if the heart is weakened to begin with.

Specific Cardiac Diseases

Congenital heart diseases, such as atrial septal defect, ventricular septal defect, mitral valve prolapse and patent ductus arteriosus, are among the more common ones found in pregnant patients. Many women will have had surgical repair of the lesions, others will not. Mitral valve prolapse rarely requires surgery. Usually these congenital disorders do not cause great problems during pregnancy, but occasionally they will trigger lung congestion, irregular heart beat, tiny blood clots, or infection.

Cardiac arrhythmias, i.e., fast, slow, or irregular heartbeats, require monitoring and often treatment during pregnancy. In addition to the drugs already mentioned, quinidine (Duraquin, Quinalan), procainamide (Pronestyl), disopyramide, phenytoin (Dilantin), verapamil (Calan, Isoptin), amiodarone (Cordarone), adenosine, and digoxin immune antibody fragment have all been used to treat arrhythmias. With the exception of quinidine, unless there are very specific indications, we prefer *not* to use these drugs to treat cardiac rhythm disorders, in part because they have not been tested adequately in pregnant women yet.

Rheumatic heart disease (rheumatic fever) can affect any or all of the heart valves - the mitral valve, the aortic valve, the tricuspid valve, or the pulmonary artery valve. Other problems can affect the heart valves as well. When tests indicate that a pregnant woman with heart valve disorders is experiencing cardiac stress, therapy consists of bed rest, plus careful use of fluid pills and digoxin (Lanoxin). Digoxin is helpful for arrhythmias (irregular heart beats), as are the so-called beta blockers (Inderal, metoprolol, labetalol).

Women with any type of heart valve disease, whether pregnant or not, must be careful about infections. Talk to your doctor or dentist about an antibiotic prescription before you have dental work done. Watch for signs of infection such as fever, sweating, chills, muscle aches and pains, and if these occur, call your doctor immediately. Rheumatic heart disease can and does flare up during pregnancy.

Coarctation of the aorta is a narrowing of the biggest artery in the body near the shoulder. It can cause chest pain, leg fatigue, and hypertension. If pregnant women with this problem develop symptoms, they need bed rest, antihypertension medication, beta blockers (such as, Inderal, labetolol) and antibiotics.

Idiopathic hypertrophic subaortic stenosis (IHSS), a thickening of the heart muscle, can produce shortness of breath and chest pain. Without medication, women, pregnant or not, risk sudden death with this disease. Inderal and the so-called calcium channel blockers (nifedipine, verapamil) are useful in the medical treatment of this disease. We also recommend that a pregnant patient with IHSS receive Holter monitoring to detect symptoms of irregular heart rhythms that might otherwise go unnoticed.

Unfortunately, drugs used to treat cardiac problems can sometimes create problems of their own. Digoxin and digitoxin can produce toxic effects such as rhythm disturbances, nausea, vomiting, headaches, and nervous symptoms. Under such circumstances, lidocaine, a local anesthetic must be given by injection or intravenously.

Artificial cardiac valves. Pregnant women with artificial cardiac valves present a special challenge for obstetricians. People with artificial heart valves must take anticoagulant drugs (blood thinners) all of their lives. Of the two common ones, warfarin (Coumadin) and heparin, heparin is by far the safer during pregnancy because it does not cross the placenta. Heparin usage must be closely monitored however, because it can cause abnormal bleeding. If heparin is prescribed and there is heavy bruising, small cuts that won't clot, or other signs of "thin" blood, a physician must be seen immediately. A drug called protamine sulfate can reverse the effects of heparin.

Special Cautions During Labor and Delivery

If there is a damaged heart valve, or if there is a high risk for bacterial endocarditis, a serious infection of the heart valves, we recommend that the patient be given antibiotics, such as penicillin and gentamicin, to protect against this infection during labor and delivery, especially in the case of a cesarean section.

Certain drugs used to *inhibit* premature labor, including ritodrine and terbutaline, can be very hard on the heart. If a cardiac disease is present, we recommend against using these drugs to stop premature labor; we prefer to use magnesium sulfate or, possibly, indomethacin (Indocin) for this problem.

If labor must be *induced*, oxytocin (Pitocin) is safe with gradually increasing doses, but a large dose all at once could create problems. Ergonovine and methylergonovine maleate (Methergine) should be avoided in women with hypertension, since they can cause severe hypertension and have even been associated with heart attack or stroke after delivery.

Intravenous fluids given to a women in labor with heart disease should be infused slowly and carefully to avoid overloading the heart. If the heart disease is serious, physicians may decide to monitor the heart with a Swan-Ganz catheter as a precaution.

Diabetes Mellitus

Diabetes is caused by a disturbance in one of the most important glands in the body - the pancreas. When affected, the pancreas does not release insulin properly and the body is unable to use the sugar in its blood for fuel. People with uncontrolled diabetes typically feel hungry and thirsty all the time, while simultaneously experiencing weakness and great fatigue. Excessive sugar can be found in both their blood and their urine.

From 2% to 3% of women who become pregnant have some form of diabetes. Diabetic pregnancies are considered high risk because so many complications can arise from a deficiency of insulin. These mothers are subject to problems with their metabolism and blood vessels and sometimes to infections. Babies of diabetic mothers are susceptible to premature delivery, birth defects, metabolic problems, being excessively large, and breathing difficulties. However, with the advances that have been made in medical science, a diabetic mother under meticulous care today has a good chance of bearing a healthy infant.

One of the key steps in averting problems is preconceptual counseling. Diabetic women who wish to complete a successful pregnancy need to plan way ahead, and that means before they get pregnant *(See Chapter 13)*.

Like high blood pressure, diabetes is often unmasked by pregnancy. Pregnancy makes great demands on the metabolism, the system the body uses to heat and cool itself and to fuel itself for action. The hormones of pregnancy change the way sugar is used by the body for energy. These changes must take place so both the unborn child and the mother can receive the nutrition they need for health. In the second half of pregnancy insulin requirements are about twice those of nonpregnant women. The extra insulin available causes pregnant women to have lower blood sugar levels than they would normally because so much of their sugar and protein is being used by the placenta and ultimately the fetus.

Despite these complex changes, most pregnant women tolerate the added demands of sugar and carbohydrate burning very well. Women with known or hidden diabetes, however, will not be so fortunate. Their blood sugar levels will rise and continue to be high during their entire pregnancy; if left untreated, these high levels may prove very dangerous to both the fetus and the mother. Therefore obstetricians must assist in controlling the blood sugar levels of pregnant diabetics very carefully through the use of insulin and diet.

In some cases a properly adjusted diet will do the trick. Caloric intake should be about 2000 to 2400 calories daily. About 45% of the calories should come from carbohydrates, 35% or less from fat, and 20% from protein. Approximately 20% of the food needed should be consumed at breakfast, 30% at lunch, 35% at dinner, and 15% as a late snack. Expectant mothers with diabetes should not go for long periods without eating.

Oral drugs to control diabetes should not be used during pregnancy. Although helpful to the mother, they cross the placenta and stimulate the fetal pancreas, which could be harmful. Subcutaneously injected insulin (insulin shots given just under the skin), on the other hand, will not cross the placenta and have no direct effect on the fetus. Most pregnant diabetics will need subcutaneous insulin, even those who have previously managed their problem with oral drugs or diet control. Since insulin must be taken every day, and often more than once, it is more convenient for a woman to administer her own insulin. While some need instructions on how to give themselves insulin injections, we have never seen a woman who was not able to learn how to do this.

The length of time it takes for insulin to act and the duration it should stay in the bloodstream must be adjusted to each patient's individual needs. Improved, more purified insulin is being marketed today, and in the future it will be easier to take insulin in lower doses with fewer side effects. Fast-acting and intermediate type insulins are preferable to long-acting insulin during pregnancy. Recombinant DNA human insulin, which was first marketed in 1983, is preferable in pregnancy, whether the pregnant woman has been using beef or pork insulin or whether she has never taken insulin before.

Usually the prospective mother's requirements for insulin will either decrease or remain unchanged during the first half of pregnancy, whereas they will almost certainly increase during the second half. Diabetics also must be managed very carefully during labor and delivery.

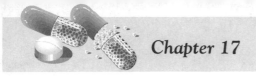

Blood sugar levels must be checked frequently so that neither too much nor too little sugar appears. Insulin may have to be administered every 4 hours and blood sugar levels adjusted with intravenous glucose injection. An alternative method is intravenous insulin diluted to 1000 cc of fluid. After delivery, insulin requirements will be lower than normal for several days.

Insulin must be used very carefully because it can have side effects. The most dangerous of these is hypoglycemia, or too little sugar in the blood. People with diabetes should always be prepared with a high-sugar food in their purses or pockets to counteract this problem. Allergic skin reactions may occur at the site where injections are administered but usually go away of their own accord. Fat just under the skin where the insulin is injected may begin to disappear. The site of injection should be changed regularly, and sometimes a more purified form of pork insulin or human insulin will need to be substituted.

The pregnant woman's need for insulin can fluctuate widely during the course of her pregnancy, which is why she must visit her doctor frequently. The increasing demands of pregnancy, acute infection, drug consumption, and overactivity of certain glands may explain this greater need for insulin. Problems with the placenta, inactivity, kidney disease, inadequate food intake, or underactivity of certain glands may decrease insulin requirements. A diabetic mother-to-be must become sensitive to the way insulin works in her body so that she can quickly report changes that may require a dosage or even an insulin type change.

The care of diabetic pregnant women has been revolutionized during the past decade. We now ask the mother to participate actively in her care by following her diet carefully and doing home blood sugar measurements by pricking her finger. Most women check their blood sugar four to six times a day, three times a week. This is the only way that tight control of blood sugar can be achieved with insulin.

In cases where women have a great deal of trouble controlling their insulin levels, insulin pumps have been used. This device, which is placed on the abdomen, supplies insulin continuously through a needle inserted just under the skin. We are not as enthusiastic now about this form of diabetes control for pregnant women as we were earlier and don't often prescribe it.

Many fetal tests are also done to assess fetal health from the thirty-fourth week of pregnancy until the baby is delivered. Currently, we deliver infants of diabetic mothers at anywhere from 37 to 40 weeks so the babies do not gain too much weight, a common problem when the mother has diabetes. Around half of these mothers will require a cesarean section because their cervixes are simply too firm and closed for an induction of labor.

New measurement tools which allow us to closely monitor fetal heart rate and fetal kicks now permit pregnant diabetics to carry their babies to term.

Thyroid Disorders

The thyroid gland, located on the lower part of the front of the neck, is one of the master glands of the body. Its job is to regulate the metabolism of the body, which includes temperature, heart rate, and use of food calories. It is intimately connected with the function of several other important glands, such as the pancreas, the pituitary, and the adrenals.

During pregnancy the two most common thyroid disorders found are hyperthyroidism and hypothyroidism.

Hyperthyroidism

Hyperthyroidism means the thyroid gland overworks itself by producing too much of the thyroid hormone called *thyroxine*. The swelling that often occurs in the neck with hyperthyroidism is known as goiter. Symptoms of an overactive thyroid are rapid heartbeat, weakness, increased appetite, shaking hands, and shortness of breath. Since these are often common complaints of pregnancy, an overactive thyroid gland may not be immediately detected during checkups.

Treatment of an overly active thyroid gland before pregnancy includes drug therapy, surgery, or radioactive iodine administration. During pregnancy drug therapy is the safest form of treatment, and, in fact, is necessary to prevent serious maternal and fetal complications, such as thyrotoxicosis, a medical emergency. The two drugs recommended for treatment of an overactive thyroid are propylthiouracil (PTU) and methimazole (Tapazole). Under no circumstances should pregnant women take radioactive iodine. It crosses the placenta readily and can have very damaging effects on the fetal thyroid, even in small doses taken for a short period of time. Propylthiouracil is preferable to methimazole in pregnancy because transfer through the placenta is probably slower. Propylthiouracil gradually lowers the amount of thyroxine stored in the body. The excess amounts are what cause the symptoms of hyperthyroidism, but it may take from 3 to 6 weeks for the full effect of the drug to be noticeable. After satisfactory thyroid hormone levels are obtained, women may be able to discontinue their thyroid medications. Daily doses should not exceed 300 mg so that side effects to the fetus can be prevented.

Because it does transfer through the placenta, propylthiouracil may affect the fetal thyroid gland. An enlarged thyroid (goiter) has been reported in up to 10% of all infants exposed to anti-thyroid medication prenatally, Fortunately, symptoms of a malfunctioning gland in newborns tend to disappear a few days after birth. From 70% to 95% of pregnancies in which thyroid medication is used have a favorable outcome with no lasting effects on the baby.

Propranolol (Inderal) can be taken to control the symptoms of an overactive thyroid, such as rapid heartbeat, shaking, and palpitations. As discussed previously, experience with its use in pregnant women has not yet been wide enough to declare its absolute safety. Up to this time, no significant problems have been associated with its use.

Hypothyroidism

Hypothyroidism (an underactive thyroid gland) is much less common in pregnancy than hyperthyroidism. Usually it occurs when a woman has had a large portion of her thyroid gland removed because it was originally overactive. Symptoms include tiring easily, intolerance to cold, slow reflexes, and general sluggishness. Once again, these overlap with many of the symptoms of pregnancy, and it may not be easy for a doctor to diagnose an underactive thyroid.

If a pregnant woman has hypothyroidism, she will have to take a thyroid hormone supplement. We recommend synthetic levothyroxine (Synthroid) because it is the drug that is best absorbed and best tolerated by pregnant women. Thyroid supplements do not pass the placental barrier in any great amounts and do not seem to affect the fetus. The only major complication with levothyroxine is overdosage, in which case the symptoms will be those of hyperthyroidism. The treatment is to check the levels of thyroid-stimulating hormone (TSH) in the mother's blood and adjust the dosage slightly.

Epilepsy

Epilepsy is a set of symptoms caused by disturbances in the brain and other parts of the nervous system that produce an altered state of consciousness. This state may be a vague feeling of withdrawal or being out of touch with the surroundings, a feeling of dread that something bad is going to happen, depression, odors or sounds or sights that aren't really there (hallucinations), or it may even be complete unconsciousness. In its worst form, epilepsy causes violent seizures, jerking, writhing, and stiffening of the body; there may even be moments when breathing comes to a temporary halt.

Epilepsy is one of the most common diseases in the world; it occurs in 0.5% of the entire world population, a number that runs into the millions. In most cases seizures start before the age of 18, so epilepsy is found widely in people of reproductive age. Advances in medicine have permitted epileptics to lead more normal lives, find partners, and bear children. Thus the likelihood of a woman with epilepsy becoming pregnant is quite high; epileptics represent between 0.33% and 1% of all pregnancies.

The combination of social problems and medical hazards means that epilepsy resulting in seizures must be treated, even during pregnancy. Seizures are not only bad for the mother, they are bad for the fetus because they can deprive it of oxygen and create high blood acid levels, a condition that is suspected to cause birth defects and perhaps brain damage. Unfortunately, some drugs used to control seizures have bad effects on the fetus, too. Minimizing their use while controlling seizures is the main challenge for doctors managing pregnant epileptics. Because of the risks of using these drugs, a woman with epilepsy should carefully evaluate how important having a child is to her and what she is willing to cope with if the infant has problems. Remember, you have to weigh risks versus benefits with almost any drug. In the case of drugs to treat epilepsy, the risks may be somewhat higher, but they don't necessarily outweigh the benefit of having a child, if that is very important to you.

Causes and Types of Epilepsy

Epilepsy has a wide range of causes. These include infections like meningitis or encephalitis; poisons like mercury, or lead; various drugs; birth injuries and injury from accidents; and heredity. If a mother has the type of epilepsy without any known specific cause, the chances of her child developing it are about 2% to 3%, five times higher than the general population.

It has many different forms, but most people have one of four major types: *(1)* grand mal epilepsy, *(2)* focal epilepsy, *(3)* psychomotor epilepsy, and *(4)* petit mal epilepsy.

Grand mal epilepsy is the most commonly recognized form of epilepsy, and it occurs either alone or in combination with petit mal or psychomotor epilepsy in more than 70% of epileptics. The violent seizures of epilepsy occur with the grand mal form. They are similar to the type of convulsion seen in eclampsia (also known as toxemia of pregnancy).

Focal epilepsy often begins with twitching of the thumb, big toe, or face and may limit itself to such a twitching episode. It can also go on to the same kind of convulsions found in grand mal epilepsy.

Psychomotor epilepsy is characterized by altered moods, disturbing thoughts, and visual distortions. The victim may also involuntarily smack her lips, chew, or make other motions. Other changes include salivation, perspiration, and dilation of the pupils.

Petit mal epilepsy is characterized by brief spells of absence from or being out of touch with the outside world. The victim may blink her eyes or roll them back, but frequently no one else even realizes that she has had a seizure. Petit mal epilepsy usually disappears after adolescence, so it is rarely seen in combination with pregnancy.

Treatment During Pregnancy

At least half of all pregnant women with epilepsy find that their seizures worsen during pregnancy. Almost everyone with grand mal epilepsy will have this happen. This is probably due to some of the physical changes of pregnancy and because the treatment drugs become diluted in the blood as its volume increases. Thus, more drugs are needed to achieve the same level of protection against seizures. Sometimes mothers-to-be stop using their anti-seizure medication because they are afraid of hurting their unborn baby. Sometimes they simply can't keep the pills down because of nausea and vomiting.

It is absolutely critical that drugs prescribed for epilepsy are taken. Otherwise there is the danger of a condition known as status epilepticus (uncontrolled seizures) which could harm the individual and the baby. We only recommend discontinuing anti-seizure medication if an individual has been free of seizures for a number of years.

Among the many problems that epilepsy and its treatment can cause are vaginal bleeding, toxemia, premature birth, low birth weight, birth defects, and vitamin D deficiency. Blood clotting problems, poor breathing, and drug withdrawal are some of the concerns for the newborn. Deaths in infants born to epileptic mothers are twice that of the general populace (although both are very low in western countries). One study of 2,000 such babies revealed that a larger than average number had defects of one kind or another in virtually every part of the body.

Since a pregnant woman with epilepsy must take her medications, the challenge to physicians is to find a way to control the seizures with as few effects on the fetus as possible. Here are his or her considerations:

1. The drug used for controlling seizures should have the best possible balance between effectiveness and potential harm to the fetus.

2. Selection of drug and treatment planning should be done *before* conception.

3. If possible, a single drug should be used in the lowest effective dosages to see if seizures can be controlled.

4. If the levels of a single drug become toxic before they become effective, then a second drug should be added, with the dosages of both drugs kept to moderate levels.

5. If the second drug accomplishes complete seizure control, then the dosage of the first should be slowly decreased but not stopped.

6. Any changes in the drugs should be made very slowly.

7. The levels of drugs should be checked with blood tests periodically.

8. In some cases, medications cannot control the seizures completely.

9. The woman and her doctor should work to prevent excessive weight gain and fluid retention since these can increase the risk of seizures.

10. Women not taking their drugs or taking too low a drug dosage are the main reasons epilepsy medications fail to control seizures.

11. Anticonvulsant or anti-epilepsy drugs must be continued during labor and delivery.

Drug used for Seizure Control

For grand mal and focal motor epilepsy phenobarbital and phenytoin (Dilantin) are the first choice drugs. Phenobarbital is less likely to affect the unborn child but may be more effective when used in conjunction with phenytoin. Primidone and carbamazepine may also be used for the grand mal and focal motor forms of epilepsy. Psychomotor epilepsy may be especially difficult to control, and primidone is the best agent to use. Phenytoin may be added, and phenobarbital, carbamazepine, and valproic acid are sometimes useful.

Although petit mal epilepsy is rare in pregnancy, if a woman suffers from this form, her number one drug choice is ethosuximide followed by clonazepam, which may occasionally be necessary.

Trimethadione (Tridione), which is used for petit mal seizures, has a high potential for producing birth defects and should not be used by women during their reproductive years. Luckily, there are good alternatives to Tridione for petit mal treatment. One of these is ethosuximide, a drug with a much lower incidence of reported associated birth defects.

Phenytoin (Dilantin) is taken by the majority of pregnant epileptics. Unfortunately, this drug sometimes produces birth defects, blood clotting problems, and mental retardation in the baby. The "Dilantin syndrome" is well known and consists of growth retardation, peculiar facial features, and mild mental retardation. It occurs in 7-10% of pregnancies where the mother is an epileptic, and the occurrence appears to be unrelated to the dosage of phenytoin received. Phenytoin does not accumulate in very great levels in breast milk; thus breast feeding can be undertaken, even if the mother is using the drug.

Phenobarbital is probably less harmful than phenytoin, but it too has some undesirable effects, such as creating a deficiency of folic acid and blood clotting problems in the newborn infant. If a pregnant woman with epilepsy takes phenytoin, phenobarbital, or primidone, she must take extra folic acid throughout her pregnancy. Her baby will need a vitamin K injection at birth. In addition, infants must often withdraw from phenobarbital at birth because it is an addictive drug and can cause respiratory depression and other drug withdrawal symptoms.

Withdrawal problems similar to phenobarbital occur with primidone. It too is associated with blood clotting abnormalities and birth defects. It hasn't been studied as thoroughly as Dilantin, so the evidence is less powerful, but, nevertheless, mothers should know that a risk is associated with this drug.

Blood Clots

Excessive blood clotting is one of the major medical problems seen during pregnancy. *Thrombosis*, *thrombophlebitis*, and *embolus formation* are terms that refer to blood clot formation, primarily in the veins. When thrombosis occurs, a cluster of blood particles of different kinds becomes stuck together to form a clot or thrombus. The danger is that the flow of blood through a vessel will be stopped and important organs like the brain or lungs might not receive enough blood. Thrombophlebitis refers to clot formation in a vein. An embolus is a clot that has moved from where it first formed to a smaller vessel where it plugs the circulation. Deep vein thrombosis of the legs and feet, pelvic vein thrombosis or thrombophlebitis, and pulmonary embolus (clots in the lungs) account for 50% of the deaths and illnesses related to pregnancy.

Physicians think that the risk of clot formation during pregnancy is particularly high because venous blood flow is not as strong in pregnant women. Their blood is thicker and more likely to clot, and blood vessels are more likely to be injured because of the added pressure put on them. In the last 3 months of pregnancy, fibrin, one of the blood particles involved in clot formation increases substantially. In the time right after delivery, women are also susceptible to clot formation.

Symptoms of clot formation include pain in the legs or feet, difficulty walking, swelling of the legs, feet, and ankles, and warmth or tenderness in a specific area. It should be mentioned that these could also be symptoms of varicose veins - veins appearing just under the skin that don't have good valve action for returning blood to the heart and thus tend to swell and get lumpy. Varicose veins are uncomfortable and at times unsightly but not dangerous unless deep vein thrombosis is also present.

Support stockings relieve some of the discomfort of leg vein problems. Elevating the feet above the waist several times a day is helpful. While standing in one place for a long time can increase leg vein discomfort, walking is beneficial because it stimulates circulation.

Women with a history of blood clots, anemic mothers, women with cancer, and women undergoing cesarean section run a higher risk of blood clot formation. For these women, we believe some attempt should be made to prevent clot formation, especially at delivery. Small doses of an anti-clot drug called heparin can be safely given to pregnant women. Heparin must be injected under the skin to work, however, so it is usually given in the hospital. If, after delivery, a woman develops a fever with no evidence of infection, we believe she has pelvic thrombophlebitis, and we administer full-dose heparin to thin the blood.

We recommend against the use of anti-clot pills such as Coumadin (warfarin) during pregnancy. The danger of hemorrhage is great with this drug, both for the mother and the baby, because it crosses the cord into the placenta.

Asthma

For reasons that physicians don't completely understand, asthma is becoming more and more common in the United States. This closing up of the bronchi (breathing tubes in the chest) is caused by allergies, sensitivity to pollutants in the air, and chronic infection. Asthma attacks can be triggered by physical or emotional stress. Right now, more than 1% of pregnant women have some form of asthma. During pregnancy, asthma remains the same for about half of those women who have it, gets better in a quarter of them, and gets worse in the other quarter.

A lot of medications have been developed to treat asthma, and most of these appear to be relatively safe for use during pregnancy. Some of them are available in inhalants of various kinds, some in tablet form. Terbutaline (Brethaire), albuterol (Ventolin, Proventil), and metaproteronol (Alupent) inhalers are the mainstays of asthma treatment. Women with stubborn, chronic asthma will need to use them on a daily basis.

Theophylline (Theo-Dur), a tablet that helps keep the airways open is also used every day by many asthmatics. However, while this drug is generally safe, it has side effects and its levels must be monitored in the blood periodically to be sure the right dosage is provided.

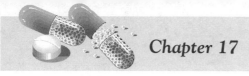

In stubborn cases of asthma, corticosteroids (prednisone) may be needed, either in pill or injectable form. Short-term use of Prednisone does not appear to harm the baby. Asthmatics may want to try the inhaled corticosteroids (Beclovent) over the long term if they need steroid therapy.

Another drug that has been recommended as a long-term preventive drug is cromolyn sodium (Intal). Intal inhalations work on certain cells in the lungs and hold back excess secretions. Intal does not work for acute asthma attacks, however.

Expectant mothers should seek emergency treatment if they have an acute asthma attack that cannot be controlled with their usual medications. Depriving the fetus of oxygen is dangerous and can have permanent effects.

Case Study

Margaret L., a young woman of 22, had not planned to become pregnant, but both she and her husband were happy when they got the news that they were to become parents. They were also worried. Margaret had had a serious problem with diabetes since she was 10, and she needed daily insulin injections along with a special low-sugar diet. During her first year in high school, she had begun to have grand mal epileptic seizures and had to take Dilantin to control them. Her doctor warned her that she had two diseases that were difficult to control during pregnancy and that there were risks to both Margaret and the baby. The doctor also assured her that medical science had come a long way in the past 20 years in helping women with problems like hers.

Because she had heard that Dilantin was a hazardous drug for unborn babies, Margaret stopped taking it right after she learned she was pregnant. Two weeks later she had a grand mal seizure. She passed out, lost her breath for almost 2 minutes and began to turn blue. She was rushed to the hospital and admitted. The doctors immediately gave her oxygen, restrained her, and started her once again on Dilantin through an intravenous line. When she returned to her normal state, her doctors urged her not to stop taking Dilantin again. They pointed out to her that depriving her fetus of oxygen during a seizure was even more dangerous than exposure to Dilantin. She reluctantly agreed to continue the drug.

For the rest of her pregnancy Margaret worked at the bank as a teller and maintained her normal activities. She was extremely careful about her diet and made sure that she ate four properly balanced meals a day. She took prenatal vitamins with extra folic acid to counteract the effects of Dilantin on her red blood cells. Because of the seriousness of her diabetes, she had to monitor her blood sugar four times each day using an Autolet system. Her insulin dosage increased gradually as her pregnancy progressed. Once a month she had blood drawn to test for the amount of Dilantin in her bloodstream. Twice the doctor had to increase the dosage of Dilantin she needed.

Case Study (continued)

At the beginning of her ninth month Margaret began to have episodes of near unconsciousness, caused by her blood sugar dropping too low during the night. Her insulin was decreased and she was admitted to the hospital so the doctors could watch her closely. Because her baby appeared to be growing very large, as fetuses of diabetic mothers often do, the doctors decided to induce labor at the beginning of her thirty-eighth week. They ascertained that the fetus's lungs were mature enough to withstand early delivery and then administered oxytocin. She had an uncomplicated 8-hour labor and gave birth to a healthy 7-pound 10-ounce girl. She was thrilled after her worrisome pregnancy, and both she and the baby did well post partum. After the delivery the doctors were able to decrease her insulin and Dilantin dosages.

Case Study

Janice, a 32-year-old African-American teacher, discovered during her first pregnancy two years previous that she had pregnancy-induced high blood pressure. During that pregnancy she received Aldomet to control the hypertension but still had to have an early delivery because her blood pressure continued to rise as her pregnancy progressed. After her daughter was born, her blood pressure dropped and remained within normal range. She was not aware of any other symptoms such as headache or chest pain.

When she first visited the clinic at the beginning of the third month of her second pregnancy, everything looked good. However, her blood pressure slowly began to rise as the weeks passed. Janice bought a home blood pressure kit to monitor her hypertension. At the beginning of her fifth month, the doctors decided she ought to take Aldomet again, which kept her blood pressure down adequately until the beginning of her seventh month. At that point she was taking the maximum allowable dosage of 2 gm per day, but the results were not satisfactory. Her doctor informed her that she would have to be hospitalized with complete bed rest to see if, along with medication, her blood pressure could be brought down. Janice objected at first because she actually felt well. After the doctor explained the dangers of high blood pressure would come to both her and the unborn baby, Janice agreed to whatever was necessary for their safety.

Janice had to lie on her left side, getting up only to use the bathroom. In addition to Aldomet, she was given hydralazine. She asked if she could be given a fluid pill, like her brother took, or Inderal, which had been prescribed for her father, since both of them suffered from hypertension too. Her doctors told her that they never prescribed fluid pills to pregnant women and that at her stage of pregnancy they did not want to start her on Inderal.

> ### *Case Study (continued)*
>
> Janice was discharged after a week and spent one more month at home, resting on her side for several hours a day. With four weeks to go until her due date, Janice began to have protein in her urine, a strong sign that she was developing preeclampsia/toxemia again. The doctors performed a repeat cesarean, and Janice and her husband both concluded that it would be wise if she had her tubes tied. She was fortunate to become the mother of a thin but otherwise healthy 5-pound 4-ounce boy.
>
> After delivery her blood pressure dropped and with the continuation of Aldomet, remained in a normal range. She currently sees her internist several times a year to keep a close eye on her hypertension.

Key Points for Medical Disorders

1. Most of the time mothers with chronic diseases will need to continue their medications during pregnancy. The general health of the mother is very important to the health of the fetus, and the harm done by discontinuing needed medications may very well outweigh the benefits.

2. Preconceptual counseling (consulting with the doctor before you are pregnant) is very important for mothers with chronic medical problems. Many problems can be avoided with advance planning, and those that remain can be managed more comfortably and safely.

3. The intake of the medications must be controlled carefully under the watchful eye of a physician, who can decide the proper dosage of a drug as pregnancy progresses.

4. Because the mother has about 2 1/2 extra quarts of blood circulating during pregnancy, she will often need higher dosages of her medication to get the same blood levels of the drug that she got when she was not pregnant.

5. A woman with a medical disorder should consult a doctor the moment she suspects she is pregnant. Until she has her first appointment, she should continue with her routine pattern of medication.

6. The pediatrician or family physician who is to care for the child should be made aware in advance of medications that the mother took during her pregnancy, so that if problems resulting from the medications occur, he or she can be prepared.

7. After delivery the medication dosages may change. Therefore a woman must return to her regular physician so that she can resume her normal course of treatment.

Notes

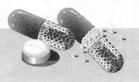

Chapter 18

Substance Abuse During Pregnancy and the Reproductive Years

Substance abuse and addiction in women of reproductive age have probably been underestimated by both the public and the medical community. While people are no longer unaware of the problem, they still may not be willing to admit how deeply it has woven itself into the fabric of society. According to the National Institute on Drug Abuse, at least *34 million women* between the ages of 15 and 44 years are currently substance abusers. Up to 2 million of these use cocaine. In fact, cocaine and marijuana are thought to be the two most commonly abused drugs during pregnancy.

The impact of substance abuse on the individual woman is the same, whether or not she is pregnant. The variable, of course, is the fetus and how drugs will affect it. In this chapter we will discuss the known (and unknown) effects of substance abuse on the unborn baby and how a woman can help herself and her baby when she is pregnant and addicted at the same time.

Profile of the Pregnant Substance Abuser

Pregnant substance abusers come from all social classes and age groups. Drug addiction and abuse encompass the crack cocaine user from an urban ghetto, the middle class teenager who has been experimenting with street drugs, and the overwrought mother of four whose drug of choice is alcohol. More and more, physicians see drug dependencies among women from every sector of society. Sometimes the prospective mother hides her habit so well that no one, including her physician, knows she is taking a drug until the baby is born and shows withdrawal symptoms.

In fact, the list of drugs to which a woman and her newborn can be habituated is quite long. A few of the well-known ones are cocaine, heroin, marijuana, hashish, alprazolam, (Xanax), pentazocine (Talwin), chlordiazepoxide (Librium), angel dust (PCP), phenobarbital, flurazepam (Dalmane), secobarbital (Seconal), amphetamines (Benzedrine, Methedrine, Dexedrine), methaqualone (Quaalude), and combinations of all these. Withdrawal symptoms have been observed in babies whose mothers used such diverse substances as phenobarbital, propoxyphene (Darvon), nicotine, LSD, and caffeine. Table 18-1 lists some of the characteristics of pregnant substance abusers and problems associated with such abuse.

From a medical standpoint, street drug use is nearly impossible to study, with the exception of heroin addicts who are followed in methadone clinics, because oftentimes users take many drugs, give unreliable information, and have other habits that confuse the issue. Sometimes it is difficult to tell if a drug user is actually pregnant. Women addicted to a single drug or combinations of drugs often have irregular periods and menstruation. Under more extreme conditions they may be ill from infection, malnutrition, and anemia, all of which produce symptoms similar to those of early pregnancy. AIDS is now commonly diagnosed in pregnant intravenous drug users. Even pregnancy tests do not work very well with addicts because of the effects of the drugs on the test materials. In some cases only ultrasound testing, feeling movement, or actually hearing the fetal heartbeat confirm that the drug user is going to be a mother.

Risks to the Mother and Fetus

Many experiments have been performed with animals in an attempt to study the effects of drug abuse on the unborn. In spite of these, it is difficult to predict what will actually happen to human babies whose mothers abuse drugs. Apparently the risk of genetic problems is no higher than in the general population. However, we are beginning to see that drug abuse has an adverse effect on growth and development, particularly brain development, especially when the drug of choice is cocaine or alcohol. For this reason and because drug abusers often have additional social and emotional problems, we believe open and sympathetic abortion counseling is very important. Many will choose to continue their pregnancies and should be supported in doing so, but abortion options - knowing that federal law permits abortion up to 24 weeks of gestation - should be considered.

Because pregnant drug abusers tend to have more medical complications than other women, their need for care as early as possible in pregnancy is compelling. Diet, treatment of infections, and management of other types of problems must be addressed. Doctors need to monitor the heart rate and growth of the fetus very carefully to be sure everything is proceeding normally. Obviously, pregnant women should curtail their drug habit, but in some cases this will be difficult and involve going through withdrawal. *Never attempt drug withdrawal from heroin, alcohol, or "downers" (phenobarbital, seconal, etc) during pregnancy without medical supervision.* Withdrawal from cocaine may not have as strong a physical effect, but psychological support may be very important.

Except for narcotics, central nervous system stimulants ("uppers"), or depressants ("downers"), symptoms are not always obvious as the drug is withdrawn. In cases of addiction to narcotics, barbiturates, or hypnotic drugs, it is important to realize that the unborn baby is addicted to the same drug as its mother. Getting the newborn infant off the drug, known as detoxification, must be done carefully and gradually. Withdrawing from a drug can be a demanding physical experience, and for an unborn or newborn baby it can be overwhelming.

Because of methadone maintenance programs, we know more about controlling heroin addiction than addiction to other drugs. Methadone must be substituted for heroin and the drug levels must be decreased slowly. Too rapid a decrease could cause the baby to be stillborn. The baby must be monitored throughout the detoxification process. If the fetus's activity seems excessive, it may be a sign that the detoxification process must be slowed down. With drugs like phenobarbital or diazepam, gradual withdrawal using decreased dosages of the same substance may also be necessary.

Overdosing is very hard on the mother and can be even worse for the unborn baby. Table 18-2 lists signs of overdose and characteristic withdrawal symptoms for the most commonly abused drugs. The most typical signs of overdose for each group of drugs involve the woman's behavior and her blood pressure and pulse.

Common Substances of Abuse

Alcohol

Alcohol has a centuries-old pattern of abuse, and it is one of the drugs whose effects we understand best. Evidence shows that between 1% and 2% of all pregnant women use alcohol to excess. Two-thirds of babies born to women alcoholics have alcohol-related effects; half of these are serious and permanent. *Fetal alcohol syndrome,* a characteristic set of problems associated with a mother's drinking occurs anywhere from 1 in 300 to 1 in 2,000 births. Babies with fetal alcohol syndrome have head and facial disfigurement, retarded growth, mental retardation, poor coordination, and extreme irritability.

Some studies suggest that 3 ounces of alcohol (6 drinks per day) will induce fetal alcohol syndrome, but we do not really know what the critical level is. We recommend that women stop drinking when they are pregnant or at least keep their consumption down to an occasional drink at a party or holiday gathering. The evidence against alcohol is too strong to ignore, and the price too high to pay for indulgence.

Cocaine

The abuse of cocaine has escalated tremendously in the last ten years, primarily due to the ready availability of cheap crack cocaine, which can be smoked. Because crack's effects don't last very long, it doesn't remain cheap for the user, however. More and more must be smoked to sustain the "high," and this is when dependency and damage to the fetus comes in.Cocaine is a dangerous drug that can cause sudden death through heart attacks, strokes, and other kinds of cardiovascular events in both the mother and the fetus or newborn. All kinds of birth complications, such as early delivery, fetal distress and even fetal death, are associated with maternal cocaine use. Malformations, particularly of the genitourinary tract, occur much more often in cocaine-exposed babies. "Cocaine babies" are miserable for days after birth with high-pitched crying, shaking, restlessness, agitation, and inability to feed properly. Evidence is mounting that this behavioral damage sometimes continues through childhood, making it very difficult for these children to learn or attend school.

Although physical withdrawal from cocaine is not as difficult for the mother and fetus as it is from drugs like alcohol or heroin, because it is so intensely addictive, we recommend that any pregnant woman with a history of cocaine abuse place herself under chemical dependency treatment both before and after delivery. Cocaine intoxication is dangerous and should be treated medically: Table18-3 details drug treatment of cocaine intoxication.

Opiates

The term *opiate* was originally used to refer to drugs derived from opium. Now it simply means any drug with an effect similar to opium, such as, drowsiness, feeling "high" and relaxed, and numbness.

Heroin, methadone, Demerol, and fentanyl are all examples of opiates, and all are very addictive. They pose constant dangers from overdose - which can throw a person into a coma - and withdrawal, which causes sweating, shaking, and abdominal cramping. Withdrawal in a pregnant woman is especially dangerous to her unborn child and can even result in its death. Because these drugs are injected intravenously, and users often share needles the risk of contracting life-threatening infections such as AIDS and hepatitis is extremely high, also.

Methadone maintenance with very gradual withdrawal of the drug is probably the best course for pregnant heroin abusers. Even then the incidence of babies with lower birth weights and smaller head sizes is quite high. Women addicted to heroin and other opiates need special medical attention during pregnancy. They must also be tested for infection, particularly for AIDS and hepatitis, and treated as much as possible for these conditions.

Marijuana

Marijuana is popular and inexpensive, and many of its advocates have asserted that it's just a fun and harmless drug. Research has since indicated that long-term usage does affect a person's ability to think, react, and concentrate. What's more the long-term effects of marijuana smoking on lungs seems to be similar to that of cigarettes, i.e., chronic bronchitis, emphysema, and other

Table 18-3	
Treatment of Acute Cocaine Intoxication	
Symptom	**Treatment**
Agitation	Diazepam (5-10 mg (IV) intravenous), lorazepam (2-4 mg (IM) intramuscular or IV), midazolam (5-10 mg IM or 3-5 mg IV), or haloperidol (10 mg IM or IV)
Hyperthermia	Tepid water or mist to skin and evaporate cooling with large fan
Seizures	Diazepam (5-10 mg IV), lorazepam (2-4 mg IM or IV), or midazolam (5-10 mg IM or 3-5 mg IV), followed loading with either phenobarbital (15-20mg/kg IV 30 or more min) or phenytoin (15 mg/kg V 30 or more min)
Hypertension	Nifedipine (10-20 mg), sodium nitroprusside (0.5-5g/kg/min IV), phentolamine (3-5 mg IV), propanolol (1-5 mg IV), or labetalol (10-20 mg IV)
Cardiac arrhythmias	Parenteral ß-blockers (propranolol, labetalol, metoprolol, or esmolol) or other standard antiarrhythmic agents
Myocardial ischemia or infarction	Nitroglycerin, other nitrates or calcium-channel blockers for coronary spasm, thrombolysis for infarction (Note: hypertension and tachycardia should be treated as above)

serious respiratory diseases. Studies have revealed that between 3% and 15% of pregnant women smoke marijuana, and the incidence may be as high as 27%. The effects of marijuana on a fetus are uncertain, mostly because marijuana use is often combined with other substance intake and the effects are hard to sort out. The lifestyle, personal habits, and social environment of many marijuana users could also contribute to problems during pregnancy.

There are indications that babies born to heavy marijuana users have increased trembling and irritability and decreased visual responses, but more work needs to be done to confirm this.

It's safe to say that the jury is still out on the hazards of marijuana smoking during pregnancy. Our feeling is that, while it may not have the devastating effects of alcohol or cocaine, marijuana contributes absolutely nothing positive to a successful pregnancy outcome and it may have some detrimental effects. We suggest that its use be minimized or better yet stopped during pregnancy.

Amphetamines

Amphetamines or "uppers" stimulate the central nervous system and give the user an illusion of great energy. Another reason women use amphetamines is for weight control because they do suppress appetite. Benzedrine, dexedrine, and methadrine are all common amphetamines. Like crack cocaine amphetamines are now available in smokable form and that product is known as "ice." The stimulation produced by amphetamines is usually short-lived and often followed by agitation, hallucinations, and paranoia, along with the urge to take more drugs so the "bad feelings" will go away. Uppers are dangerous and can cause life-threatening heart rhythm problems, strokes or even heart attacks in pregnant women.

Amphetamines have been associated with birth defects, preterm labor, fetal growth retardation, ruptured placenta, and blood vessel rupture in the mother. Babies born to amphetamine users have experienced withdrawal characterized by trembling, jitteriness, poor feeding, and abnormal sleep patterns.

In summary, we recommend that pregnant women with an amphetamine habit withdraw from it during pregnancy, seeking help from a chemical dependency program if they need to. The drugs are dangerous and could do serious damage. As we have stated earlier, pregnancy is not a time to be on a diet or to be using drugs that help lose weight. What's more, using the drugs to diet can cause a dependency on their other effects without even realizing it.

Needs of the Pregnant Drug Abuser

We make the following recommendations to the pregnant drug abuser:

1. Avoid physical and emotional stresses that cause drug use (including alcohol) for relief.

2. Attend prenatal classes and groups designed specifically to help work through issues related to drug use during pregnancy.

3. Use crisis intervention programs staffed by professionals and paraprofessionals (former drug addicts) to assist with marital and family conflicts during pregnancy.

4. Make sure the diet is balanced and nutritious; include recommended vitamin supplements containing iron and folic acid.

5. Go to childbirth preparation classes given either in the community or at a hospital.

6. Do not seek to relieve symptoms with other drugs. Using multiple drugs can make things even worse for the fetus.

Physical Problems

Among the medical complications created by drug abuse are anemia, bacteremia (bacteria in the blood), endocarditis (an infection in the heart, often found in people with defective heart valves), dental infections, retaining water in the tissues, hepatitis (liver infection), phlebitis and poor veins, pneumonia, water in the lungs, septicemia (blood poisoning), tetanus (lockjaw), tuberculosis, bladder and urinary tract infections, and a wide variety of sexually transmitted diseases, including the most dangerous of all - the presence of HIV virus eventually leading to AIDS. Several visits to the doctor's office might be necessary before these problems are completely diagnosed and treated. The pregnant substance abuser may need frequent medical appointments even in the early months of her pregnancy.

Emotional Problems and Rehabilitation

When under the influence of their drug of choice, many women maintain an artificial sense of well-being and stay out of touch with their real problems and ways of coping with them. Once in a rehabilitation program, the pregnant addict is apt to come up against the fear, guilt, and shame she had been previously masking with drugs. Many drug abusers have emotional, psychological and psychiatric problems that they have been self-medicating with drugs or alcohol. Unless these underlying problems are addressed through treatment, they may revert back to their habits, unable to cope with the reality unmasked by going off drugs.

In other cases, frightened for her child's well being, a pregnant drug user will go "cold turkey," that is, abstain suddenly and completely from drugs, regardless of the discomfort it causes her. The safety of going cold turkey depends on the drug, and a woman should seek help from a physician before she attempts any sudden withdrawal. Besides, the results of going cold turkey are often temporary, with the woman going right back to using her drugs of choice after she recovers from the initial shock.

People with the urge to use addictive drugs may attempt almost anything to acquire the substances they want. Often they will substitute more easily acquired drugs for the ones they are trying to give up. Women who actually are using other drugs (particularly alcohol) concurrently with methadone comprise between 15% and 40% of pregnant addicts. When multiple drug abuse is involved in a pregnancy, fetal death rises as high as 90%, and the multiple drug user should be aware that she is taking this level of risk for her unborn child.

Nutrition

Malnutrition is a frequent complication of drug abuse. Nutritional counseling, diet supplements, and assurance that the woman has enough money for food (and that she spends it on food, not drugs!) are all necessary. Since many women abusing drugs eat so poorly, their diets often need to be of even higher quality than in a normal pregnancy. If possible they should see nutrition counselors to help them achieve a diet that includes at least 100 gm of protein a day. Supplementary vitamins and minerals are also a must. At least 25% of drug addicts are anemic and will need iron supplementation twice a day plus additional folic acid.

Delivery Considerations

While the incidence of delivery complications in drug dependent women is not a lot higher than for women who don't use drugs, there are some unique problems. In general, women on drugs have a premature delivery rate two to three times higher than other women. The placenta will tear away from the wall of the uterus prematurely more often in cocaine users. Premature rupture of the membranes (water bag) occurs three times more often in pregnant substance abusers, according to some studies, most likely because of chronic vaginal infections. This latter problem may occur in as much as 20% of pregnancies where the mother has been addicted to drugs. The babies themselves are often smaller than normal. The nursery team must be alert to the symptoms of withdrawal in the newborn. These include shaking, sweating, excessive yawning, unstable temperature, vomiting, diarrhea, rapid respiration, irritability, sleeplessness, a shrill high-pitched cry, and seizures. After delivery the babies may need to receive the drug their mothers were taking in gradually decreasing amounts to help them withdraw with less discomfort.

Case Study

Lisa L, divorced, jobless, and pregnant, was a street-drug abuser. Looking considerably older than her 23 years, the thin, stringy-haired blonde admitted to her obstetrician that she had been using PCP (angel dust), crack cocaine, and heroin when she conceived. Now about 4 months pregnant, she was still shooting heroin. She told her doctor that, in spite of her drug habit, she very much wanted her baby. The doctor reassured Lisa that she would do everything in her power to help her deliver a healthy infant, but she needed Lisa's commitment to follow her recommendations. Lisa agreed to go on a decreasing methadone maintenance program to help her get off heroin.

Case Study (continued)

Fortunately Lisa did not have HIV positivity (early AIDS), gonorrhea, hepatitis, or any of the other infections often found among street-drug abusers. She told the doctor she had made it a policy never to share needles with fellow drug users. She was, however, anemic and badly nourished. Her doctor referred her to a government-funded community service agency, where a team of physicians, nurses, nutritionist, and social workers worked with her almost daily. With her food stamps she was able to purchase fresh fruit, vegetables, meat, milk, and prenatal vitamins. Even though she didn't keep her medical appointments regularly, Lisa managed to gain 25 pounds, Her anemia remained stable, neither improving nor worsening.

Lisa wanted to try to kick her heroin habit, but her doctors informed her that, if she attempted to quit too quickly, it could harm her baby. She enrolled at a methadone clinic and started on a program where she received a daily dose of 80 mg of methadone. Her dosage was gradually decreased until it was at 15 mg daily at the end of her pregnancy.

Because Lisa's periods had been irregular since she began using drugs, the date of her conception was uncertain. Her doctor used ultrasonic imaging to determine the age of her fetus, and she continued ultrasound testing throughout the pregnancy to check on the baby's development. Just about the time of the predicted due date, Lisa went into spontaneous labor and delivered what appeared to be a healthy 6-pound 5-ounce girl. The baby was watched carefully in the nursery for symptoms of drug withdrawal. She appeared to be slightly groggier and less responsive than would be expected of a baby from a normal mother, but she ate well, and her alertness was increasing at the time Lisa left the hospital with her.

Lisa was in reasonably good physical health at the time of her discharge. Her parents had decided to let her and the baby come back home with them. Lisa remained on methadone maintenance for four more months, and then the drug was stopped. She continued to see her social worker twice weekly and enrolled in vocational training classes at the local community college.

Key Points for Substance Abuse

1. Despite drug addiction, many women get pregnant and want to have their babies. They usually need extra support and assistance in completing a successful pregnancy, compared to other pregnant women.

2. Apparently there are no obvious risks of birth defects or genetic damage associated with drug abuse in the mother. At this time we believe that drugs like alcohol and cocaine can have permanent effects on growth and brain development in the baby. We do not know how such damage will affect the future children of these babies.

3. Intravenous drug usage carries a high risk of infection from often fatal diseases such as hepatitis and AIDS. Pregnant intravenous drug users should be tested for these diseases and counseled on the risks of transmission to their infant.

4. Diagnosis of early pregnancy in a drug abuser may not be easy. Because of the potential risks to the unborn baby, the option of abortion should be discussed in an open and sympathetic manner.

5. The extent of drug abuse or addiction at conception or throughout pregnancy is sometimes difficult to assess. The mother-to-be may hide her habit so well that she cannot receive adequate care.

6. The chances of an addict completing a successful pregnancy will be much higher if she is totally honest with her physician about the substances she is taking, and if she is willing to work at controlling her habit for the sake of the baby and herself.

7. Pregnant drug addicts often have many health problems. They need good medical attention, a highly nutritious diet, and supplemental prenatal vitamins containing iron and folic acid.

8. Not all pregnant women should go off their drugs "cold turkey." Depending on the drug and the doctor's care plan, they may need to go on a maintenance program with gradually decreasing amounts of the drug administered to them.

9. Pregnant drug abusers often need psychiatric attention, vocational counseling, and moral support, as well as good medical care.

10. Babies of addicted mothers may need a staged withdrawal program shortly after birth.

Table 18-1
Characteristics Associated With Substance Abuse

Behavioral and Personal

Noncompliance with appointments	Domestic violence
Difficulty concentrating and remembering things	Alcohol- or drug-abusing partner
	Family history of substance abuse
Slurred speech or staggering gait	Prostitution
Bizarre or inappropriate behavior	Incarceration
Psychiatric history	Frequent emergency department visits
Child abuse or neglect	Chronic unemployment

Medical

Drug overdose or withdrawal	Pancreatitis
Cellulitis, abscesses, or phlebitis	Lymphedema
Septicemia	Anemia
Bacterial endocarditis	Stroke
Sexually transmitted diseases	Heart Attack
HIV positivity	Poor dental hygiene
Tuberculosis	Poor nutritional status
Hepatitis	

Obstetric

No or little prenatal care	Fetal growth retardation
Spontaneous abortion	Fetal distress
Preterm delivery	Intrauterine fetal death
Preterm rupture of the membranes	Congenital anomalies
Birth outside hospital	Fetal alcohol syndrome
Abruptio placentae	Neonatal abstinence syndrome
Sudden infant death syndrome	

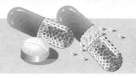

Table 18-2 Drug Abuse			
Drug Group	**Overdose Signs and Symptoms**	**Withdrawal Symptoms**	**Fetal Effects**
Alcohol	Unusual behavior, mostly depressant with stupor, loss of memory, hypotension	Agitation, tremors	Microcephaly mental retardation, altered facial expressions
Anticholinergics Atropine Belladonna Scopolamine	Pupils-dilated & fixed Heart rate--increased Temperature--increased; flushed skin	None	None
Cannabis Marijuana THC Hashish Hash oil	Pupils--normal but conjunctiva injected BP--decreased in standing Heart rate--increased sensorium--clear, dreamy, fantasy state, time & space distorted	None	None known
CNS Sedatives Barbiturates Chlordiazepoxide Diazepam Flurazepam Glutethimide Meprobamate Methaqualone, etc.	Pupils--unchanged BP--decreases ± shock Respiration--depressed Tendon reflexes--decreased Drowsiness, coma, lateral nystagmus, Ataxia, slurred speech, deliriums, convulsions	Tremulousness, insomnia, chronic blink reflex, agitation toxic psychosis	None
CNS Stimulants Antiobesity drugs Amphetamines Methylphenidate Phenmetrazine	Pupils--dilated and reactive Respiration--shallow BP--increased Tendon reflexes--hyperactive Cardiac arrhythmias Dry mouth, tremors, hyperactivity, sensorium hyperacute	Muscle aches, abdominal pain, hunger, prolonged sleep, sometimes suicidal	Hyperactivity with increased kicks

Table 18-2 (continued)
Drug Abuse

Drug Group	Overdose Signs and Symptoms	Withdrawal Symptoms	Fetal Effects
Hallucinogens LSD Psilocybin Ketamine Mescaline 2.S-Dimethoxy-4- Methylamphetamine Dimethyltryptamine Phencyclidine (PCP)	Pupils--dilated BP--elevated Heart rate--increased Tendon reflexes--increased Face flushed, euphoria, anxiety, inappropriate effect, illusions, hallucinations, realization	No withdrawal symptoms	No known fetal effects
Narcotics Codeine Heroin Hydromorphone Meperidine Morphine Opium	Pupils--constricted Respiration--depressed BP--decreased Reflexes--hyperactive Sensorium-obtunded	Flu-like syndrome agitation, dilated pupils, abdominal pain	Intrauterine withdrawal increased fetal activity; newborn withdrawal
Cocaine	Hypertension, rapid pulse convulsion, paranoia, cardiovascular collapse intracerebral bleed (stroke) respiratory failure separation placenta death		Small gestational age, preterm delivery, behavior abnormalities, congenital malformations: cardiac CNS genibumary fetal distress, still birth

Pain Relief During Labor

Kathryn Zuspan, M.D.

One thing we know for sure about labor it is painful. In fact, studies show that labor pain hurts worse than the pain of a toothache, a broken leg, or chronic cancer pain. Medical advances now allow us better control of labor pain, but in the past, women had to suffer during childbirth. Even after pain relief techniques had been developed, many cultural and religious beliefs prevented a woman from using drugs or other methods to obtain pain relief. During the 1500's, midwives using labor pain relief techniques were burned at the stake as witches. People took literally the passage in Genesis that read, "In sorrow thou shalt bring forth children."

Sir James Simpson first used chloroform in 1848 to ease labor pain, defending his actions by showing how the original Hebrew word for "sorrow" really translated to "labor" or "toil". Anesthetic techniques, he said, eased the pain but not the labor of childbirth. Obstetrical pain relief was finally accepted after Queen Victoria of England received chloroform during the birth of her eighth child, Prince Leopold.

Today a variety of methods are available to a woman about to give birth. They include drugs that tranquilize and narcotize, techniques employing specific breathing patterns, auto-suggestion, relaxation, positive visualization, and numbing medications. Under the guidance of her obstetrician and anesthesiologist, a woman can have major input into the choice of techniques for her labor pain management.

A woman should do all she can to prepare for childbirth. Hospitals and clinics frequently offer preparatory courses. Many communities have prenatal education classes that teach the mother-to-be and her support person about the process of labor and delivery, including pain relief options. Studies have shown that mothers who attend childbirth classes actually experience less severe labor pain. The mechanisms of childbirth can be overwhelming. If a woman feels she has some control and can ask for pain relief if she needs it, the process will seem less painful and frightening.

Some women are able to go through labor and delivery without drugs, but many women giving birth will ask for and need some form of pain relief before the baby actually arrives. A woman not feel guilty if she needs some assistance. Enduring agony so you won't have to use a drug does not help you or your baby. We now know that certain hormones are produced when a person feels pain. These hormones, called catecholamines, put both the mother and baby under additional stress. Childbirth and labor go much more smoothly when the mother is as comfortable as possible under the circumstances.

If a woman wishes to use one of the nondrug techniques, she should work out a plan with her doctor that allows for an alternate method of pain relief if it is needed. Preplanning allows her to be involved in the choice of labor management when she is not in pain and can consider her options objectively. This helps prevent the guilt and upset that some women feel later in labor when they find they need more pain control than first anticipated. This is especially true for first babies, when the mother typically has a longer labor and can't easily predict how her body is going to respond to the demands of labor.

Many women worry that labor pain relief techniques will make them sleepy or less in control, slow the progress of labor or delivery, or be detrimental to their babies. As will be discussed, present methods of pain control minimize or negate these problems.

No single method is perfect for everyone. The most updated national statistics were gathered in 1981. These revealed that about 32% of women used a non-drug technique such as Lamaze or no pain control method at all; 49% used some form of intravenous pain medication; 16% used epidural anesthesia; and 5% received a paracervical block. Since 1981, the trend has been more toward epidural anesthesia and less toward Lamaze and intravenous drugs. Paracervical blocks are rarely used these days.

Some General Points About Labor

Labor must be established before an obstetrician can can consider pain relief methods. This means that a woman should be having contractions with the cervix dilating or effacing (thinning).

Once labor is underway, it is very important that a woman protect herself by avoiding all food, drink, gum, candy, or popsicles. Ice-chip chewing should be kept to a bare minimum. This is done to decease the risk of vomiting and possibly inhaling stomach contents into the lungs (aspiration). Even today, aspiration is the cause of one-third of all obstetrical anesthesia-related deaths. Some recent articles have appeared in obstetricians' and midwives' journals indicating that "no eating or drinking during labor" is an unnecessary precaution. This is incorrect. Eating and drinking do present major hazards for a woman in labor.

Although the risk of aspiration is low during a vaginal delivery, an unexpected cesarean section may be needed. These are sometimes done under general anesthesia, where the risk of aspiration is at its highest. Thus it is always safest to stop eating and drinking once labor begins. Necessary fluids and nutrition during labor can be provided by intravenous solutions (IVs) given through an IV catheter, placed in the arm. While IVs may seem like a hassle, they are very helpful during labor. They provide food and liquid for both mother and baby; pain relief or other medication can be injected through them, thus avoiding the need for shots; they are necessary for most pain relief options and are required for all forms of anesthesia for a cesarean section (C-section).

Most deliveries go smoothly, but no one can predict who may or may not need a C-section. Emergencies can arise that endanger both mother and baby, and the C-section must often be performed as quickly as possible. If the IV is not in place, this can unnecessarily delay the start of the operation.

Labor Pain Relief Options

Lamaze

Lamaze is a form of psychoprophylaxis, a technique that assists a person in controlling pain without medication. It stresses education in ways to deal with pain. Parents attend several class sessions prior to delivery to learn Lamaze techniques, which include special patterns of breathing, massage, and coaching by a delivery support person, visualization of positive images, counting through contractions, and positioning the body for maximum comfort.

Use of the Lamaze techniques was once considered the very best thing a mother could do for her baby because there were no drugs involved. The problem with this thinking is that Lamaze alone does not provide enough pain relief for many women, although it works well for some. Often women find that Lamaze is effective in the early stages of labor, but, as labor progresses, they need an additional technique, such as an epidural or spinal or IV pain medication.

In the past, prenatal classes would sometimes convey the message that Lamaze was the only good option and that women requiring other techniques were not good mothers. This is not true. The best thing a mother can do for her unborn child during labor is to decrease her own stress and pain.

Every woman and every labor is different. Thus, there is no one best way to provide labor pain relief for all women. Fortunately, there are several options available, and these are discussed below.

Intravenous Pain Medications

Intravenous drugs are medications injected through the IV line. These enter the blood stream and spread throughout the body.

Narcotics and narcotic-like drugs are the most widely used intravenous medications for reduction of pain during the first stage of labor. They block the pain messages going from your uterus and pelvic area to the pain "message centers" in your brain. The drugs commonly used during labor are meperidine (Demerol), fentanyl (Sublimaze), butorphanol (Stadol), and nalbuphine (Nubain).

Narcotics given in the small-to-moderate dosages appropriate for labor usually produce drowsiness and mental fuzziness, but not unconsciousness. They provide a degree of pain relief by raising the pain threshold (level at which a person can tolerate pain) and reducing the feeling of pain. Sometimes they have side effects such as nausea or even vomiting. Narcotics easily cross the placenta and can affect the fetus by causing breathing slowdowns. The major concern is that the baby will be sleepy and not breathe deeply at the time of delivery. In low dosages, however, narcotics are considered safe and have little affect on the fetus. Naloxone (Narcan) can be given to a baby who is sleepy at delivery to reverse the effect of the narcotic.

Sedatives and tranquilizers may be used to help reduce anxiety, promote sleep, and make the narcotic drugs more effective. Vistaril is the most commonly used drug for this purpose. Typically given with the narcotic, Vistaril helps reduce nausea and vomiting that may be caused by a narcotic.

Paracervical Block

Once a popular method, this technique is seldom used. The problem is that it has a significant incidence of complications in the fetus (anywhere from 1 to 30%) where the baby's heart rate drops to dangerously low levels. This occurs about 2-10 minutes after the block is given and lasts from 15 to 30 to 45 minutes. The baby does not tolerate this condition well, and often the result is an emergency C-section.

The paracervical block is performed by the obstetrician who places a speculum (a device that holds the vagina open) in the mother's vagina while she lies in bed. The obstetrician injects local anesthetic into several spots next to the mother's cervix, and the medication dulls the pain of contractions.

Spinal Anesthesia

Spinal anesthesia is a relatively new method for labor pain relief. These particular spinals go under a variety of names, including intrathecal morphine or narcotics, subarachnoid morphine or narcotics, or spinal morphine or narcotics. These are used for labor only.

To receive a spinal, the mother is placed in a fetal position laying either on her side or sitting on the side of the bed. The anesthesiologist numbs the skin in the middle of her back at hip level with a little local anesthetic. A very thin needle is placed through that area and advanced into the patient's spinal fluid sac. The spinal cord actually ends above this level, so women should not worry that their spinal cord will be "skewered." The doctor injects a small amount of medication through the needle, which is then removed. Typically this medication is a very small amount of narcotic drug, smaller than that given using the IV pain relief technique. Mothers will get pain relief in less than 5 minutes, and this lasts about three hours or until the cervix dilates to 8 centimeters, whichever comes first. This is a good technique, especially for women who have short labors and who have no problem in the second stage of labor when they are pushing the baby out. This technique works less well for women having their first baby who are in early labor; for those who are likely to have a long labor; or for those who need a forceps or C-section delivery. It works poorly for women receiving oxytocin (Pitocin) to improve their labor contractions.

Some of the benefits of spinal anesthesia are that laboring mothers can get some consistent pain relief yet still be clear-headed and able to walk around or sit up in a chair. There is no decrease in muscle strength, so they can still push well. One drawback is the slight risk of a spinal headache. This is a severe, intense headache that typically appears 24-48 hours after a spinal is given. Young pregnant women seem to be at special risk for spinal headaches, but the anesthesiologist can try to minimize such risk by using a small-sized needle or one with a special tip.

When a spinal headache does occur, there are several types of treatment available. The oldest includes bed rest, pain medication, and increased fluid consumption. Sometimes caffeine will be given through an intravenous line or by mouth. The most effective treatment is the epidural blood patch, which is done just like a labor epidural. With this technique, however, no catheter is used. Instead, a small amount of the woman's own blood is put in the epidural space. Relief is quick and success occurs about 95% of the time.

Other drawbacks to spinals include the limited time interval of relief and the fact that additional relief requires that a second procedure be done.

All in all, the spinal method for labor pain relief provides more pain relief than Lamaze or IV pain medication, but typically less than an epidural.

Epidural Anesthesia

Epidural anesthesia is the most effective and popular technique for labor pain control. It provides pain relief for the duration of labor and may also be used for spontaneous vaginal delivery, forceps delivery, or C-section.

The epidural is placed in a manner similar to the spinal. The laboring mother is placed in the fetal position, either on her side or sitting on the side of her bed. The skin on the middle of her back at hip level is numbed with a local anesthetic. An epidural needle is placed through this spot and advanced carefully into the epidural space, a tiny cavity that lies just outside of a sac filled with spinal fluid. This sac extends up the back and at a higher level it surrounds the spinal cord. The epidural needle enters the epidural space below the lower level of the spinal cord so there is no risk of "sticking the needle in the spine."

After the epidural needle enters the epidural space, the epidural catheter, a tiny clear tubing, is threaded through the center of the needle. The anesthesiologist then removes the needle, while leaving the catheter in place. He or she then tapes the part of the catheter extending outside the skin to the woman's back. Because it is flexible, she can lie on it or feel free to move around in bed without causing problems.

Finally, the anesthesiologist injects a local anesthetic through the epidural catheter, and it is the presence of this drug in the epidural space that provides pain relief during labor. Occasionally a small dose of narcotic may be used to supplement the anesthetic.

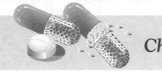
After the initial dose is given, the anesthesiologist may decide to connect the epidural catheter to an IV pump that dispenses a small amount of the pain relief medication continuously. This allows the pain relief to remain constant throughout labor and delivery. Or, the anesthesiologist may give additional medication through the catheter when the first dose starts to wear off.

An epidural provides the most effective pain relief of any of the options available to a woman in labor, that is, about 75-100% of the pain will be relieved. Even so, she should not expect to simply doze off and wake up a mother. She will not be numb from the waist down. She will fall asleep only if she is sleepy. Usually, women report feeling a pressure sensation in their abdomen with contractions, their legs may take on a "rubbery" or "tingly" feeling and will be less strong. To avoid falls or stumbling, women must stay in bed once the epidural is initiated.

Having an epidural is an option as soon as active labor begins and the mother is uncomfortable with her contractions - provided of course the obstetrician and anesthesiologist agree with the choice of pain relief. It may be performed all the way up to delivery, taking into account that time is needed to talk with the anesthesiologist, have the procedure done, and get some effect from the medication.

However, not all people are candidates for epidural anesthesia. The anesthesiologist will determine who does not qualify. For example, those who are bleeding or have blood-clotting problems will not be able to undergo epidural anesthesia. Women with fevers or infections at the site where the epidural needle enters the back are not candidates. Patients with progressive neurologic problems such as multiple sclerosis often do not qualify. Chronic back problems may or may not prevent a patient from having an epidural, and these should be evaluated during pregnancy well before delivery.

Problems with an epidural include the following:

1. It may not work. This is unusual, but normally can be corrected by having the epidural catheter replaced.

2. There may be a spot on the abdomen that doesn't get adequate pain relief. Often the anesthesiologist can correct this by repositioning the woman right before giving an additional dose of medication through the catheter.

3. One side of the body may get more pain relief than the other. This common problem is handled by placing the woman with the painful side lying closest to the bed and giving an additional dose of epidural medication.

4. The patient's blood pressure may drop. This is the most common complication and it won't harm the patient or her baby as long as it is corrected immediately. In order to avoid a blood pressure drop, patients receive a bolus dose of IV fluids (usually about one full bag of solution) prior to placement of the epidural. Once the epidural dose is given, the anesthesiologist monitors the patient's blood pressure for about 20 minutes and corrects any blood pressure drops that might occur.

5. Once in awhile, the epidural needle or catheter may end up in one of the many blood vessels in the epidural space. The anesthesiologist will have to start over and redo the catheter placement at a point either higher or lower on the patient's back.

6. Even rarer is the chance that the epidural needle might puncture the spinal fluid sac. If this does happen, there is about a 50/50 chance of getting a spinal headache. Several tests are routinely done to recognize this complication. If these tests show that the catheter is in the spinal fluid sac, then the catheter is removed and the procedure is repeated a little higher or lower on the patient's back. The final test by the anesthesiologist is to inject a small test dose of medication into the epidural catheter. If this catheter is in the spinal fluid sac, the patient will become very numb up to the breast level or higher. The patient would feel no pain. This would wear off in time and then the epidural could be reattempted.

Epidurals are sometimes accused of slowing labor, distressing fetuses, or causing forcep deliveries or C-sections. These accusations are all false and reflect outdated and unproven information.

Epidural anesthesia for labor actually has many benefits. It does <u>not</u> slow labor or decrease labor contractions. As a matter of fact it has been proven that epidural anesthesia may even speed up labor in patients that are having dysfunctional labor. Epidurals do not cause any problems with the fetus. Actually this technique reduces labor pain and stress so effectively that the baby has been shown to benefit. When local anesthetics are used with or without a tiny dose of narcotic there is no worry about depressing the baby's breathing at birth.

Epidural anesthesia does not increase the patient's risk of a forceps delivery. Some muscle relaxation from the waist down does occur so mothers may take a little longer to "push" out the baby. Pushing is possible and effective even if your contractions are not painful. Good coaching from the labor nurse and determination on the mother's part is all that are needed. Most new mothers have no idea how much work is involved in the "pushing" part of labor. Women should know that with or without an epidural, the pushing stage of labor is some of the hardest physical work that they will ever do.

Finally, epidurals do not increase the risk of getting a C-section. Good controlled studies have proven this. The benefits of an epidural for labor are many. It is an excellent form of pain relief. It can be easily supplemented and redosed so that it will last through labor and delivery. It works well for C-sections or forceps deliveries and can also be kept in place to use for a post partum tubal ligation done a day or two later. And finally, in emergencies, the epidural can often be quickly redosed and used for a C-section, thus avoiding the need for a general anesthetic which is less safe for mother and baby.

Vaginal Delivery Pain Relief Options

Mothers often require some extra form of anesthesia at the time of delivery. The most recent statistics (from 1981) show that 15% of mothers received no anesthesia or used Lamaze, 59% had the perineum and or vagina numbed with local anesthetics by their obstetrician, 14% had their labor epidural continued through delivery, 9% received a spinal, 6% inhaled a mixture of gases, and 3% received general anesthesia. Nowadays we use few spinals and almost never have women inhale gases or undergo general anesthesia.

When the epidural is used for vaginal delivery, often a larger, stronger dose of local anesthetic is given. This increases the pain relief in the vagina and on the perineum and the mother feels quite numb from the waist or hips on down. She will have some difficulty moving her legs at this point, although some pressure sensations may persist. The epidural can be used for a spontaneous vaginal delivery or a forceps delivery.

Spinal anesthesia for delivery differs from that used for labor. For a vaginal delivery the anesthesiologist injects local anesthetics instead of narcotics into the spinal fluid sac. The mother becomes completely numb below the waist or hips and is unable to move her legs. The possible complications of delivery spinals and epidurals are similar to those mentioned for a labor epidural. Spinals are typically used for a forceps delivery.

Few women breath gas mixtures or receive general anesthesia for vaginal delivery nowadays because these techniques are less safe. The major concern is that the mother or baby can become too sleepy. This leads to a baby who doesn't breathe deeply enough at delivery and a mother at high risk for vomiting and aspiration.

Another popular technique involves injecting local anesthetics into the area surrounding the vaginal outlet called the perineum, right before the baby comes out. This well-known application of delivery-related local anesthesia is done just before the doctor does an episiotomy (a cut in the tissue surrounding the vaginal opening). An episiotomy is a minor surgical procedure performed to prevent tearing of the tissues as the baby's head emerges and is done in 85% of the deliveries in the United States. A local anesthetic, commonly lidocaine, is injected into the region below the vaginal opening so the doctor can perform the episiotomy without pain to the mother. This technique is reasonable for spontaneous vaginal deliveries. For a forcep delivery, additional local anesthetic is injected by the obstetrician into the upper vagina in the area surrounding the pudendal nerve. This provides pain relief in the vaginal area as well.

C-Section Anesthesia Options

No one can be guaranteed a vaginal delivery. Yet, we see many women undergoing C-sections who say they skipped prenatal class on the night that C-sections were discussed because they were sure they wouldn't need one. Every pregnancy is different. There is always the possibility of a C-section, even when a woman has had previous successful vaginal deliveries. Unexpected difficulties or emergencies (example: fetal distress) may arise during pregnancy or labor that require a C-section. The best advice is to prepare by considering your anesthesia options ahead of time.

The 1981 statistics on C-Sections show that 21% of patients received an epidural, 34% got a spinal, and 41% received general anesthesia. Currently, epidurals and spinals are more popular, and more epidurals than spinals are done. General anesthesia is reserved for women that don't qualify for a spinal/epidural or when there is an emergency requiring an immediate C-section.

Some General Points About C-Sections

Before the surgery begins, the mother drinks a small amount of a clear antacid which neutralizes the acids present in her stomach. this is done as a precaution in case the mother vomits during the surgery and aspirates some vomit into her lungs.

During surgery mothers must lay flat on their backs on the operating room table. A pregnant woman knows that such a position makes her feel dizzy. This is because the baby is essentially lying on top of the mother's major blood vessels and slowing the blood flow back to her heart. As a result the mother's blood pressure drops and the blood flow to the baby is decreased. To prevent this problem during pregnancy most women lay on their sides. However, this isn't possible during surgery. During a C-section this problem is corrected by placing a soft wedge under the mother's right hip and abdomen. This shifts her pregnant abdomen to the left and thereby shifts her uterus off of her major blood vessels. This avoids the stress to mother and baby that a drop in the mother's blood pressure could produce.

During the C-section mothers need lots of oxygen. The more oxygen the mother gets, the better it is for the baby. With a spinal or epidural, mothers breathe additional oxygen through a mask over their nose and mouth. During general anesthesia mothers receive as much oxygen as possible through a breathing tube. This is especially important right before delivery of the baby. Once the obstetrician cuts into the mother's uterus the blood supply carrying oxygen and nutrients to the baby is disrupted. Thus the baby is essentially "holding its breath" until it is delivered and takes its own first breaths. This period of time is typically 1-3 minutes. If the mother is breathing additional oxygen, this essentially boosts the baby's oxygen supply so it can better tolerate this stress.

The anesthesiologist will discuss several variables that go into the choice of the best anesthetic for a C-section. These include past medical health, any possible complications with pregnancy or labor, how close a woman is to her due date, her baby's present condition, and whether or not there is peril to the mother or child that indicates the need for an emergency C-section.

Epidural and Spinal Anesthesia

Most non-emergency C-sections are done with epidural or spinal anesthesia. With these two techniques, the patient is numb from about nipple level down to her toes. They involve local anesthetics, which allow mothers to be awake and alert throughout the procedure. Mothers can see their babies at delivery and hold the baby while the obstetrician completes the C-section. Even though, like most drugs, local anesthetics cross the placenta and get into the baby, they do not make it sleepy or cause any significant problems. Following delivery, patients may request some sedation. However, this is not routinely given unless requested.

During the C-section under spinal or epidural anesthesia, the mother's legs will be very heavy and she will be unable to lift or move them. This numbness typically wears off over the hour following the operation. Some women dislike the postop numbness because they can't move their legs. It's worth remembering that, while they are numb following anesthesia, women do not feel pain and they can be clear-headed to greet family, hold the baby, or make phone calls from the recovery area.

The procedures for these C-section spinals and epidurals are the same as those prescribed for spinals or epidurals for labor. For a C-section, an epidural is dosed with a larger amount and a stronger concentration of local anesthetic than that used for labor. The medication is typically given through the epidural catheter and additional doses can be administered throughout the C-section to keep the mother comfortable. The epidural catheter is removed easily and painlessly at the end of the C-section.

For a C-section spinal, local anesthetics instead of narcotics are injected through the spinal needle. One of several different local anesthetics can be chosen by the anesthesiologist, depending upon how long the C-section is expected to last.

General Anesthesia

Sometimes a general anesthetic is the best method for a C-section. In order to limit the amount of time the baby is exposed to anesthetic drugs that might make it sleepy at delivery, many things will be done before a woman is anesthetized. An nurse will scrub and shave her abdomen then place sterile drapes over it. The obstetrician will scrub his or her hands, put on a sterile gown and gloves and be poised ready to begin. At this time the anesthesiologist injects medication into the intravenous line, which puts the patient to sleep in about 20 seconds. Sometimes women notice a pressure sensation on the front of their neck as they lose consciousness. This is due to someone in the operating room pressing on the front of the mother's neck in order to help prevent aspiration of any stomach contents that might come up as the patient loses consciousness with the anesthetic. A breathing tube is then placed through the mouth and into the windpipe. This breathing tube further helps prevent aspiration of stomach contents into the lungs. It also assures that both mother and baby get plenty of oxygen during surgery. Women generally don't remember the breathing tube because it is placed after they are unconscious and removed as they are waking up from anesthesia and in control of their gag reflex.

The amount of drugs used in a C-section is limited, in order to decrease the risk of making the baby sleepy at delivery and help the mother make a faster, safer recovery from anesthesia. Despite this fact, the mother will typically feel tired and groggy for a few hours after the operation.

Pain Relief Options After Delivery

A woman may or may not need further pain relief after her baby is born, but if she does, there are several options. For mothers who have had an uncomplicated vaginal delivery, Tylenol (acetaminophen) for a day or two may be all that is necessary. For more complicated deliveries or C-sections, traditionally, women are offered medications either through their IV line or as an intramuscular injection or "shot". These are usually narcotics such as Demerol or morphine. When women are able to eat or drink, they receive oral medications such as Tylenol with codeine.

Although reasonably effective, these narcotic drugs all have unpleasant side effects such as grogginess, nausea, and vomiting. Breast-feeding mothers are often reluctant to use medication even though this short term use has essentially no effect on the baby.

A second option is epidural narcotics. Women who have had surgery with an epidural anesthetic can receive narcotics through the epidural catheter after delivery of the baby. Morphine, which is commonly used, provides 17-20 hours of consistent pain relief. Side effects from this technique include itching, nausea and vomiting, difficulty urinating and, very rarely, respiratory depression. Because of this last complication, these mothers are watched more closely for their first 24 hours after surgery.

A third option is patient controlled analgesia or PCA. More and more, obstetricians are introducing their patients to PCA to help with post=cesarean section pain. This method allows the mother to have more direct control over her own pain relief.

The mother's intravenous line is connected to a PCA machine that gives out a small dose of medication, usually a narcotic, when she pushes a button. The PCA machine is programmed to dispense no more than a predetermined maximum dose so that a mother can't overdose herself. Mothers tend to be less sleepy and less nauseated with this method as compared to shots, since smaller more frequent doses are given. Women are often very satisfied with this method because they feel they have some control, they don't need to ask a nurse for pain medication, it's instantly available, and they receive good pain relief. All these options help diminish pain, but none totally relieve all the pain.

Anesthesia for Post-Partum Tubal Ligation

Postpartum tubal ligations are usually done using spinal, epidural, or general anesthesia. The techniques would be similar to those used for a C-section. If a mother had an epidural for labor, the epidural catheter can be left in place and used at the time of her tubal ligation, even if it takes place as long as 48-72 hours after delivery. For mothers who are breast-feeding, special care is taken to limit the medications used, since these drugs can be transmitted in breast milk to the babies.

To lower risk from anesthesia, the post-partum tubal ligation should not be done until at least 8 hours after delivery. The mother should not eat or drink anything for 8 hours prior to the procedure. Precautions to prevent aspiration are still needed, including the use of a clear antacid before surgery and use of a breathing tube for a general anesthetic.

Case Study

Sarah R, a 27-year -old computer programmer, had worked hard during her first pregnancy to prepare for her delivery. Both she and her husband attended childbirth education classes, toured the hospital's labor and delivery areas, and discussed the birth process with her doctor. They were initially interested in childbirth without drugs, but, after hearing about the options that are now available, they became open to other techniques, as well. Eventually they decided they were willing to use whatever measures were necessary to ensure a safe and comfortable delivery.

Sarah's membranes (bag of waters) ruptured 3 days before her due date while watching TV with her husband. She called her obstetrician who advised her to come to the hospital. By the time she arrived, she was having a few contractions. While she was being admitted to labor and delivery and an IV was being placed in her arm, she noticed her contractions getting stronger.

Sarah initially used her Lamaze breathing techniques to relieve the pain. This worked well for about 2 hours with her husband massaging her lower back as he coached her through the increasingly intense contractions. When she felt that this technique alone was not providing enough relief, she asked for additional help. Because she was well informed, she knew the hospital offered epidural anesthesia and she specifically requested it. Her obstetrician was contacted and gave the "okay" for the procedure to be done. Next, an anesthesiologist talked with her and determined that she was a good candidate for an epidural. They discussed the risks and benefits and Sarah gave the "go ahead."

The anesthesiologist inserted an epidural catheter in Sarah's back, local anesthetics were given through the catheter, and her pain was relieved within 10 minutes. Her anesthesiologist then connected her to an apparatus which allowed her to get a continuous small dose of epidural medication throughout labor and delivery. Sarah began to relax. She felt only a mild pressure sensation during contractions. She continued to dilate and was comfortable and anxious to push when the time came. Sarah knew she would have to push extremely hard at this point, even though she did not have pain. With contractions, she concentrated on bearing down hard like she was having a large bowel movement. As a result, she pushed effectively for 45 minutes ending in the delivery of an 8-pound boy with a 1-minute Apgar score of 9 and 5-minute Apgar of 10.

Case Study (continued)

Just before delivery the obstetrician used local anesthesia to numb Sarah's perineum (the area surrounding the vagina). Because she still had her epidural working, Sarah did not feel the needle used to numb her. She was also much more comfortable during delivery and repair of the episiotomy. A half hour later, she was relaxing in bed and able to move her legs well. The anesthesiologist easily and painlessly removed Sarah's epidural catheter, as she admired her lovely new son.

Key Points for Labor Pain Relief

1. Childbirth preparation is extremely important. Methods of massaging pain and other aspects of delivery should be discussed with your obstetrician well in advance of delivery. We recommend that everyone become well informed about pregnancy, labor, childbirth, and care of the newborn.

2. The major methods of labor pain control are: psychoprophylaxis (Lamaze), injections of narcotics, spinal narcotics, and epidural anesthesia.

3. Try to remain flexible and be willing to consider more than one pain relief option, since no one method is best for everyone. Contact the anesthesiologist at your hospital to answer questions in advance. Remember, once you are in active labor, you will be less able to ask questions and consider the answers well.

4. Don't feel guilty about requesting some form of pain relief. Remember that, if you are in pain and stressed, this also stresses your baby.

5. Avoid eating or drinking once you go into labor. Instead depend on your intravenous line (IV) to provide fluid and nutrition for you and your baby and a safety mechanism for emergencies.

6. All pain relief techniques help decrease the pain of labor, but none can take it away completely. You should expect to participate actively in labor, and you should not expect to fall asleep and wake up a mother.

7. No one is guaranteed a vaginal delivery. Examine your anesthesia options in advance, should the need for a C-section arise while you're in labor. Several methods are available for post C-section pain control including intramuscular injections of narcotics, epidural narcotics, and patient controlled analgesia.

8. A post partum tubal ligation is safest when done at least 8 hours after delivery.

Notes

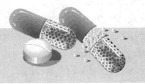

Chapter 20

Drugs and Breast Milk: Lactation and Lactation Suppression

Shortly after delivery of a baby, nature produces yet another marvel in the ongoing sequence of marvels that began with conception. This early postpartum phenomenon is called *lactation* or breast milk production. Nowadays, obstetricians and pediatricians strongly encourage women to breast-feed even if only for a few weeks. Despite this increasing interest in breast-feeding today, however, many new mothers still choose not to breast-feed or cannot do so for medical reasons. (For example, mothers who are HIV-positive probably should not breast-feed, since we believe the virus can be transmitted this way.) It is certainly possible to meet an infant's nutritional needs with a good formula, and no woman should feel pressured to nurse her baby. In this chapter we discuss the role of drug therapy for women who choose to breast feed and also for those who choose to suppress lactation.

Maintaining Lactation

Right after delivery, rapidly fluctuating hormone levels (a sharp decrease in estrogen and progesterone and a rise in the hormone of breast-feeding, prolactin) cause the 15-25 ducts in the breast to secrete a nutritious substance called colostrum. Quite different from breast milk, colostrum is thought to give the baby an important dose of fats, proteins, and maternal anti-bodies to help him adjust to a radical change of environment.

In two to three days, the colostrum will give way to normal breast milk, one of nature's more perfect foods. Guided by an intricate series of physiological, neurological, and psycho-logical events, breast milk, once established, can continue to nourish your baby for many months or even years.

Breast-feeding is popular and has been on the rise since the middle 1960s. In some commu-nities it is difficult to find a formula-fed baby. The upsurge in breast-feeding coincides with the natural foods and holistic health movement along with growing public sentiment against artificially manufactured foods. Psychologists and pediatricians have demonstrated the importance of the maternal-infant bond in the early days of life and emphasized the role that breast-feeding plays in this bonding process.

Breast-feeding is pleasurable for both the infant and the mother. Nursing an infant publicly is viewed less negatively than it was 20 years ago. It is a more convenient way of feeding a baby because there is no fuss with bottle and formula preparation and no cleaning up. Nursing is cheaper than buying formula, so it should be attractive to families with limited incomes. Ironically, it seems to be more popular among the high income families.

From both the obstetrician's and pediatrician's point of view, there is no doubt that breast-fed babies are healthier. They have fewer infections, allergies, and digestive upsets. Breast milk is tailor-made for human babies and very different in composition from cow's or goat's milk. It takes over where the placenta left off. In some cultures breast milk is called "white blood," an accurate term if you consider that it contains antibodies against all kinds of infec-tions, enzymes that destroy bacteria, virus-inhibiting substances, lactose (milk sugar, which promotes the growth of necessary/helpful bacteria in the intestines, and growth-stimulating molecules that assist the development of cells lining the infant's intestinal tract. Human breast milk has a high concentration of fat and lactose compared with cow's milk, which has a much higher protein component. The milk proteins are casein and whey: in cow's milk casein is the predominant protein; in human milk whey predominates, and it is much easier to digest especially for small infants.

Effects of Drugs and Other Substances in Breast Milk

Much of what a mother eats, drinks, and even breathes will find its way into breast milk. Breast milk has a large amount of fat, and body fat tends to be a depository for chemical substances ingested by humans. This includes undesirable materials - certain drugs, dangerous minerals such as lead or mercury, and environmental pollutants. Physicians are conducting ongoing research on the action of drugs in breast milk and how they transfer to and affect infants. At the moment we do not know a great deal; much of our information comes from reports on studies of one or two patients. The most significant large study to date has found that women who ingested the chemical compound PCB in breast milk as infants have continued to show high levels of the chemical in their body fat and breast milk. Researchers have not, however, concluded that the presence of these chemicals have been harmful either to the women or the infants they are now nursing.

We know that infants in the first two months of life are not equipped to digest or metabolize drugs the way an older child can; therefore certain drugs may accumulate to undesirably high levels in their tiny bodies. Conversely because of their immature digestive systems, some drugs may be excreted with few or no side effects - fewer even than older children who may digest them more thoroughly. Each drug behaves in a unique fashion. Because mothers are concerned about the effect of pollutants, chemicals, and drugs on their babies, they frequently ask their doctors if breast-feeding should be stopped when they take medication. They also want to know which drugs are safe to take and if breast-feeding ought to be avoided for short periods after a drug has been swallowed.

In most cases the concentrations of drugs in breast milk are low enough that a mother need not stop breast-feeding, unless her baby shows definite symptoms of being affected by the drug. When drug therapy is essential for a mother, consideration should be given to the drug alternative (providing there is one) that is least likely to concentrate in breast milk. Scheduling drug doses immediately after an infant has breast fed or just before he is likely to sleep for a long time can avert this problem to some extent.

Some drugs actually affect milk production itself. Stimulants and decongestants may decrease blood flow to the breast and therefore milk yield. Large amounts of nicotine (more than 2 packs of cigarettes a day) can decrease milk supply. Levodopa, ergocryptine, bromocriptine, pyridoxine, and monoamine oxidase inhibitors (MAOs) cause decreases in prolactin production and therefore breast milk. Drugs like the phenothiazines, cimetidine, metoclopramide, methysergide, and some high-blood pressure medications (reserpine, clonidine, and methyldopa) stimulate prolactin (and breast milk) production. (Table 20-1 outlines the effects on the infant of many common drugs in the mother's breast milk.) Certain drugs are not often used by nursing mothers, so our information is sparse. Table 20-1 notes what information does exist in the medical literature.

Table 20-1
Drugs Excreted in Breast Milk, and
Their Effects on Newborns

Drug (Brand)	Neonatal Effect at Maternal Therapeutic Dose
Analgesics and anti-inflammatory agents	
Acetaminophen	Maximum dose ingested by infant after a 650-mg dose = 0.23% of maternal dose. Amount ingested after a 1 g dose = 1.85% of maternal dose. Acetaminophen and metabolites were detected in infant's urine. Once case report of an infant developing a rash due to acetaminophen ingested while breast-feeding. This was confirmed by rechallenge. Considered compatible with breast-feeding.
Aspirin	One case report of a 16-day-old infant who developed salicylate poisoning with serum levels of 24 mg/dL (milk and maternal serum levels were not obtained). It is very doubtful that these levels could have resulted from breast-feeding, but parents denied administering any salicylates to infant. In a case report of a mother taking aspirin, 2.4 g/day, infant plasma levels = 0.47 mmol/L. Normally infant would ingest very small quantities via breast milk, but concern of relationship of aspirin and Reye's syndrome cause us to advise mothers to use caution in taking aspirin while breast-feeding.
Butophanol (Stadol)	Estimated dose ingested by infant = 4µg/day. Probably not significant.
Codeine	Not significant.
Fenoprofen (Nalfon)	Probably not significant.
Fentanyl (Sublimaze)	Due to very small amounts excreted in milk, doses ingested by infant would probably be too small to cause adverse effects.
Flurbiprofen (Ansaid)	Due to extremely small amounts excreted in milk, it is doubtful that the infant would receive an amount that would cause

	adverse effects. Probably not significant.
Heroin	Can cause addiction. Levels in milk not high enough to prevent withdrawal in addicted infants.
Ibuprofen (Motrin, Advil)	Not significant.
Indomethacin (Indocin)	Case report of convulsions in breast-fed infant. Used to close patent ductus arteriosus. Insufficient data on the effect on other vessels. May be nephrotoxic.
Ketoprofen (Orudis)	Probably not significant.
Ketoralac (Toradol)	Maximum dose ingested by infant = 3.16-7.9 μg or 0.16-0.4% of maternal dose. Probably not significant.
Mefenamic acid (Ponstel)	Not significant.
Methadone (Dolophine)	Breast-feeding permissible during methadone maintenance. Up to 80 mg/day, no ill effects on infant. Not significant.
Meperidine (Demerol)	No adverse effects noted in any infants. Probably not significant.
Morphine	Maximum dose ingested by infant after 4 mg epidurally was calculated to be 8 μg/100 mL milk. Maximum amount ingested after 15 mg IV/IM = 50 μg. Usually not significant. Compatible with breast-feeding.
Naproxen (Naprosen)	Total cumulative amount excreted in infant urine is 0.26% of maternal dose. Not significant.
Oxycodone (Percocet, Tylox)	No adverse effects noted. Probably not significant.
Oxyphenbutazone (Tandearil)	No known effect. Oxyphenbutazone is a metabolite of phenylbutazone; caution is advised.
Phenylbutazone (Butazoldin)	Infant serum levels 3-20 μg/mL after 750-mg IM dose. Risk to infant not well defined. May accumulate in infant. Caution due to possible idiosyncratic blood dyscrasias.
Piroxicarn (Feldone)	Maximum daily dose ingested by infant calculated to be 6.3% of maternal dose. No adverse effects noted in any infant. Probably not significant.
Propoxyphene (Darvon, Darvocet)	Only symptoms detectable would be failure to feed and drowsiness. If mother ingests maximum recommended dosage in a 24-hr period, the infant could receive 1 mg/day, a significant dose in a neonate.

Tolmentin (Tolectin)	Calculated dose ingested by infant = 27.7μg. Extremely small amounts excreted. Probably not significant.

Anti-arthritic agents

Cloroquine (Aralen)	Maximum daily dose ingested = 0.7% of the maternal dose. Effects on infant unknown.
Gold compounds (auranofin, gold sodium thiomalate, aurothioglucose)	Estimated infant dose ingested in the gold sodium thiomalate case = 20% of maternal dose. In the second case when mother's serum level = 9.97 μg/mL gold levels detected in infant red blood cells = 0.354 μg/mL and infant serum = 0.712 μg/mL. This may cause rashes, nephritis, hepatitis, and hematologic abnormalities.
Hydroxychloroquine (Plaquenil)	Estimated dose ingested by infant = 2% of maternal dose per day. Effect on infant unknown.
Penicillamine (Cuprimine, Depen)	Unknown.

Antibiotics

Amantadine (Symmetrel	May cause vomiting, urinary retention, skin rash.
Amoxicillin (Amoxil, Polymox, Larotid)	May alter oral and GI flora and cause thrush. May interfere with interpretation of culture results. No systemic adverse reactions.
Ampicillin	Possibility of allergic sensitization exists. Can produce candidiasis and diarrhea in infant. Not significant.
Ampicillin/Sulbactam (Unasyn)	No adverse effects noted. Same precautions as ampicillin.
Aztreonam (Azactam)	No adverse effects noted. May alter mouth and GI flora and produce candidiasis. May interfere with interpretation of culture results
Carbenicillin (Geopen)	Not significant.
Cephalosporins	No significant systemic effects. As with other cephalosporins, may alter GI flora and result in candidiasis. May interfere with interpretation of culture results. Risk of allergic sensitization.
Cefaclor (Ceclor)	Same as cephalosporins.
Cefamandole (Mandol)	No infant data available. Due to very small amounts excreted in breast milk, probably not significant. Same precautions as with other cephalosporins.
Cefazolin (Ancef, Kefzol)	Not absorbed well by mouth 0.075% of maternal dose excreted in milk. Not significant.

Cefotaxime (Claforan)	Same precautions as for cephalosporins.
Cefoxitin (Mefoxin)	Infant could receive 0.7 mg/day. Not significant. Peak milk concentration occurs at 4-7 hr after IM injection in most subjects.
Ceftizoxime (Cefizox)	Same precautions as for cephalosporins
Ceftriaxone (Rocephin)	Despite long half-life, very small amounts could be ingested by infant. Same precautions as for cephalosporins.
Cephalexin (Keflex)	Only very small amounts could be ingested by infant. Same precautions as for cephalosporins.
Cephalothin (Keflin)	Same precautions as for cephalosporins.
Chloramphenicol (Chloromycetin)	Reported adverse effects include refusal to feed, falling asleep while feeding, intestinal gas, and vomiting after feeding. Although ingested amounts are low, the theoretical risk of bone marrow suppression causes us to classify it as an agent whose effect is unknown and may be of concern.
Clindamycin (Cleocin)	Not significant.
Colistin (Coly-Mycin)	Not well absorbed orally. Not significant.
Ciprofloxacin (Cipro)	Infant could ingest up to 1.33 μmol after this single dose. Ciprofloxacin is currently not recommended for infants secondary to risk of arthropathy.
Cycloserine (Seromycin	No adverse effects reported in infants. 0.6% of maternal dose excreted in milk..
Demeclocycline (Declomycin)	Same precautions as for tetracycline.
Doxycycline (Vibramycin)	Same precautions as for tetracycline.
Erythromycin (E.E.S. E-Mycin)	Most recent reports indicate minimal risk to the infant; compatible with breast feeding. Not significant.
Ethambutol (Myambutol)	Not significant. Compatible with breast feeding.
Gentamicin (Garamycin)	Not well absorbed from GI tract. May change gut flora. If GI inflammation or diarrhea exists, monitor infant's serum levels to avoid ototoxicity and nephrotoxicity.
Isoniazid (INH)	Acetyl-INH thought to cause liver toxicity. Infant could ingest significant amounts (25% of maternal dose) if receiving chronic therapy.
Kanamycin (Kantrex)	Probably not significant. (Same precautions as for gentamicin.)
Lincomycin (Lincocin)	Not significant.

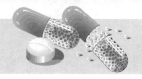

Mandelic acid (methenamine mandelate— Mandelamine is 50% mandelic acid)	Drug detectible in urine of all infants. Estimated daily dose ingested = 86 mg/kg/day. Significance unknown.
Methacycline (Rondomycin)	Same precautions as for tetracycline.
Methenamine hippurate (Hiprex)	Infant would receive 0.05-0.1 mg/kg. No untoward effects.
Metronidazole (Flagyl)	Use during breast-feeding remains controversial. Some sources still cite animal carcinogenic studies. At maternal doses of 600-1,200 mg/day infant plasma levels 20% of mother's. No adverse effects noted in these infants. If a single 2-g oral dose is administered, hold breast-feeding 12-24 hr to reduce infant drug exposure.
Minocycline (Minocin)	Same precautions as for tetracycline.
Moxalactam (Moxam)	Infant could ingest 2 mg/day in 550 mL/milk. Theoretical risk of enterocolitis from altered GI flora.
Nalidixic acid (NegGram)	One case of hemolytic anemia reported in G6PD-deficient infant. Not significant.
Nitrofurantoin (Macrodantin)	Not significant, except in G6PD-deficient infants. No adverse effects reported in normal infants.
Nystatin (Mycostatin)	None
Oxacillin (Prostaphlin)	Not significant, same precautions as penicillin.
Oxytetracycline (Terramycin)	Same precautions as for tetracycline.
Penicllin, benzathine	Same precautions as for penicillin.
Penicillin G	Not significant. May alter GI flora. Risk of candidiasis and allergic sensitization. May interfere with interpretation of culture results.
Penicillin VK	Not significant. Same precautions as for penicillin.
Piperacillin (Pipracil)	Not significant. Same precautions as for penicillin.
Pyrimethamine (Daraprim)	Quantity excreted not sufficient to treat malaria in infants less than 6 mo old, although there have been cases where this has been accomplished via drug in milk.
Quinine/Sulfate	Probably not significant. Caution in infants at risk for G6PD deficiency. Maximum total daily dose ingested by infant 2-3 mg/kg/day. Monitor for hypersensitivity reactions, thrombocytopenia
Rifampin	0.05% of maternal dose excreted in milk. Probably not significant.
Streptomycin	Not significant. Due to small amount excreted in milk and negligible oral absorption, risk to infant is minimal.

Sulfonamides	Rare reports of averse reactions: diarrhea, rash, oral and GI candidiasis. Breast-feeding while taking sulfonamides remains controversial, but risk is thought to be very low for healthy full-term infants. Avoid use in sick premature infants with hyperbilirubinemia or infants at risk of G6PD deficiency. Sulfonamides considered compatible with breast-feeding.
Sulfacetamide	Probably not significant.. Neonatal jaundice due to displacement of bilirubin from protein-binding sites. Hemolytic anemia in G6PD-deficient infants. Rash.
Sulfadiazine	Probably not significant. (Same precautions as for sulfacetamide.)
Sulfamethazine	Same as sulfacetamide.
Sulfamethoxazole (Gantanol)	Caution during first 2 weeks of life. Same precautions as for sulfacetamide.
Sulfanilamide	Greater risk of hyperbilirubinemia, encephalopathy because of high concentration in milk.
Sulfapyridine	Same as for sulfanilamide.
Sulfathiazole	Probably not significant. (Same precautions as for sulfacetamide.)
Sulfisoxazole (Gantrisin)	Not significant. Amount absorbed from milk too small to cause displacement of bilirubin from protein binding sites in healthy term neonate.
Tetracycline (Sumycin)	The risk of dental staining and delayed bone growth that exists with its use during pregnancy is remote during breast-feeding. Infant serum levels are undetectable (<0.05 µg/mL) and the drug has low bioavailability due to chelation with milk calcium. Probably not significant. Compatible with breast-feeding.
Ticarcillin (Ticar)	Not significant. Same precautions as for penicillin.
Tobramycin (Nebcin)	Due to small amount excreted in milk and negligible oral absorption, risk to infant is minimal. Same precautions as for gentamicin.
Trimethoprim (Trimpex; also in combination with sulfamethoxazole in Bactrim and Septra)	Small amounts excreted, probably not significant. May alter GI flora. Candidiasis, rash, risk of allergic sensitization. May interfere with interpretation of culture results. We considers it compatible with breast-feeding

Vancomycin	Due to negligible oral absorption, risk to infant is minimal. May alter GI flora.

Anticoagulants

Bishydroxycoumarin (dicumarol)	Usually not significant. Monitor infant. Vitamin K may be given to infant if blood clotting tests warrant or if infant to undergo surgery
Ethyl biscoumacetate (Tromexan)	Avoid use due to reported episodes of hemorrhage of umbilical stump and cephalohematoma.
Heparin	None
Phenindione (Hedulin)	Case report of increased blood clotting problems in infant and incisional and scrotal hemorrhage after inguinal herniotomy.
Warfarin (Coumadin)	May safely breast-feed. Not significant.

Anticonvulsants

Carbamazepine (Tegretol)	A 4-kg infant would receive approximately 0.5 mg/kg. Infant serum levels in range of 1.0 µg/mL. Peak serum level of 4.7 µg/mL reported in one infant. Long-term effects unknown. Monitor for poor sucking, sedation, and vomiting.
Clonazepam (Klonopin)	Infant plasma level after 7 days of nursing = 2.9 ng/mL which may have resulted primarily from in utero exposure. Persistent apnea noted, not known whether this was due to clonazepam. Caution due to long half-life in neonates.
Ethosuximide (Zarontin)	6% of maternal dose excreted in milk, infant plasma levels may reach 25% of maternal plasma levels. Monitor infant closely.
Phenobarbital	Due to long half-life (156 hr) in neonates, accumulation of drug in infant plasma has been shown to occur in some cases. Infant plasma levels 2-13 µg/mL. Reports of sedation. Use with caution in breast-feeding.
Phenytoin (Dilantin)	Usually no effect at maternal doses of 300 mg/day. Calculated infant dose ingested, 0.03-0.47 mg/kg/day. Infant phenytoin clearance usually high. In one study 2 infants had low but detectable plasma levels. None of the infants exhibited adverse effects. Possibility of enzyme induction. One case report of methemoglobinemia and cyanosis in infant whose mother was taking phenytoin and phenobarbital.

Primidone (Mysoline)	Infant plasma levels 2.5 µg/mL. Half-life in infant 23.0 ± 8.6 hr. Drowsiness and decreased feeding reported. Use with caution in breast-feeding.
Valproic acid (Depakene)	Infant serum level 7.6% of maternal serum level. No adverse effects noted in any of the reported cases.

Antihistamines and Decongestants

Clemastine (Tavist)	One case report of drowsiness, irritability, refusal to feed, high-pitched cry, neck stiffness.
Dexbrompheniramine maleate, 6 mg, with d-isophedrine, 120 mg (sustained-release tablets) (Drixoral)	One case report of irritability, excessive crying, and disturbed sleeping patterns of 5 days' duration. Avoid long-acting preparations.
Diphenhydramine (Benadryl)	Not significant. May cause sedation, decreased feeding.
Pseudoephrine/ triprolidine (Actifed)	Estimated infant dose ingested = 0.25-0.33 mg, or 0.5%-0.7% of the maternal dose. We consider it compatible with breast-feeding.
Trimeprazine (Temaril)	Not significant. (Same precautions as for diphenydramine.)
Tripelennamine (Pyribenzamine)	Not significant. (Same precautions as for diphenhydramine.)

Antivirals

Acyclovir (Zovirax)	Acyclovir was detected in infant urine at concentration of 1.06 1.08 µg/mL. Since acylovir is used to treat infants with herpes infections and no adverse effects were noted in this case, we consider it compatible with breast feeding.

Autonomic Drugs

Atropine	No adverse effects reported. We consider it compatible with breast-feeding.
Carisoprodol (Soma, Rela)	CNS depression, GI effects.
Ergotamine (Cafergot	Signs of ergotism; vomiting, diarrhea, weak pulse, and unstable blood pressure. Short courses probably not significant. High doses inhibit prolactin.
Menpenzolate bromide (Cantil)	None
Methocarbamol (Robaxin)	Not significant.

Neostigmine	Not significant.
Propantheline bromide (Pro-Banthine)	Drug is rapidly metabolized in maternal system to inactive metabolite. Avoid long-acting preparations.
Scopolamine (Hyoscine)	Not significant.

Cardiovascular drugs

Acebutolol (Sectral)	Pharmacologically active amounts of drug may be ingested by infant. Symptoms of ß-blockade (hypotension and bradycardia) reported in one infant; mother's dose was 400 mg/day.
Amiodarone (Cordarone)	Estimated drug ingested by infant approximates a low maintenance dose. Not recommended during breast-feeding.
Atenolol (Tenormin)	Infant may ingest 5.7-9.2% of maternal dose. Plasma concentration of 2 µg/mL measured 48 hr after feeding. Symptoms of ß-blockade included bradycardia, cyanosis, and hypothermia
Captopril (Capoten)	Amount of captopril in milk not sufficient to cause adverse effects.
Clonidine (Catapres)	Infant's serum concentration half of that of mother. No hypotension or other side effects occurred. Nearly therapeutic levels in infant of concern.
Digoxin (Lanoxin)	Due to large volume of distribution the total daily excretion of digoxin in milk of mothers with therapeutic serum concentrations would not exceed 1-2 µg, not sufficient to affect child.
Disopyramide (Norpace)	Not detectable in infant serum at maternal dose of 450 mg q8h. Maximum calculated infant dose = 3.7 mg/day (<2 mg/kg/day). No detectable side effects in infants in case reports.
Enalapril (Vasotec)	No adverse effects noted in 3 infants reported at maternal doses of 5-10 mg 2 x daily.
Encainide (Enkaid)	Unknown.
Flecainide (Tambocor)	Unknown. Infant in case report not breast-fed
Guanethidine (Ismelin)	No adverse effects noted; 1 infant breast-fed by mother receiving chronic therapy.
Hydralazine (Apresoline)	Calculated infant dose 0.013 mg per feeding.
Labetalol (Normodyne, Trandate)	Measurable plasma levels found in only 1 infant: 21 ng/mL at 8 hr postdose. Percent maternal dose likely to be ingested = 0.07%. No adverse effects noted in any case reports.
Methyldopa (Aldomet)	Infant plasma levels not detectable. Urine level in 1 infant 3.8 µg/mL. No adverse effects noted in any reports.

Metoprolol (Lopressor)	Concentrates in milk.
Mexiletine (Mexitil)	One case report of an infant breast-fed for 3 mo at maternal doses of 250-mg t.i.d. Infant began formula supplementation at 17 days for poor weight gain. No other adverse effects noted.
Minoxidil (Loniten)	No adverse effects noted.
Nadolol (Corgard)	Infant could ingest 2-7% of adult therapeutic dose. Caution in breast-feeding.
Nifedipine (Procardia)	Less than 5% of maternal dose excreted in milk. Optimum time to breast-feed $= \geq 4$ hr after dose. Infant in this study not breast-fed.
Prazosin (Minipress)	Unknown.
Procainamide (PA)	Amount consumed by infant < 1.0% of maternal dose, probably not significant.
Propranolol (Inderal)	Preferred ß-blocker in breast-feeding. Maximum dose ingested by infant (21 µg/day) less than 0.1% of maternal dose. No adverse effects in infants noted
Quinidine	Approximately 1% of maternal dose appears in milk.
Reserpine	May cause nasal stuffiness, lethargy, diarrhea, increased tracheobronchial secretions with difficulty breathing. Also reported to cause galactorrhea.
Timolol	Calculated infant dose 2.4 µg/kg/day when maternal dose 5 mg t.i.d. can accumulate in milk. Monitor infant for apnea, bradycardia.
Tocainide (Tonocard)	Infant in this report not breast-fed. Caution since drug concentrates in breast milk. Effects unknown.
Verapamil (Isoptin, Calan)	Infant serum levels not detectable. Percent maternal dose likely to be ingested $= 0.01\%$. No adverse effects noted.

Chemotherapeutic Agents

Cisplatin (Platinol)	Unknown. Breast-feeding contraindicated.
Cyclophosphamide (Cytoxan)	Contraindicated. One report of infant developed neutropenia.
Doxorubicin (Adriamycin)	Infant not breast-fed in this case. Considered contraindicated secondary to concern for possible immunosuppression, carcinogenesis, neutropenia, and unknown effect on growth.
Hydoxyurea (Hydrea)	Infant not breast-fed in this case. Calculated dose likely to be ingested = 3-4 mg/day.

	Effects on infant unknown. Considered contraindicated during breast-feeding.
Methotrexate	Infant could receive 0.26 µg/100 mL, which researchers consider nontoxic for infant.

Diuretics

Acetazolamide (Diamox)	Infant plasma level 0.6 µg/mL. Estimated infant dose 0.6 mg/day. Percent maternal dose likely to be ingested, 0.06%. Probably not significant.
Bendroflumethiazide (Rauzide, Naturetin)	Lactation suppressed.
Chlorothiazide (Diuril)	Amount ingested by infant insignificant. May suppress lactation due to dehydration of mother. Possibility of thrombocytopenia (rare).
Chlorthalidone (Hygroton)	Baby may ingest 0.18 mg/day when maternal dose is 50 mg/day. Effect on infant unknown. Caution due to long half-life (60 hr).
Furosemide (Lasix)	No reports of adverse effects. May suppress lactation due to dehydration of mother.
Hydrochlorthiazide (HydroDiuril)	Estimated dose ingested by infant, 0.05 mg. Probably not significant. Infant electrolytes normal
Spironolactone (Aldactone)	Electrolytes normal in infant. Approximately 0.2% of maternal dose transferred to infant. Effects on infant unknown. Probably not significant.

Environmental agents

Aldrin	Not a reason to wean. No need to test milk, unless inordinate exposure.
Dichlorodiphenyl dichloroethane (DDE)	In survey of 858 infants followed from birth to 1 yr, bottle-fed infants were heavier. Mothers with higher DDE levels breast-fed shorter times.
Dieldrin	Not a reason to wean. Also, found in permanently mothproofed garments. Avoid.
DDT*	No need to test milk unless inordinate exposure.
Halothane	Possibility of hepatic and renal damage. No reports of effects on infants.
Heptachlorepoxide	Not a reason to wean. No need to test milk unless inordinate exposure.
Hexachlorobenzene	Severe porphyria and some deaths occurred in nursing infants whose mothers had eaten wheat seed contaminated with hexachlorobenzene in Turkey in 1956.
Kepone	70 documented cases of poisoning of persons working with Kepone. No need to test milk unless inordinate exposure.

Mercury	Several outbreaks of mercury poisoning have occurred in Japan, Iraq, Pakistan, and Guatemala. Poisoning of nursing infants has been documented.
Polybrominated biphenyl (PBB)	PBB entered animal food chain when cattle feed was contaminated in Michigan; effects unknown.
Polychlorinated biphenyl (PCB)	If mother at high risk from environment or diet (usually contaminated fish), measure milk level. Breast-fed infants of Japanese women who ingested PCBs in contaminated rice oil appeared enervated, expressionless, apathetic, and hypotonic, and lacked endurance. Three presented with abnormalities 5 yr later. Induction of microsomal liver enzymes.
Texachlorethylene	Obstructive jaundice.
Gastrointestinal drugs	
Aloe (found in over-the-counter laxative combinations)	Possible diarrhea.
Bisacodyl (Dulcolax)	Not significant.
Casanthranol (in combination with stool softener in Dialose Plus and PeriColace)	Possible diarrhea and colic. Usually not significant.
Cascara sagrada	Possible diarrhea and colic. Usually not significant.
Castor oil	Not significant.
Cimetidine (Tagamet)	Estimated dose ingested by infant = 6 ng/day. Decreased gastric acidity. Effects on infant unknown. High levels may cause CNS stimulation and inhibit cytochrome P-450 enzymes. We consider its use compatible with breast-feeding.
Docusate sodium (Colace)	None
Danthron (Modane, Doxidan)	Possible diarrhea and colic. Usually not significant.
Magnesium citrate	Not significant.
Mesalamine (Rowasa)	Appears to be safe during breast-feeding. Does not cause bilirubin binding displacement reactions. Effect of high metabolite levels unknown.

Metoclopramide	Estimated infant dose ingested at maternal dose of 30 mg/day = 1-45 µg/kg/day. Drug detected in infant plasma in 1 of 5 infants at this dose. Two reports of abdominal discomfort at maternal doses of 30-45 mg/day. Caution at higher doses due to possible CNS EPS reactions.
Mineral oil	None
Phenolphthalein (Correctol, ex-Lax Feen-A-Mint	Not significant.
Psyllium hydrophilac mucilloid (Metamucil)	None
Ranitidine (Zantac)	Diffusion into milk promoted by low plasma protein-binding (15%), weak base and lipid solubility. Concentrates in milk. Peak milk concentration occurred before maternal dose.
Senna (Senokot)	Possible diarrhea and colic. Senokot appears to have no effect on infant
Sulfasalazine (Azulfidine).	Detected in serum in 2 of 8 infants. No adverse reactions noted in any infant in this One report of bloody diarrhea in an report. exclusively breast-fed infant whose mother took 3 g/day. Infants serum level = 5.3 µg/mL. Bloody diarrhea stopped 72 hr after drug treatment discontinued. Drug should be used with caution in breast-feeding.
Heavy metals	
Aluminum	Report of 2 uremic infants who developed sever e lethal encephalopathy due to high aluminum content in infant formula. Caution in severe renal failure.
Arsenic	Can accumulate in infant's blood. Check level if there is reason to suspect exposure.
Copper	Unknown.
Fluorine	Monitor infant for excessive dose (excessive salivation and GI disturbances).
Iron	Intake of iron is beneficial to mother and infant.
Lead	Nursing contraindicated if maternal serum 40 µg/mL. Bone meal or dolomite in natural calcium/phosphorus supplements contains up to 20 ppm lead. Maximum recommended daily intake of lead for infants is 100 µg/day.

Hormones and synthetic substances

Contraceptives, oral	Reports of decreased weight gain, decreased milk production and decreased nitrogen and protein composition of milk in malnourished mothers. No adverse effects on infant or milk composition or yield if mother is healthy and well-nourished and pills are instituted after milk is well established (12 wk postpartum).
Ethinyl estradiol	At maternal doses ≤ 50 µg/day, estimated infant dose ingested = 10 ng/day, approximately the same amount of natural estrogens received by infants of mothers not taking contraceptive pills.
Lynestenol	Not significant.
Mestranol	Not significant if daily dose is 100 or less.
Medroxyprogesterone (Depo-Provera)	No significant effect on infant or milk yield.
Progestins (19-nortestosterone derivatives norethindrone)	Not significant if maternal daily dose is 2.5 mg or less. No effect on milk yield.
Norgestrel Noresthindrone acetate Norethynodrel	Infant dose ingested at maternal dose of 30 µg/day = 0.03 µg/day. At maternal dose of 250 µg/day, infant dose = 0.3 µg/day. Not significant.,
Methylprednisolone (Medrol)	No adverse effects noted in report of 3 infants whose mothers were receiving long-term therapy of 6-8 mg/day.
Prednisolone	Not significant at maternal doses ≤ 20 mg/day. Use of prednisolone rather than prednisone may expose infant to less active drug, especially in patients requiring high doses or prolonged therapy.
Prednisone	Not significant. at maternal dose ≤ 20 mg/day.

Immunosuppressive agents

Azathioprine (Imuran)	Unknown.
Cyclosporine (Sandimmune)	Contraindicated because it is secondary to potential for immunosuppression, neutropenia, unknown effect on growth, and possible association with carcinogenesis.

Psychoactive substances

Alcohol (ethanol)	Not significant in moderation. Chronic alcohol exposure may impair psychomotor development. At maternal blood alcohol levels of 300 mg/dL mild sedation occurs in the baby.

Antidepressants

Amitriptyline (Elavil, Endep)	No detectable level in infant serum. Estimated amount ingested by infant is 1% of maternal dose. No adverse effects noted. Effect on infant unknown.
Amoxapine (Asendin)	No reports of breast-fed infants. Effects on infant unknown but may be of concern.
Desipramine (Norpramin, Pertofrane)	No detectable level in infant serum. No adverse effects noted. Effects on infant unknown but may be of concern.
Dothiepin (Prothiaden)	Effects on infant not reported and are unknown but may be of concern.
Doxepin (Adapin, Sinequan)	Infant in first case was found limp, pale, and near respiratory arrest. Infant plasma level was < 3 ng/mL and metabolite concentration was 58-66 ng/mL, demonstrating marked accumulation. Infant in second case had metabolite serum concentration of 15 ng/mL. Doxepin levels were undetectable. No adverse effects noted.
Fluoxetine (Prozac)	No adverse effects noted in infant.
Imipramine (Tofranil)	Infant daily dose ingested estimated to be 0.2 mg. Effect on infant unknown but may be of concern.
Nortriptyline (Aventyl, Pamelor)	No adverse effects noted in infant in this case. Normal motor development. Long-term effects unknown but may be of concern.
Tranylcypromine (Parnate)	Not significant. May inhibit lactation.

Barbiturates — Usually not significant. May induce liver microsomal enzymes.

Barbital	Not significant. One case of sedation.
Butabarbital (Butisol)	Not significant.
Pentobarbital (Nembutal)	Not significant.
Phenobarbital (see	2 of 11 infants became difficult to awaken and

Anticonvulsants)	slept excessively after mother received hypnotic doses (90 mg) for 5 days. NS in maternal antiepileptic doses (60-200 mg/day). May induce liver microsomal enzymes.
Secobarbital (Seconal)	Not significant.
Thiopental (Pentothal)	Not significant.
Benzodiazepines	
Alprazolam (Xanax)	Breast-fed infant whose mother took alprazolam for 9 mo after delivery exhibited symptoms of withdrawal while mother was tapered off drug therapy. Symptoms of irritability, crying, and sleep disturbances resolved after 2 wk.
Chlordiazepoxide (Librium)	Amount secreted usually insufficient to affect infant, although CNS depression has been reported.
Clorazepate (Tranxene)	Drowsiness. Infant younger than 2 mo may have prolonged drug half-life due to immaturity of drug-metabolizing enzymes. Possibility of accumulation on chronic administration. Caution because of long half-life.
N-Desmethyldiazepam	Infant plasma levels in this case 20-21 ng/mL. No adverse effects noted in this case. Caution in breast-feeding due to unknown long-term effects.
Diazepam (Valium)	Reports of lethargy and weight loss, infant most susceptible during first 4 days of life. Hyperbilirubinemia. Most sources do not advise its use during breast-feeding. Drug accumulation may occur.
Flurazepam (Dalmane)	Some sedation, but usually not significant.
Lorazepam (Ativan)	No adverse effects noted in reported cases.
Oxazepam (Serax)	Infant plasma level = 7.5-9.1 ng/mL. No adverse effects noted. Caution during breast-feeding.
Temazepam (Restoril)	Infant plasma level = 7 ng/mL. No adverse effects noted. Caution during breast-feeding.
Bromides	Drowsiness and rash. Possibility of allergic reactions.
Caffeine	Estimated dose ingested by infant 0.5-1/64 mg after a single cup of coffee. Another study found at maternal ingestion of 500 mg/day that the infant ingested 0.3-1.0 mg/kg/day. Infant plasma levels after 5 days of maternal

	dose of 500 mg/day. 0.8-2.8 µg/mL. Caffeine has an extremely long half-life in neonates 100-200 hr. May accumulate in infant. No adverse effects noted in infants in this study. Irritability and poor sleeping patterns have been observed in infants after heavy coffee consumption by mother.
Chloral hydrate (Noctec)	Sedation, usually not significant..
Chloroform	Deep sleep.
Cocaine	Cocaine and its metabolite benzoylecgonine have been found in urine of breast-fed infants whose mothers used cocaine. Symptoms observed in infants include irritability and tremulousness, increased startle responses, hyperactive Moro reflex, hyperactive deep tenson reflexes, and marked lability of mood. Symptoms may persist for 60 hr after exposure. Cocaine contraindicated during breast-feeding.
Dextroamphetamine (Dexedrine)	Found in infant's urine. No adverse effects noted. Contraindicated during breast-feeding.
Ether	Sedation.
Glutethimide (Doriden)	Some sedation, usually not significant.
Haloperidol (Haldol)	No adverse effects noted in infant. Effects on infant unknown but may be of concern
Lithium (Eskalith, Lithobid)	Measurable lithium in infant's serum. Infant kidney can clear lithium. Reports of cyanosis, hypothermia, poor muscle tone, and ECG changes in nursing infants. Contraindicated during breast-feeding.
Marijuana	High levels of THC and its metabolites found in fecal sample from infant. When infants who had been exposed to THC by breast-feeding during first year of life were compared with infants not exposed, no significant differences were found in terms of mental or motor development at 1 year. Long-term effects unknown. Contraindicated during breast-feeding.
Meprobamate	Monitor infant for drug intoxication since drug accumulates in milk.
Phenothiazines	
Chlorpromazine (Thorazine)	One infant showed signs of lethargy and drowsiness at milk level of 92 ng/mL. May be of concern.

Mesoridazine (Serentil)	Since the effects of the drug on the infant are unknown but may be of concern, risks vs benefits must be seriously considered before prescribing it to breast feeding mothers.
Perphenazine (Trilaton)	Since the effects of the drug on the infant are unknown but may be of concern, risks vs. benefits must be seriously considered before prescribing it to breast-feeding mothers.
Prochlorperazine (Compazine)	None known.
Thioridazine (Mellaril)	None known.
Trifluoperazine (Stelazine)	None known.

Radiopharmaceuticals and Diagnostic Materials

Barium	None.
^{131}I (Iodine)	Breast-feeding contraindicated after large therapeutic dose and should be withheld for up to 14 days after diagnostic doses. Check milk before resuming feeding.
[(^{131}I)]-labeled (Iodine) macroaggregated albumin	Discontinue breast-feeding for 10-12 days. Extreme avidity for iodine by the thyroid of young infants. 1/10 of the limit of the International Commission on Radiological Protection (ICRP) for drinking water reached 10 days after IV dose of 200 mCi.
Iopanoic acid (Telepaque)	No averse effects. Iodine excretion can cause rash. Probably no problem with just one dose.
Gallium citrate	Discontinue nursing until 2 wk after 5^{69}Ga has usually cleared.
^{90}Sr	Not significant. Less than in cow's milk
^{99}TcO$^-_4$	Breast-feeding contraindicated for 32-72 hr after 10-mCi dose. Breast-feeding can be resumed 24 hr after 2-mCi dose for lung scanning.
Tuberculin test	Tuberculin-sensitive mothers can passively immunize their infants through breast milk. Immunity may last several years.

Respiratory agents

Dyphylline (Lufyllin)	Probably not significant.
Terbutaline (Brethine, Bricanyl)	Estimated infant dose 0.4-0.6 µg/mL or 0.2-0.7% of maternal dose. Not detectable in infant plasma. No adverse effects reported.
Theophylline	Usually not significant. Some reports of irritability and insomnia in infants. Premature infants 3-15 days old have average half-lives of 30.2 hr. Maximum amount of theophylline

that an infant could ingest is 8 mg/L milk per day. Avoid nursing at time of peak serum level.

Thyroid drugs

Levothyroxine (Synthroid)
Milk levels are too low to adequately treat a hypothyroid infant, although breast-feeding offers better protection to infants with congenital hypothyroidism than formula does.

Liothyronine (Cytomel)
Maximum dose ingested, 2.1-2.6 µg/day, much less than amount required to treat congenital hypothyroidism. In a study comparing T_3 levels in 22 breast-fed and 29 formula-fed infants, significantly higher levels were found in the breast-fed infants. These levels (2.24 and 1.79 ng/mL) were of doubtful clinical significance. Milk T_3 levels are too low to interfere with neonatal thyroid screening programs.

Methimazole (Tapazole)
Maximum dose ingested 16-39 µg. Maternal doses of 10-15 mg/day do not pose a major risk to the infant if thyroid function is monitored biweekly.

Potassium iodide
May alter thyroid function in infant. May cause goiter.

Propylthiouracil (PTU)
Percent maternal doses likely to be ingested is 0.07%. No change in thyroid function tests in any of the reported cases.

Thyroid
Not significant.

Miscellaneous

DPT vaccine
Does not interfere with immunization schedule.

Ergonovine (Ergotrate)
Causes lowered prolactin levels in postpartum patients. Multiple doses may suppress lactation.

Fluoride
Fluoride intake 5-10 µg/day in both 0.2-ppm and 1-ppm areas.

Lindane (Kwell)
Estimated infant dose ingested is 30 µg/day, about the same as a would be absorbed from one direct application to the infant. Probably not significant.

Magnesium sulfate
Breast-fed infant would receive only 1.5 mg more magnesium than non-treated mothers. Not significant.. Milk calcium not affected.

Poliovirus vaccine
Live virus taken orally. Not necessary to withhold nursing 30 minutes before and after dose. Provide booster after infant no longer nursing.

Rh antibodies	Destroyed in GI tract.
Rubella vaccine	Usually not significant. One report of isolation of live attenuated vaccine from throat of breast-fed infant. No detectible serologic response and no adverse effects. One case report of a 13 day-old breast-fed infant who contracted rubella 11 days after maternal vaccination. It could not be determined whether the infant was infected by virus shed in mother's milk.
Theobromine	No adverse effects observed in infants. 4 oz . chocolate contains 240 mg theobromine.
Tolbutamide	Unknown

Drugs Commonly Taken While Nursing

Alcohol

Almost every source of information dealing with the presence of alcohol in breast milk recounts a case report published in 1936 in the medical literature. A nursing mother drank a bottle of port wine over a 24-hour period. Her baby could not be aroused from sleep. It snored, breathed slowly and deeply, and showed no reaction to pain. Such a tale may be enough to frighten nursing mothers into complete abstention from alcohol. However, an occasional alcoholic drink will produce insignificant effects on the baby. Mild sedation can occur in infants whose mothers have consumed about eight or nine drinks, probably the maximum a woman could drink and still be conscious enough to nurse her child. Obviously, a heavy drinker or chronic alcoholic or a woman who is intoxicated should not be nursing.

A 1991 study of lactating women did show that infants actually can smell minute quantities of alcohol in breast milk. When they detect the presence of alcohol, babies evidently nurse more vigorously at first, but for a shorter time than they normally would. While this information is interesting, we don't believe it means that women cannot take an alcoholic drink when nursing. Most physicians and nurses believe that drinking liquids, regardless of whether they contain alcohol, is the most important nutritional factor in good breast milk production.

Caffeine

Although caffeine concentrates in very low quantities in breast milk, it can accumulate in the baby's body. If a nursing mother drinks six to eight cups of caffeine-containing beverages (coffee, tea, or colas) per day or goes overboard on chocolate, her baby is likely to show signs of caffeine stimulation such as hyperactivity and wakefulness. We recommend that nursing mothers limit their intake of caffeine-containing beverages to no more than one or two cups or glasses per day. Many caffeine-free coffees, teas, and colas are available in the supermarket.

Nicotine and smoke

Nicotine reaches very low levels in breast milk. It is not easily absorbed by the infant's intestines and is metabolized quickly. We do not worry a great deal about infants being poisoned by nicotine received through breast milk, but nicotine does have an impact on breast milk production. Women who smoke 20 to 30 cigarettes per day may produce significantly less milk than their infant needs, causing their baby to have nausea, vomiting, diarrhea, and abdominal cramping. More importantly, it is now clear that babies of parents who smoke have more respiratory difficulties, such as irritation and infection of the lungs, asthma, and allergies. We strongly recommend that if you continue to smoke after your baby is born, do not do it in the same room where you are nursing the baby or caring for it. The best policy is to smoke out of doors where the smoke will not reach the air that the baby breathes.

Pain Relief Medications

Aspirin, ibuprofen (Motrin, Advil), and acetaminophen (Tylenol) in normal doses do not appear to affect a breastfeeding infant. If a mother must take large doses of aspirin for treatment of arthritis, for example, it could interfere with the baby's blood-clotting abilities. Your doctor may recommend blood tests for the baby to be sure this is not happening.

Narcotics such as morphine, codeine, Demerol, and methadone do not reach high levels in human breast milk and do not appear to affect nursing infants. Mothers addicted to heroin can be maintained on 50 to 80 mg of methadone per day and still breast-feed their babies. Propoxyphene (Darvon) may be inadvisable during nursing if the maximum doses are being taken by the mother. One infant was reported to have unusually poor muscle tone when its mother was taking Darvon every 8 hours on a regular basis.

Antibiotics

Most antibiotics appear in breast milk, and their concentration depends mainly on their particular chemical properties. Commonly prescribed antibiotics such as amoxicillin, Ceclor, and Keflex almost never cause problems for breastfeeding infants. Rare reactions to the presence of sulfas in milk have been reported An allergic reaction has been reported in an infant whose mother was being treated for syphilis with penicillin, but this reaction is highly unlikely to occur. Even women who develop breast infections while nursing can normally continue breast-feeding concurrently with antibiotic therapy, unless a severe abscess develops.

Tetracycline should never be taken during pregnancy because it can cause a reaction which stains the baby's teeth brown. Although there are no reports of this happening during breast-feeding, there is still a theoretical possibility that it could so an alternative to tetracycline is probably wise.

The aminoglycoside antibiotics (gentamicin, clindamycin) are generally considered safe during breast-feeding because they are not well absorbed through the intestinal tract. If the baby has a gastrointestinal inflammation or diarrhea, he or she may absorb the drug more efficiently, in which case side effects from the drug might occur. As far as we know, this is only a hypothetical problem.

Chloramphenicol reaches higher levels in breast milk than do many other antibiotics. It should not be used right after birth because it can interfere with bone marrow production in the baby. Antibiotics concentrate in breast milk in higher levels than in the mother's blood. These include erythromycin, metronidazole (Flagyl), isoniazid (INH), and trimethoprim sulfamethoxazole (Bactrim, Septra). Isoniazid is typically given to individuals with tuberculosis in combination with one or two other drugs. It has been thought to be responsible for liver toxicity in breast-feeding babies. Mothers with active tuberculosis should not be breast-feeding, in any case; babies have a very low resistance to tuberculosis and can contract it readily when in close contact with someone who already has the disease.

If, for some reason, a woman must take erythromycin, Flagyl, or Bactrim during breast-feeding, short courses of the drugs will probably not hurt the baby. It may be wise to withhold breast-feeding for 24 hours at the beginning of drug therapy and substitute a formula. However, she should continue to pump milk to maintain a sufficient supply.

Blood Thinners

The most popular anticoagulants (blood thinners) are safe during breast-feeding. Heparin molecules are too large to pass into breast milk. Warfarin (Coumadin), a smaller molecule, reaches very low levels in breast milk, although its effects have been known to cause bruising of the nipple.

Laxatives

The safest laxatives for a nursing mother are the bulk formers, which include bran, cellulose, and psyllium hydrophyllic mucilloid. These go under the trade names of Metamucil and Serutan. Milk of magnesia also seems to be safe and does not enter the mother's bloodstream or her breast milk. Stool softeners like dioctyl sodium sulfosuccinate (Colace) are also safe since they are not absorbed into the mother's system.

Strong laxatives such as senna, cascara sagrada, danthron, and casanthranol may cause diarrhea in small, nursing infants - a situation to be avoided without doubt. We recommend that you not use these laxatives during breast-feeding, especially since there are many others to choose from.

Birth Control Pills

The hormones found in birth control pills do reach breast milk in very low concentrations. Pill usage during breast-feeding has the potential to decrease the milk supply, change the composition of milk, and create some undesirable side effects in the baby - although these are very rare these days. For the most part, concern about oral contraceptive use during nursing centers around their ability to change the composition of breast milk unfavorably. Doctors have found that if birth control pill use is resumed after an adequate milk supply has been established usually several weeks after delivery, it is less likely to influence milk production.

Twenty years ago, when the dosage of hormones in contraceptive pills was much higher, babies had more problems. These included changes in the vagina in baby girls, unusual breast development in boys, and excessive production of bilirubin, a by-product of liver metabolism. Today, with the low-dosage birth control pills we see fewer problems with milk production and no apparent long-term hazards to the children.

Even so, our preference is to keep our patients off birth control pills while they are nursing, if they can use another form of contraception satisfactorily. If this is not possible, then we recommend staying off the pill for at least 12 weeks after delivery.

Breast Milk Suppressants

When a woman decides not to nurse, measures may need to be taken after delivery to help stop the flow of milk and make the mother as comfortable as possible in the process.

Traditional methods of stopping lactation, such as breast binding, ice packs, and fluid restrictions have seen a comeback recently. Many women prefer to use these techniques over drug suppression of lactation.

Ice-packs should be applied on the day engorgement (filling of the breasts) occurs. For 2-4 days, the woman will need to restrict fluid intake. For about 10 days she should bind her breasts tightly, both day and night.

When a woman prefers the convenience of a drug that helps to stop the flow of milk comfortably in a relatively short period of time, she can use bromocriptine. Bromocriptine mesylate (Parlodel) is a nonhormonal agent that quickly abolishes the rise in prolactin levels and prevents the lactation process from continuing. This drug is taken by mouth twice a day for 14 days.

An advantage to bromocriptine is that it will also work in women whose breast milk has already been established. Bromocriptine is also used to treat amenorrhea (lack of menstruation), premenstrual discomfort, galactorrhea (spontaneous milk production), and microadenoma of the pituitary gland, which can result in a failure to ovulate and ensuing infertility *(See Chapter 14)*.

Other hormone-type lactation suppressants, such as chlorotrianisene (TACE) and combined estradiol and testosterone (Deladumone OB), that were popular in the past, are no longer used.

Mild to moderate recurrence of milk production has been reported in up to 40% of women who discontinue bromocriptine use. The problem is usually handled by continuing the course of the drug for another 7 days. Uncommon side effects include headache, dizziness, and nausea. Recent studies have indicated that bromocriptine should not be given to women who have had hypertension or other heart disease, since it may aggravate these conditions.

Case Study

Shannon M. was pregnant for the first time at the age of 31. She gained 40 pounds during her pregnancy, and the doctors predicted that she would bear a large child. Shannon herself was a petite 5 feet 2 inches, and before pregnancy she had weighed 110 pounds. Her pregnancy stretched over an entire summer, including the hay fever season. She had always had problems with allergies and finally her doctor prescribed Seldane, an antihistamine, to relieve her severe sneezing and runny nose.

After 30 hours in labor, Glenda's doctor realized that the baby's head was too large to come through the pelvis, and she decided to perform a cesarean section. Using epidural anesthesia, the doctor delivered a healthy 9-pound 2-ounce boy surgically. After the operation Shannon ran a fever and experienced a pain in her lower abdomen. Her doctor diagnosed a pelvic infection and prescribed two intravenous antibiotics, penicillin and gentamicin. She took Tylenol with codeine every 6 hours or so to relieve her pelvic pain. Shannon had to continue taking Seldane as well because the ragweed season was not yet over.

Shannon had thought she would like to to nurse her baby, but she was concerned that the number of drugs she was taking would enter her breast milk and harm her baby. The doctor reassured her that, in spite of the medications she was taking the baby could still be nursed safely. She went ahead with breast-feeding and the baby suffered no apparent ill effects.

Before her pregnancy Glenda had used low-dose birth control pills for contraception. She wanted to resume using them as soon as possible but her doctor persuaded her to wait until she was through nursing even though a low-dose pill would probably be safe. She was fitted with a diaphragm and instructed about its use at her 6 weeks postpartum checkup.

Chapter 20

Key Points for Breast-Feeding

1. The vast majority of drugs do get into breast milk, but most of the time the levels of drugs in breast milk are very low and do not affect the baby.

2. Drugs prescribed for specific medical disorders should be continued because, as in pregnancy, the mother's good health is highly important to successful breast-feeding.

3. A few drugs tend to accumulate in infants because they have immature digestive and elimination systems. These drugs should be avoided when several daily doses are necessary. Commonly used ones include metronidazole, trimethoprim-sulfamethoxazole, tetracycline and chloramphenicol.

4. Most of the drugs commonly used by nursing mothers should not prevent her from breast-feeding. The advantages of breast-feeding usually outweigh any drug effects on the baby.

5. If a baby shows definite symptoms of being affected by a drug and the mother cannot discontinue it or find an acceptable drug substitute careful scheduling of nursing and drug-taking may be tried. The mother can express milk to be put in a bottle for future feedings or a formula can be substituted when the levels of drug in her bloodstream are likely to be high. The most advantageous time to take a drug when breast-feeding is just before or just after feeding, since gastrointestinal absorption does not begin for at least an hour or two. Many mothers elect not to continue breast-feeding when a drug they are taking upsets the baby.

6. Women who do not wish to nurse may use a drug-free method of suppressing lactation with ice-packs, fluid restriction, and breast-binding.

7. Bromocriptine is an effective drug for those women who wish to suppress lactation quickly. Women with high blood pressure should not use this drug.

Notes

Cost Comparisons Between Commonly Prescribed Drugs

Prices listed in this appendix are wholesale prices based on 100 tablet or capsule doses, unless otherwise noted. The data were gathered from *Drug Topics Redbook*, Oradell, N.J., Medical Economics Data Incorporated. 1991. These prices are for relative cost comparison only; the actual cost to the patient will vary from one pharmacy to another. This table does not consider the frequency of administration or the duration of therapy.

Product	Wholesale Cost per 100 ($)
β-Adrenergic Tocolytic Agents	
Brethine 2.5 mg tab	22.35
Bricanyl 2.5 mg tab	25.50
Isoxsuprine HC1 10 mg tab	3.50 - 9.00
Vasodilan 10 mg tab	27.84
Yutopar 10 mg tab (UD; no bulk)	232.89
Antianxiety Drugs	
Atarax 25 mg tab	73.80
Ativan 2 mg tab	94.04
Chlordiazepoxide HC1 25 mg cap	3.00 - 8.00
Halcion .125 mg	59.18
Hydroxyzine HC1 25 mg tab	3.30 - 13.60
Librium 25 mg cap	77.70
Serax 15 mg cap	69.20
Tranxene 7.5 mg	118.00
Valium 5 mg tab	53.47
Vistaril 25 mg cap	73.80
Xanax 1 mg	86.60
Antibiotics	
Ampicillin 500 mg cap	9.95 - 22.00
Anspor 500 mg	170.00
Bactrim tab	60.50
Ceclor 500 mg cap	365.47
Amoxicillin 250 mg	3.75 - 24.97
500 mg	15.91 - 39.41
Ciprofloxacin 250 mg	244.00
500 mg	282.37
750 mg	489.78
Dicloxacillin 250 mg	12.60 - 42.02
500 mg	49.14 - 75.63
Doxycycline hyclate	13.96 - 141.72
Duricef 500 mg cap	284.50
Erythrocin 250 mg tab	14.00
Erythromycin base 250 mg	11.42

Product	Wholesale Cost per 100 ($)
Erythromycin stearate 250 mg tab	4.11 - 14.50
Gantrisin 500 mg tab	21.20
Keflex 500 mg cap	242.20
Macrodantin 50 mg cap	63.00
Metronidazole 250 mg	3.93 - 22.25
Flagyl 250 mg tab	119.26
Protostat 250 mg	103.85
Norfloxacin 400 mg	228.30
Polycillin 500 mg cap	33.26
Septra tab	60.60
Septra DS tab	99.70
Sulfisoxazole 500 mg tab	3.45 - 10.50
Tetracycline HC1 500 mg cap	5.18 - 9.25
Velosef 500 mg	162.39
Vibramycin 100 mg cap	314.00

Anticholinergics/Antispasmodics

Product	Wholesale Cost per 100 ($)
Bentyl 10 mg cap	21.78
Dicyclomine HC1 10 mg cap	2.50 - 6.50
Ditropan 5 mg tab	39.81
Probanthine 15 mg tab	57.95
Propantheline HBr 15 mg tab	3.50 - 24.00
Urispas 100 mg tab	66.00

Anticonvulsants

Product	Wholesale Cost per 100 ($)
Depakene 250 mg cap	95.00
Dilantin 100 mg cap	21.22
Phenobarbital sodium 32 mg tab	1.50 - 5.00
Tegretol 200 mg tab	31.45
Zarontin 250 mg cap	63.45

Antidepressants

Product	Wholesale Cost per 100 ($)
Amitriptyline 50 mg tab	2.09 - 10.68
Elavil 50 mg tab	61.27
Imipramine HCI 50 mg tab	2.76 - 10.18
Tofranil 50 mg tab	65.90

Antiemetics

Product	Wholesale Cost per 100 ($)
Compazine 25 mg suppos	30.00/12
Phenergan 25 mg suppos	24.50/12

Antihistamines/Decongestants

Product	Wholesale Cost per 100 ($)
Actifed tab	12.90
Entex-LA	62.58

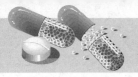

Product	Wholesale Cost per 100 ($)
Dimetapp tab	28.50
Drixoral tab	30.00
Histatab Plus	2.50
Ornade cap	74.60
Pseudoephedrine HC1 60 mg tab	1.90 - 4.07
Sudafed 60 mg tab	18.50

Antihypertensives

Aldomet 250 mg tab	30.70
Apresoline 25 mg tab	25.92
Chlorothiazide 500 mg tab	6.30 - 10.09
Diuril 500 mg tab	19.41
Dyazide cap	35.20
Hydralazine 25 mg tab	2.00 - 5.50
Hydrochlorothiazide 50 mg tab	1.50 - 5.00
HydroDiuril 50 mg tab	19.41
Inderal 40 mg tab	46.70
Lasix 40 mg tab	18.25
Lopressor 50 mg	46.06
Minipress 2 mg	51.26
Tenormin 50 mg	80.20

Estrogen

Diethylstilbestrol 1 mg tab	8.75
Estinyl 0.05 mg tab	40.48
Estrace 1 mg tab	28.06
Estraderm 0.05 mg	15.15/8
0.1 mg	16.50/8
Ogen 0.625 mg tab	44.53
Premarin 0.625 mg tab	34.54

Insulin

Humulin-N 10 mL	16.30
Humulin-R 10 mL	16.30
Ilentin II Regular Beef 100U	18.14
Ilentin II Regular Pork 100U	21.50
Ilentin II Lente Beef 100U	18.14
Ilentin II Lente Pork 100U	21.50
Ilentin II NPH Beef 100U	18.14
Ilentin II NPH Pork 100U	21.50
Lente 100U	13.19
NPH 100U	12.68
Regular 100U vial	13.19
Semilente 100U	13.19

Product	Wholesale Cost per 100 ($)
Oral Contraceptives	
Brevicon 20 or 28	20.01
Demulen 21 or 28	23.94
Demulen 1/35 28	21.56
Loestrin 1/20 21	22.33
Loestrin 1.5/30	22.33
LoOvral 1/35 21 or 28	22.26
Modicon 21 or 28	22.33
Norlestrin 2.5/50	22.33
Norlestrin 1/50 21 or 28	22.33
Norinyl 1/50 21 or 28	19.40
Norinyl 1/35 21 or 28	19.40
Ortho Novum 1/35 21 or 18	20.15
Ortho Novum 7/7/7	20.15
Ortho Novum 10/11 28	22.20
Ortho Novum 1/50 21 or 28	20.15
Ovcon 35 21 or 28	21.02
Ovcon 50 21 or 28	23.20
Ovulation Induction	
Clomid 50 mg	6.50 ea.
Factrel 100 μg/mL	56.26
500 μg/mL	93.75
Lutrepulse 0.8 mg	270.00/liter
3.2 mg	450.00/liter
Parlodel 2.5 mg	133.60
5 mg	214.80
Pergonal 75 IU	55.24/liter
	516.27/10
150 IU	106.05/liter
Serophene 50 mg	55.53/10
Pelvic Pain Relief	
Acetaminophen 325 mg tab	1.50 - 2.90
Advil 200 mg	7.87
Anaprox 275 mg tab	67.35
Aspirin 325 mg tab	1.00 - 2.50
Bayer Aspirin 325 mg tab	5.10
Clinoril 150 mg tab	86.11
Danocrine 100 mg cap	141.59
Indocin 25 mg cap	48.48
Motrin 400 mg tab	18.60
Naprosyn 250 mg tab	71.50
Nuprin 200 mg 100s/doz	7.07
Ponstel 250 mg cap	84.60

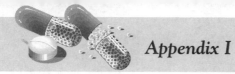

Product	Wholesale Cost per 100 ($)
Rufen 400 mg	17.50
Spironolactone	6.00 - 9.50
Tylenol 325 mg tab	5.70

Urologic Disorders

Bethanechol HC1 10 mg tab	2.50 - 8.50
Dibenzyline 10 mg cap	54.75
Urecholine 10 mg tab	60.50

Vulvovaginal Candidiasis Preparations

Fluconazole 50 mg	131.25/30
100mg	206.25/30
Gyne-Lotrimin 100 mg tab	13.14/6
Gyne-Lotrimin vag cr 45 gm	15.70/7 day
Monistat 3 tab	21.00
Monistat 7 tab	20.10
Monistat 7 vag cr 45 gm	18.50
Mycelex-G 100 mg tab	14.70/7
Mycelex-G 500 mg	12.28
Mycelex vag cream 45 gm	14.40
Mycostatin vag tab 100,000U	13.90/15
Nilstat vag tab 100,000U	6.65
Nystatin vag tab 100,000U	3.50 - 5.50
Terazol 7 cream	20.25
Terazol 3 suppos	20.25

Notes

Generic and Brand Name Drug Cross-Reference Guide

Drugs or drug type	Brand Names	Generic name
Acetaminophen	Datril Liquiprin Phenaphen Panadol SK-APAP Tempra Tylenol Tylenol Extra Strength Valadol	Acetaminophen
Acetaminophen and codeine	Aceta with codeine Capital with codeine Empracet with codeine Papa-Deine Pavadon Phenaphen with codeine Proval SK-APAP with codeine Tylenol with codeine	
Adrenocorticoids (topical)	Cyclocort Benisone Celestone Valisone Tridesilon Topicort Aeroseb-Dex Decaderm Decadron Decaspray Hexadrol Florone Locorten Fluonid Flurosyn Synalar	Amcinonide Betamethasone Desonide Desoximetasone Dexamethasone Diflorasone Flumethasone Fluocinolone

*Drugs listed are all systemic (taken for internal use unless otherwise indicated.

Drugs or drug type	Brand Names	Generic name
	Lidex	Fluocinonide
	Topsyn	
	Oxylone	Fluorometholone
	Cordran	Flurandrenolide
	Halciderm	Halcinonide
	Halog	
	Cortaid	Hydrocortisone
	Cort-Dome	
	Cortef	
	Cortisol	
	Cortril	
	Dermacort	
	Hydrocortone	
	Hytone	
	Texacort	
	Medrol	Methylprednisolone
	Meti-Derm	Prednisolone
	Aristocort	Triamcinolone
	Aristogel	
	Kenalog	
	Spencort	
	Triacet	
Adrenocorticoids	Celestone	Betamethasone
	Cortone	Cortisone
	Decadron	Dexamethasone
	Dexasone	
	Hexadrol	
	Alphadrol	Fluprednisolone
	A-Hydrocort	Hydrocortisone
	Cortef	
	Cortenema	
	Hydrocortone	
	Solu-Cortef	
	Betapar	Meprednisone
	A-MethaPred	Methylprednisolone
	Duralone	
	Medralone	
	Medrol	
	Methylone	
	Haldrone	Paramethasone
	Delta-Cortef	Prednisolone
	Hydeltrasol	
	Meticortelone	
	Sterone	

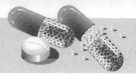

Drugs or drug type	Brand Names	Generic name
	Predoxine	Prednisolone, buffered
	Deltasone	Prednisone
	Meticorten	
	Orasone	
	Sterapred	
	Aristocort	Triamcinolone
	Aristospan	
	Cinonide	
	Kenacort	
	Kenalog	
	Tramacort	
	Doca	Desoxycorticosterone
	Percorten	
	Florinef	Fludrocortisone
Alcohol and acetone (topical)	Seba-Nil	
	Sebasum	
	Tyrosum	
Alcohol and sulfur (topical)	Acne Aid	
	Acnomead	
	Epi-Clear	
	Liquimat	
	Postacne	
	Transact	
	Xerac	
Allopurinol	Lopurin	Allopurinol
	Zyloprim	
Aminoglycosides	Amikin	Amikacin
	Apogen	Gentamicin
	Bristagen	
	Garamycin	
	U-Gencin	
	Kantrex	Kanamycin
	Klebcil	
	Mycifradin	Neomycin, Streptomycin
	Nebcin	Tobramycin
Amphetamines	Benzedrine	Amphetamine
	Dexampex	Dextroamphetamine
	Dexedrine	
	Diphylets	
	Ferndex	
	Obotan	
	Oxydess	

Drugs or drug type	Brand Names	Generic name
	Spancap	
	Desoxyn	Methamphetamine
	Methampex	
Anticoagulants	Miradon	Anisindione
	Hedulin	Phenindione
	Liquamar	Phenprocoumon
	Athrombin-K	Warfarin potassium
	Coumadin	Warfarin sodium
	Panwarfin	
Antidiabetics, oral	Dymelor	Acetohexamide
	Diabinese	Chlorpropamide
	Tolinase	Tolazamide
	Orinase	Tolbutamide
Antihistamines	Optimine	Azatadine
	Ambodryl	Bromodiphenhydramine
	Bromphen	Brompheniramine
	Dimetane	
	Puretane	
	Symptom 3	
	Clistin	Carbinoxamine
	Chloramate	Chlorpheniramine
	Chlor-Trimeton	
	Hismanal	Astemizole
	Histaspan	
	Phenetron	
	Seldane	Terfenadine
	Teldrin	
	Tavist	Clemastine
	Cyprodine	Cyproheptadine
	Periactin	
	Polaramine	Dexchlorpheniramine
	Dramamine	Dimenhydrinate
	Eldodram	
	Dimethpyrindene	Dimethindene
	Forhistal	
	Triten	
	Benadryl	Diphenhydramine
	Bendylate	
	Eldadryl	
	Valdrene	
	Diafen	Diphenylpyraline
	Hispril	
	Decapryn	Doxylamine
	Allertoc	Pyrilamine
	Mepyramine	
	Thylogen	

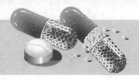

Drugs or drug type	Brand Names	Generic name
	PBZ	Tripelennamine
	Pyribenzamine	
	Actidil	Triprolidine
Antithyroid agents	Tapazole	Methimazole
	Thiamazole	
	Propacil	Propylthiouracil
	Propyl-Thyracil	
APC (Aspirin, phenacetin, and caffeine)	Acetophen	
	Aidant	
	APAC	
	A.S.A. Compound	
	Asalco No. 1	
	Asphac-G	
	P-A-C Compound	
	Phencaset	
	Sal-Fayne	
	Salphenine	
	Tabloid APC	
APC and codeine	Empirin Compound with Codeine	
	A.S.A. and Codeine Compound	
	P-A-C Compound with Codeine	
	Salatin with Codeine	
	Tabloid APC with Codeine	
Appetite suppressants	Didrex	Benzphetamine
	Pre-Sate	Chlorphentermine
	Voranil	Clortermine
	Tenuate	
	Tepanil	
	Sanorex	Mazindol
	Bontril PDM	Phendimetrazine
	Phendiet	
	Plegine	
	Preludin	Phenmetrazine
	Fastin	Phentermine
	Ionamin	
Barbiturates	Amytal	Amobarbital
	Buticaps	Butabarbital
	Butisol	

Drugs or drug type	Brand Names	Generic name
	Sombulex	Hexobarbital
	Mebaral	Mephobarbital
	Gemonil	Metharbital
	Sedadrops	Phenobarbital
	SK-Phenobarbital	
	Solfoton	
	Seconal	Secobarbital
	Tuinal	Secobarbital and amobarbital
	Lotusate	Talbutal
Belladonna alkaloids and barbiturates	Minabel	Atropine, hyoscyamine, scopolamine, and butabarbital
	Omnibel	
	Palbar	
	Cyclo-Bell	Atropine, hyoscyamine, scopolamine, butabarbital, pentobarbital,
	Barbidonna	Atropine, hyoscyamine, scopolamine, and phenobarbital
	Donna-Sed	
	Donnatal	
	Donphen	
	Hasp	
	Hybephen	
	Hyosophen	
	Kinesed	
	Sedralex	
	Setamine	
	Spalix	
	Spasmolin	
	Spasmophen	
	Spasmorel	
	Tri-Spas	
	Alised	Atropine and phenobarbital
	Antrocol	
	Atrobarb	
	Amobell	Belladonna and amobarbital
	Butibel	Belladonna and butabarbital
	Belap	Belladonna and phenobarbital
	Bellophen	
	Bello-Phen	
	Chardonna	
	Donabarb	
	Donnabarb	
	Oxoids	

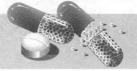

Drugs or drug type	Brand Names	Generic name
	Phenobel	Phenobella
	Sedajen	
	Valaspas	
	Hybar	Hyoscyamine, scopolamine, and phenobarbital
	Cystospaz-SR	Hyoscyamine and butabarbital
	Anaspaz PB	Hyoscyamine and phenobarbital
	Levsin-PB	
	Levsin w/ Phenobarbital	
	Levsinex w/ Phenobarbital	
Benzodiazepines	A-poxide	Chlordiazepoxide
	Librium	
	SK-Lygen	
	Tranxene	Clorazepate
	Valium	Diazepam
	Dalmane	Flurazepam
	Ativan	Lorazepam
	Serax	Oxazepam
	Verstran	Prazepam
Anti-acne medications (topical)	Benoxyl	Benzoyl peroxide
	Benzac	
	Benzagel	
	Clear By Design	
	Dermodex	
	Desquam-X	
	Epi-Clear	
	Fostex BPO	
	Oxy-10	
	Panoxyl	
	Persadox	
	Persa-Gel	
	Porox 7	
	Teen	
	Topex	
	Xerac BP	
Beta-adrenergic blocking agents	Lopressor	Metoprolol
	Corgard	Nadolol
	Inderal	Propranolol
Urinary stimulants	Duvoid	Bethanecol
	Myotonachol	
	Urecholine	

Drugs or drug type	Brand Names	Generic name
Bleomycin	Blenoxane	Bleomycin
Lactation suppressant	Parlodel	Bromocriptine
Expectorant/decongestants	Dimetane expectorant Midatane expectorant Normatene expectorant Puretane expectorant Spentane expectorant	Brompheniramine, guaifenesin, phenylephrine, and phenylpropanolamine
	Dimetane expectorant-DC Midatane DC expectorant Normatane DC expectorant Puretane Expectorant DC Spentane DC expectorant	Brompheniramine, guaifenesin, phenylephrine, phenylpropanolamine, and codeine
	Brompheniramine Compound Bromatapp Dimetapp Eldatapp Puretapp	Brompheniramine phenylephrine, and phenylpropanolamine
Busulfan	Myleran	Busulfan
Butalbital and APC	Fiorinal	
Butalbital, APC, and codeine	Fiorinal with Codeine	
Butorphanol	Stadol	Butorphanol
Calcitonin	Calcimar	Calcitonin
Carboprost	Prostin/15 M	Carboprost
Carisoprodol	Rela Soma Soprodol	Carisoprodol
Cephalosporins	Ceclor Ceftin Duricef Ultracef Mandol Ancef Kefzol Mefoxin Keflex	Cefaclor Cefuroxime Cefadroxil Cefamandole Cefazolin Cefoxitin Cephalexin

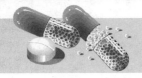

Drugs or drug type	Brand Names	Generic name
	Kafocin	Cephaloglycin
	Loridine	Cephaloridine
	Keflin Neutral	Cephalothin
	Cefadyl	Cephapirin
	Anspor	Cephradine
	Velosef	
Charcoal, activated (oral)	Charcocaps	
	Charcodote	
	Charcotabs	
Chloral hydrate	Acquachloral	
	Cohidrate	
	Noctec	
	Oradrate	
Chlorambucil	Luekeran	Chlorambucil
Chloramphenicol	Amphicol	Chloramphenicol
	Chloromycetin	
Chloramphenicol (topical)	Chloromycetin	Chloramphenicol
Chlordiazepoxide and amitriptyline	Limbitrol	
Chlordiazepoxide and clidinium	Librax	
Chlorpheniramine, phenylpropanolamine, and isopropamide	Allernade	
	Capade	
	Ornade	
Cholestyramine (oral)	Questran	Cholestyramine
Cimetidine	Tagamet	Cimetidine
Cisplatin	Platinol	Cisplatin
Clindamycin (topical)	Cleocin T	Clindamycin
Clofibrate	Atromid-S	Clofibrate
Clomiphene	Clomid	Clomiphene
Clonidine	Catapres	Clonidine

Drugs or drug type	Brand Names	Generic name
Clonidine and chlorthalidone	Combipres	
Clotrimazole (topical)	Lotrimin	Clotrimazole
	Mycelex	
Clotrimazole (vaginal)	Gyne-Lotrimin	Clotrimazole
Colchicine	Colsalide Improved	Colchicine
Colistin, neomycin, and hydrocortisone (otic)	Coly-Mycin S	
Cyclobenzaprine	Flexeril	Cyclobenzaprine
Cyclophosphamide	Cytoxan	Cyclophosphamide
Cycloserine	Seromycin	Cycloserine
Cytarabine	Cytosar-U	Cytarabine
Dacarbazine	DTIC-Dome	Dacarbazine
Dactinomycin	Cosmegen	Dactinomycin
Danazol	Danocrine	Danazol
Dantrolene	Dantrium	Dantrolene
Dapsone	Avlosulfon	Dapsone
Dexbrompheniramine and pseudoephedrine	Disophrol	
	Drixoral	
Diazoxide (oral)	Proglycem	Diazoxide
Dicyclomine	Bentyl	Dicyclomine
	Dyspas	
Digitalis medicines	Cedilanid-D	Deslanoside
	Digifortis	Digitalis
	Pil-Digis	
	Crystodigin	Digitoxin
	Purodigin	
	Lanoxin	Digoxin
	Gitaligin	Gitalin
	Cedilanid	Lanatoside C
	Strophanthin-G	Ouabain
Dinoprost (intraamniotic)	Prostin F2 Alpha	Dinoprost

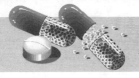

Drugs or drug type	Brand Names	Generic name
Dinoprostone (vaginal)	Prostin E2	Dinoprostone
Dione-type anticonvulsants	Paradione Tridione	Paramethadione Trimethadione
Diphenoxylate and atropine	Colonil Lomotil SK-Diphenoxylate	
Dipyridamole	Persantine	Dipyridamole
Disopyramide	Norpace	Disopyramide
Disulfiram	Antabuse	Disulfiram
Doxapram	Dopram	Doxapram
Drocode, promethazine, and APC	Synalgos-DC	
Ephedrine	Ectasule Minus Ephedsol	
Epinephrine	Adrenalin AsthmaHaler Bronitin Bronkaid Medihaler-Epi Primatene AsthmaNefrin microNEFRIN Vaponefrin	Epinephrine Racepinephrine
Ergoloid mesylates	Hydergine	
Ergonovine	Ergotrate Methergine	Ergonovine Methylergonovine
Ergotamine	Ergomar Ergostat Gynergen Medihaler Ergotamine	Ergotamine tartrate
Ergotamine, belladonna alkaloids, and phenobarbital	Bellergal Bellergal-S	
Ergotamine and caffeine	Cafergot Cafermine	

Drugs or drug type	Brand Names	Generic name
	Cafetrate	
	Ergocaf	
	Ergocaffeine	
	Lanatrate	
	Migrastat	
Ergotamine, caffeine, belladonna alkaloids, and phenobarbital	Cafergot-PB	
Erythromycin	E-Mycin	Erythromicin
	Ilotycin	
	Robimycin	
	RP-Mycin	
	Hosone	Erythromycin estolate
	E.E.S.	Erythromycin ethylsuccinate
	E-Mycin E	
	Pediamycin	
	Wyamycin E	
	Ilotycin	Erythromycin gluceptate
	Erythrocin	Erythromycin lactobionate
	Bristamycin	Erythromycin stearate
	Erypar	
	Ethril	
	Pfizer-E	
	SK-Erythromycin	
	Wyamycin S	
Estrogens	TACE	Chlorotrianisene
	DES	Diethylstilbestrol
	Stilphostrol	
	Delestrogen	Estradiol
	Estrace	
	Progynon	
	Premarin	Conjugated estrogens
	Amnestrogen	Esterified estrogens
	Theelin	Estrone
	Ogen	Estropipate
	Piperazine Estrone Sulfate	
	Estinyl	Ethinyl estradiol
	Feminone	
	Estrovis	Quinestrol

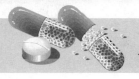

Drugs or drug type	Brand Names	Generic name
Estrogens (vaginal)	DV Cream	Dienestrol
	DES	Diethylstilbestrol
	Premarin	Conjugated estrogens
	Ogen	Estropipate
	Piperazine estrone sulfate	
Estrogens and progestins-oral contraceptives	Demulen	Ethynodiol diacetate and ethinyl estradiol
	Ovulen	Ethynodiol diacetate and mestranol
	Ovcon	Norethindrone and
	Brevicon	ethinyl estradiol
	Norinyl	Norethindrone and
	Ortho-Novum	mestranol
	Norlestrin	Norethindrone acetate
	Loestrin	and ethinyl estradiol
	Enovid	Norethynodrel and mestranol
	Ovral	Norgestrel and ethinyl
	10-Ovral	estradiol
Ethacrynic acid	Edecrin	Ethacrynic acid
Ethambutol	Myambutol	Ethambutol
Ethchlorvynol	Placidyl	Ethchlorvynol
Ethinamate	Valmid	Ethinamate
Ethionamide	Trecator-SC	Ethionamide
Ethylnorepinephrine	Bronkephrine	Ethylnorepinephrine
Fenfluramine	Pondimin	Fenfluramine
Fenoprofen	Nalfon	Fenoprofen
Flucytosine	Ancobon	Flucytosine
	Adrucil	Fluorouracil
Furosemide	Lasix	Furosemide
	Neo-renal	
Gentian violet (vaginal)	Genapax	Gentian violet
	Hyva	
Glutethimide	Doriden	Glutethimide
	Dormtabs	
Glycerin	Glyrol	
	Osmoglyn	

Drugs or drug type	Brand Names	Generic name
Griseofulvin	Fulvicin P/G Fulvicin-U/F Grifulvin V Grisactin GrisOwen Gris-PEG	Griseofulvin
Guaifenesin	2/G Anti-Tuss Breonesin Genetuss Glycotuss Glytuss Hytuss Malotuss Nortussin Proco Robitussin	Guaifenesin
Guaifenesin and codeine	Cheracol Nortussin w/ Codeine Robitussin A-C Tolu-Sed	
Guaifenesin and dextromethorphan	Anti-Tuss DM Cheracol D Dextro-Tuss GG 2 G-DM G-Tuss DM Guaiadex Neo-Vadrin Queltuss Robitussin-DM Silexin Tolu-Sed DM Trocal Unproco	
Guanethidine	Ismelin	Guanethidine
Guanethidine and hydrochlorothiazide	Esimil	
Haloperidol	Haldol	Haloperidol
Heparin	Heprinar Lipo-Hepin Liquaemin Panheprin	Heparin

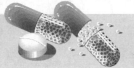

Appendix II

Drugs or drug type	Brand Names	Generic name
Hydantoin-type anti-convulsants	Peganone Mesantoin Dilantin Di-Phen Diphenylan Diphenylhydantoin	Ethotoin Mephenytoin Phenytoin
Hydralazine	Apresoline	Hydralazine
Hydrocortisone (rectal)	Cortifoam Cort-Dome Proctocort	Hydrocortisone
Hydrocortisone, bismuth, benzyl benzoate, peruvian balsam, and zinc oxide (rectal)	Anusol-HC	
Hydroxyurea	Hydrea	Hydroxyurea
Hydroxyzine	Atarax Vistaril	Hydroxyzine
Ibuprofen	Motrin Nuprin	Ibuprofen Advil
Indomethacin	Indocin	Indomethacin
Insulin	Actrapid Regular Insulin Regular Iletin II (new) Velosulin	Insulin injection
	Globin Insulin	Globin zinc insulin injection
	Insulatard NPH NPH Iletin II	Isophane insulin suspension
	Mixtard	Isophane insulin suspension and insulin injection
	Lentard Lente Insulin Lente Iletin II Monotard	Insulin zinc suspension
	Ultralente Ultralente Iletin Ultratard	Extended insulin zinc suspension
	Semilente Semilente Iletin Semitard	Prompt insulin zinc suspension

Drugs or drug type	Brand Names	Generic name
	Protamine Zinc & Iletin II PZI	Protamine zinc insulin suspension
Iodoquinol	Moebiquin Yodoxin	Iodoquinol
Isoetharine	Bronkometer Bronkosol	Isoetharine
Isometheptene, dichloralphenazone, and acetaminophen	Midrin	
Isoniazid	INH Nydrazid	Isoniazid
Isoproterenol	Aerolone Iprenol Isuprel Medihaler-Iso Norisodrine Aerotrol Proternol Vapo-Iso	Isoproterenol
Isoproterenol and phenylephrine	Duo-Medihaler	
Isoxsuprine	Vasodilan Vasoprine	Isoxsuprine
Kanamycin	Kantrex	Kanamycin
Kaolin and pectin	Kaomead Kaopectate Pargel	
Kaolin, pectin, belladonna alkaloids, and opium	Donnagel-PG	
Kaolin, pectin, and paregoric	Parepectolin	
Laxatives, bulk-forming	Maltsupex Cellothyl Cologel Hydrolose	Malt soup extract Methylcellulose
		Polycarbophil
	Mitrolan	Polycarbophil calcium
	Effersyllium	Psyllium mucilloid

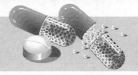

Drugs or drug type	Brand Names	Generic name
	Konsyl	Psyllium seed
	L.A. Formula	Psyllium
	Metamucil	
	Modane Bulk	
	Mucilose	
	Plova	
	Serutan	
	Siblin	
Laxatives, emollient	Surfak	Docusate calcium
	Kasof	Docusate potassium
	Afko-Lube	Docusate sodium
	Colace	
	Colax	
	Comfolax	
	Dioctyl Sodium Sulfosuccinate	
	Alaxin	Poloxamer 188
	Magcyl	
Laxatives, hyperosmoticlactulose and saline	Chronulac	Lactulose
	Citrate of Magnesia	Magnesium citrate
	Adlerika	Magnesium sulfate
	Epsom Salt	
	Phospho-Soda	Sodium Phosphate (or phosphates)
	Sal Hepatica	Effervescent sodium phosphate
Laxatives, lubricant	Liquid Petrolatum	Mineral oil
	Nujol	
	Neo-Cultol	Mineral oil (jellied)
Laxatives, stimulant	Cenalax	Bisacodyl
	Codylax	
	Dulcolax	
	Theralax	
	Cascara Sagrada	Cascara
	Cas-Evac	
	Alphamul	Castor oil
	Neoloid	
	Dorbane	Danthron
	Modane	
	Cholan-DH	Dehydrocholic acid
	Decholin	
	Neocholan	

Drugs or drug type	Brand Names	Generic name
	Alophen	Phenolphthalein
	Espotabs	
	Evac-U-Gen	
	Evac-U-Lax	
	Ex-Lax	
	Feen-A-Mint	
	Phenolax	
	Prulet	
	Black Draught	Senna
	Casa Fru	
	Dr. Caldwell's Senna Laxative	
	Fletcher's Castoria	
	Senokot	
	Swiss Kriss	
	X-Prep	
	Glysennid	Sennosides A and B
	Senokot	
	X-Prep	
Levodopa	Sinemet	Carbidopa and levodopa
	Bendopa	Levodopa
	Dopar	
	Larodopa	
Lincomycins	Cleocin	Clindamycin
	Lincocin	Lincomycin
Lindane (topical)	Kwell	Lindane
Lithium	Eskalith	Lithium carbonate
	Lithonate	
	Lithobid	
	Lithonate-S	
	Lithane	
Loperamide	Imodium	Loperamide
Loxapine	Daxolin	Loxapine
	Loxitane	
Magnesia, milk of	Magnesia	
	Magnesium hydroxide	
Mechlorethamine	Mustargen	Mechlorethamine
Meclizine	Bucladin-S	Buclizine
	Marezine	Cyclizine

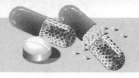

Drugs or drug type	Brand Names	Generic name
	Antivert Bonine	Meclizine
Meclofenamate	Meclomen	Meclofenamate
Melphalan	Alkeran	Melphalan
Meperidine	Demerol Pethadol	Meperidine
Meprobamate	Equanil Meprospan Miltown SK-Bamate Tranmap	Meprobamate
Meprobamate, ethoheptazine, and aspirin	Equagesic Heptogesic Mepro Compound Meprogesic	
Mercaptopurine	Purinethol	Mercaptopurine
Metaproterenol	Alupent Metaprel	Metaproterenol
Methadone	Dolophine Westadone	Methadone
Methaqualone	Mequin Parest Quaalude Sopor	Methaqualone
Methenamine	Hiprex Urex Mandelamine Prov-U-Sep	Methenamine hippurate Methenamine mandelate
Methocarbamol	Delaxin Forbaxin Marbaxin-750 Metho-500 Robamol Robaxin Spinaxin Tumol	Methocarbamol
Methotrexate	Mexate	Methotrexate

Drugs or drug type	Brand Names	Generic name
Methoxsalen	Oxsoralen	Methoxsalen
Methyldopa	Aldomet	Methyldopa
Methyldopa and thiazide diuretics	Aldoclor	Methyldopa and chlorothiazide
	Aldoril	Methyldopa and hydrochlorothiazide
Methylphenidate	Ritalin	Methylphenidate
Methyprylon	Noludar	Methyprylon
Methysergide	Sansert	Methysergide
Metronidazole	Flagyl	Metronidazole
Metyrosine	Demser	Metyrosine
Miconazole	Monistat	Miconazole
Miconazole (topical)	Micatin	Miconazole
Miconazole (vaginal)	Monistat	Miconazole
Minoxidil	Loniten Rogaine	Minoxidil
Mithramycin	Mithracin	Mithramycin
Mitomycin	Mutamycin	Mitomycin
Mitotane	Lysodren	Mitotane
Monoamine oxidase (MAO) inhibitors	Marplan Nardil Parnate Prozac	Isocarboxazid Phenelzine Tranylcypromine Fluoxetine
Nalbuphine	Nubain	Nalbuphine
Nalidixic acid	Neg Gram	Nalidixic acid
Naproxen	Anaprox Naprosyn	Naproxen
Neomycin	Mycifradin Neobiotic	Neomycin
Neomycin, polymyxin B, and bacitracin (topical)	Mycitracin Neo-Polycin Neosporin	
Neomycin, polymyxin B, and gramicidin (ophthalmic)	Neo-Polycin Neosporin	

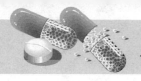

Appendix II

Drugs or drug type	Brand Names	Generic name
Nicotinyl alcohol	Roniacol	Nicotinyl alcohol
Organic nitrates (other than nitroglycerin)	Cardilate	Erythrityl tetranitrate
	Dilatrate-SR Iso-Bid Isordil Isotrate Sorate Sorbide Sorbitrate	Isosorbide dinitrate
	Duotrate Kaytrate Pentraspan Pentritol Peritrate	Pentaerythritol tetranitrate
Nitrofurantoin	Cyantin Furadantin Macrodantin	
Nitroglycerin	Glyceryl trinitrate Nitro-Bid Nitroglyn Nitrol Nitrong Nitrospan Nitrostat	Nitroglycerin
Nylidrin	Arlidin	Nylidrin
Nystatin	Mycostatin Nilstat	Nystatin
Nystatin (topical)	Candex Mycostatin Nilstat	Nystatin
Nystatin (vaginal)	Korostatin Mycostatin Nilstat	Nystatin
Nystatin, neomycin, gramicidin, and triamcinolone (topical)	Mycolog Myco Triacet Mytrex Triamcinolone NNG	
Orphenadrine	Flexojet	

Drugs or drug type	Brand Names	Generic name
	Flexon	
	Marflex	
	Myolin	
	Neocyten	
	Norflex	
	Ro-Orphena	
	Tega-Flex	
	X-Otag	
Orphenadrine and APC	Norgesic	
	Norgesic Forte	
Oxolinic acid	Utibid	Oxolinic acid
Oxtriphylline and guaifenesin	Brondecon	
	Brondelate	
Oxycodone and acetaminophen	Percocet-5	
	Tylox	
Oxycodone and aspirin	Percodan	
	Percodan-Demi	
Oxymetazoline (nasal)	Afrin	Oxymetazoline
	Duration	
	St. Joseph Decongestant for Children	
Papaverine	Cerebid	Papaverine
	Cerespan	
	Dipav	
	Dylate	
	Hyobid	
	Kavrin	
	Myobid	
	Orapav	
	P-A-V	
	Pavabid	
	Pavacap	
	Pavacon	
	Pavadur	
	Pavakey	
	Pavased	
	Pavasule	

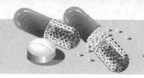

Drugs or drug type	Brand Names	Generic name
	Pavatest	
	Pavatran	
	Paverolan	
	Ro-Papav	
	Sustaverine	
	Vasal	
	Vasospan	
Paraldehyde	Paral	
Pargyline	Eutonyl	
Pemoline	Cylert	
Penicillamine	Cuprimine	
	Depen	
Penicillins	Amoxil	Amoxicillin
	Larotid	
	Polymox	
	Robamox	
	Sumox	
	Trimox	
	Utimox	
	Amcill	Ampicillin
	Omnipen	
	Penbritin	
	Pensyn	
	Polycillin	
	Principen	
	Supen	
	Totacillin	
	Geocillin	Carbenicillin
	Geopen	
	Pyopen	
	Cloxapen	Cloxacillin
	Tegopen	
	Cyclapen-W	Cyclacillin
	Dycill	Dicloxacillin
	Dynapen	
	Pathocil	
	Veracillin	
	Versapen	Hetacillin
	Versapen-K	
	Azapen	Methicillin
	Celbenin	
	Staphcillin	

Drugs or drug type	Brand Names	Generic name
	Nafcil	Nafcillin
	Unipen	
	Bactocill	Oxacillin
	Prostaphlin	
	Bicillin	Penicillin G
	Crysticillin	
	Duracillin	
	Pentids	
	Permapen	
	Wycillin	
	Betapen-VK	Penicillin V
	Penapar VK	
	Pen-Vee K	
	Uticillin VK	
	V-Cillin	
	Veetids	
	Ticar	Ticarcillin
Pentazocine	Talwin	Pentazocine
Pentazocine and aspirin	Talwin Compound	
Pentobarbital and carbromal	Carbrital	
Perphenazine and amitriptyline	Etrafon	
	Triavil	
Phenazopyridine	Azo-100	Phenazopyridine
	Azodine	
	Azo-Standard	
	Di-Azo	
	Phen-Azo	
	Phenazodine	
	Pyridiate	
	Pyridium	
	Pyrodine	
Phenothiazines	Tindal	Acetophenazine
	Repoise	Butaperizine
	Proketazine	Carphenazine
	Chloramead	Chlorpromazine
	Promapar	
	Thorazine	
	Permitil	Fluphenazine
	Prolixin	

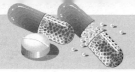

Appendix II

Drugs or drug type	Brand Names	Generic name
	Serentil	Mesoridazine
	Trilafon	Perphenazine
	Quide	Piperacetazine
	Compazine	Prochlorperazine
	Stemetil	
	Sparine	Promazine
	Mellaril	Thioridazine
	Stelazine	Trifluoperazine
	Vesprin	Triflupromazine
Phenoxybenzamine	Dibenzyline	
Phenylbutazone	Oxalid	Oxyphenbutazone
	Tandearil	
	Azolid	Phenylbutazone
	Butazolidin	
	Azolid-A	Buffered phenylbutazone
	Butazolidin Alka	
	Phenylzone-A	
Phenylephrine (nasal)	Alcon-Efrin	
	Allerest	
	Contac	
	Coricidin	
	Isophrin	
	Neo-Mist	
	Neo-Synephrine	
	Pyracort-D	
	Rhinall	
	Sinarest	
	Super Anahist	
	Synasal	
	Vacon	
Phenylpropanolamine	Coffee-Break	
	Control	
	Delcopro	
	Diadax	
	Dietac	
	Obestat	
	Pro-Dax 21	
	Propadrine	
	Rhindecon	
Phenylpropanolamine, phenylephrine, phenyltoloxamine, and chlorpheniramine	Naldecon	

Drugs or drug type	Brand Names	Generic name
Potassium iodide	K1-N Pima	Potassium iodide
Potassium phosphates	K-Phos Original	Monobasic potassium phosphates
	Neutra-Phos-K	Potassium phosphates

**Potassium and sodium
  phosphates**
	Uro-KP-Neutral	Dibasic potassium
		  and sodium phosphates

	K-Phos M. F. K-Phos Neutral K-Phos No. 2	Monobasic potassium and sodium phosphates
	Neutra-Phos	Potassium and sodium phosphates

Potassium supplements	Potassium Triplex
	Tri-K
	Trikates
		Potassium acetate,
		  potassium bicarbonate,
		  and potassium citrate

	K-Lyte	Potassium bicarbonate and citric acid

	KEFF	Potassium bicarbonate,
		  potassium carbonate,
		  and potassium chloride

	Klorvess	Potassium bicarbonate and potassium chloride

	K-Lyte/C1	Potassium bicarbonate,
		  potassium chloride,
		  and citric acid

	Kaochlor-Eff	Potassium bicarbonate,
		  potassium chloride,
		  and potassium citrate

	Kaochlor Kaon-C1 Kato Kay-Ciel K-Lor KLOR-10% KLOR-CON Klorvess Klotrix K-Lyte/C1 Slow-K	Potassium chloride
	Kolyum	Potassium chloride and potassium gluconate
	Twin-K	Potassium citrate and potassium gluconate

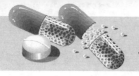

Drugs or drug type	Brand Names	Generic name
	Kaon	Potassium gluconate
Prazosin	Minipress	Prazosin
Primidone	Mysoline	Primidone
Probenecid	Benemid	Probenecid
	Probalan	
Probucol	Lorelco	Probucol
Procainamide	Procamide	Procainamide
	Procan	
	Procan SR	
	Procopan	
	Pronestyl	
	Sub-Quin	
Procarbazine	Matulane	Procarbazine
Prochlorperazine and isopropamide	Combid	
Progestins	Duphaston	Dydrogesterone
	Delalutin	Hydroxyprogesterone
	Provera	Medroxyprogesterone
	Megace	Megestrol
	Micronor	Norethindrone
	Nor-Q.D.	
	Norlutin	
	Norlutate	Norethindrone acetate
	Ovrette	Norgestrel
	Proluton	Progesterone
	Lipo-Lutin	
Promethazine	Historest	Promethazine
	Phenergan	
	Remsed	
Propantheline	Pro-Banthine	Propantheline
Propoxyphene	Darvon	Propoxyphene
	Dolene	
	Pargesic 65	
	Proxagesic	
	Proxene	
	SK-65	

Drugs or drug type	Brand Names	Generic name
Propoxyphene and acetaminophen	Darvocet-N Dolacet Dolene AP-65 SK-65-APAP Wygesic	
Propoxyphene and APC	Darvon Compound Dolene Compound-65 SK-65 Compound	
Propoxyphene and aspirin	Darvon with A.S.A. Darvon-N with A.S.A.	
Pseudoephedrine	Afrinol D-Feda Neobid Novafed Ro-Fedrin Sudafed Sudrin	Pseudoephedrine
Pyrilamine and pentobarbital	Eme-Nil Wans	
Pyrithione zinc (topical)	Danex Head and Shoulders Zincon	
Pyrvinium	Povan	Pyrvinium
Quinidine	Cardioquin Cin-Quin Duraquin Quinaglute Dura-Tabs Quinidex Extentabs Quinora	
Quinine	Coco-Quinine Quine	Quinine
Quinine and aminophylline	Quinamm Quinite Strema	
Rauwolfia alkaloids	Harmonyl Raudixin Raulfia Raupoid Rauserpa	Deserpidine Rauwolfia serpentina

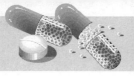
Drugs or drug type	Brand Names	Generic name
	Rau-Sed	
	Reserpine	
	Reserpoid	
	Sandril	
	Serpasil	
Rauwolfia alkaloids and thiazide diuretics	Oreticyl	Deserpidine and
	Oreticyl Forte	hydrochlorothiazide
	Enduronyl	Deserpidine and
		methyclothiazide
	Rauzide	Rauwolfia serpentina
		and bendroflumethiazide
	Exna-R	Reserpine and benzthiazide
	Diupres	Reserpine and chlorothiazide
	Demi-Regroton	Reserpine and chlorthalidone
	Regroton	
	Hydropres	Reserpine and
	Reserpazide	hydrochlorothiazide
	Serpasil-Esidrix	
	Salutensin	Reserpine and
	Salutensin-Demi	hydroflumethiazide
	Diutensen-R	Reserpine and
		methylclothiazide
	Renese-R	Reserpine and polythiazide
	Hydromox-R	Reserpine and quinethazone
	Metatensin	Reserpine and
	Naquival	trichlormethiazide
Reserpine and hydralazine	Serpasil-Apresoline	
Reserpine, hydralazine, and hydrochlorothiazide	Ser-Ap-Es	
	Tri-Hydroserpine	
Resorcinol and sulfur (topical)	Acne-Dome	
	Acnomel	
	Cenac	
	Exzit	
	pHisoAc	
	Sulforcin	
Rifampin	Rifadin	Rifampin
	Rimactane	
Rifampin and isoniazid	Rifamate	

Drugs or drug type	Brand Names	Generic name
Salicyclates	Bayer Aspirin	Aspirin
	Ecotrin	
	Empirin Analgesic	
	Measurin	
	St. Joseph Aspirin	
	Ascriptin	Buffered aspirin
	Bufferin	
	Calurin	Carbaspirin
	Arthropan	Choline salicylate
	Parbocyl	Sodium salicylate
	Uracel	
Salicylic acid and sulfur **(topical)**	Acne-Dome	
	Acno	
	Antiseb	
	BUF	
	Exzit	
	Fostex	
	Klaron	
	Meted	
	Pernox	
	Rezamid	
	SAStid	
	Sebex	
	Sebulex	
	Therac	
	Vanseb	
Salicylic acid, sulfur, **and coal tar** **(topical)**	Antiseb-T	
	Sebex-T	
	Sebutone	
	Vanseb-T	
Selenium sulfide **(topical)**	Exsel	
	Iosel	
	Selsun	
	Selsun Blue	
	Sul-Blue	
Sodium fluoride	Denta-Fl	
	Flo-Tab	
	Fluorident	
	Fluoritab	
	Fluorodex	
	Flura	
	Karidium	
	Luride	

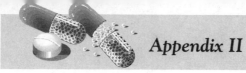

Drugs or drug type	Brand Names	Generic name
	Luride-SF	
	Nafeen	
	Pedi-Dent	
	Pediaflor	
	Stay-Flo	
	Studaflor	
Spironolactone	Aldactone	Spironolactone
Spironolactone and hydrochlorothiazide	Aldactazide	
Succinimide-type anticonvulsants	Zarontin	
	Celontin	
	Milontin	
	Ethosuximide	
	Methsuximide	
	Phensuximide	
Sulfasalazine	Azulfidine	Sulfasalazine
	S.A.S.-500	
Sulfinpyrazone	Anturane	Sulfinpyrazone
	Zynol	
Sulfonamides	Renoquid	Sulfacytine
	Gantanol	Sulfamethoxazole
	Methoxal	
	Methoxanol	
	Bactrim	Sulfamethoxazole and trimethoprim
	Septra	
	Gantrisin	Sulfisoxazole
	Lipo Gantrisin	
	Sosol	
	Sulfalar	
	Sulfizin	
Sulfonamides (vaginal)	AVC	Sulfanilamide, aminacrine, and allantoin
	Femguard	
	Nil	
	Tricholan	
	Vagidine	
	Vagimine	
	Vagitrol	
	Sultrin	Sulfathiazole, sulfacetamide, and sulfabenzamide
	Trysul	

Drugs or drug type	Brand Names	Generic name
	Koro-Sulf	Sulfisoxazole
	Vagilia	Sulfisoxazole, aminacrine, and allantoin
Sulfonamides and phenazopyridine	Azo Gantanol	Sulfamethoxazole and phenazopyridine
	Azo Gantrisin	Sulfisoxazole and phenazopyridine
	Azo-Soxazole	
	Azosul	
	Azo-Sulfizin	
	Suldiazo	
Sulindac	Clinoril	Sulindac
Tamoxifen	Nolvadex	Tamoxifen
Terbutaline	Brethine	Terbutaline
	Bricanyl	
Terpin hydrate and codeine	Cortussis	
Testolactone	Teslac	Testolactone
Tetracyclines	Declomycin	Demeclocycline
	Doxychel	Doxycycline
	Doxy-Tabs	
	Vibramycin	
	Vibra-Tabs	
	Rondomycin	Methacycline
	Minocin	Minocycline
	Oxlopar	Oxytetracycline
	Oxy-Kesso-Tetra	
	Terramycin	
	Tetramine	
	Achromycin	Tetracycline
	Bristacycline	
	Cyclopar	
	Panmycin	
	Retet	
	Robitet	
	Sumycin	
	Tetracyn	
Theophylline, ephedrine, and barbiturates	Asminyl	
	Asma-lief	
	Phedral	
	Tedfern	
	Tedral	

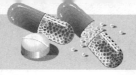
Drugs or drug type	Brand Names	Generic name
	Thalfed	
	Thedrizem	
	Theodrine	
	Theofed	
	Theofenal	
	Theoral	
	Theotabs	
Theophylline, ephedrine guaifenesin, and barbiturates	Broncholate	
	Bronkolixir	
	Bronkotabs	
	Duovent	
	Luftodil	
	Mudrane GG	
	Quibron Plus	
	Verequad	
Theophylline, ephedrine, and hydroxyzine	Asminorel	
	E.T.H. Compound	
	Hydrophed	
	Marax	
	Theophozine	
	Theozine	
Theophylline and guaifenesin	Asbron G	
	Asma	
	Cerylin	
	Dialixir	
	Glybron	
	Glyceryl T	
	Hylate	
	Lanophyllin-GG	
	Quibron	
	Slo-Phyllin GG	
	Synophylate-GG	
	Theo-Col	
	Theo-Guaia	
Thiazide diuretics	Naturetin	Bendroflumethiazide
	Aquastat	Benzthiazide
	Aquatag	
	Exna	
	Hydrex	
	Diuril	Chlorothiazide
	SK-Chlorothiazide	
	Hygroton	Chlorthalidone
	Uridon	

Drugs or drug type	Brand Names	Generic name
	Anhydron	Cyclothiazide
	Esidrix	Hydrochlorothiazide
	Hydro-Aquil	
	HydroDIURIL	
	Oretic	
	Diucardin	Hydroflumethiazide
	Saluron	
	Aquatensen	Methyclothiazide
	Duretic	
	Enduron	
	Diulo	Metolazone
	Zaroxolyn	
	Renese	Polythiazide
	Hydromox	Quinethazone
	Metahydrin	Trichlormethiazide
	Naqua	
Thioxanthenes	Taractan	Chlorprothixene
	Navane	Thiothixene
Thyroid hormones	Levothroid	Levothyroxine
	L-T-S	
	Ro-Thyroxine	
	Synthroid	
	Cytomel	Liothyronine
	Ro-Thyronine	
	Tertroxin	
	Euthroid	Liotrix
	Proloid	Thyroglobulin
	S-P-T	Thyroid
	Thyrar	
	Thyrocrine	
Thyrotropin	Thyrotron	Thyrotropin
	Thytropar	
Tolmetin	Tolectin	Tolmetin
Tolnaftate (topical)	Aftate	Tolnaftate
	Tinactin	
Tretinoin (topical)	Retin-A	Tretinoin
Triamterene	Dyrenium	Triamterene
Triamterene and hydrochlorothiazide	Dyazide	
Triazolam	Halcion	Triazolam

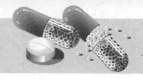

Drugs or drug type	Brand Names	Generic name
Tricyclic antidepressants	Amitid	Amitriptyline
	Amitil	
	Elavil	
	Endep	
	Norpramin	Desipramine
	Pertofrane	
	Adapin	Doxepin
	Sinequan	
	Imavate	Imipramine
	Janimine	
	SK-Pramine	
	Tofranil	
	Aventyl	Nortriptyline
	Pamelor	
	Vivactil	Protriptyline
	Surmontil	Trimipramine
Trimethobenzamide	Tigan	Trimethobenzamide
Triprolidine and pseudoephedrine	Actifed	
	Allerphed	
	Tagafed	
Undecylenic acid compound (topical)	Decylenes	
	Desenex	
	Medaped	
	Quinsana Plus	
Urea	Ureaphil	
Valproic acid	Depakene	Valproic acid
Vinblastine	Velban	Vinblastine
Vincristine	Oncovin	Vincristine
Vitamins and fluoride	Vita-Flor	Multiple vitamins and fluoride
	Adeflor	
	Mulvidren-F	
	Novacebrin with Fluoride	
	Vi-Penta F	
	Poly-Vi-Flor	
	V-Daylin with Fluoride	

Drugs or drug type	Brand Names	Generic name
	Cari-Tab	Vitamins A, D, and C
	Tri-Vi-Flor	and fluoride
Methyl-Xanthines	Aminodur	Aminophylline
	Lixaminol	
	Mini-Lix	
	Somophyllin	
	Airet	Dyphylline
	Dilin	
	Dilor	
	Lufyllin	
	Neothylline	
	Choledyl	Oxtriphylline
	Accurbron	Theophylline
	Aerolate	
	Bronkodyl	
	Elixicon	
	Elixophyllin	
	Physpan	
	Slophyllin	
	Somophyllin-T	
	Theobid	
	Theoclear	
	Theodur	
	Theolair	
	Theolixir	
	Theophyl	
	Theospan	
Xylometazoline (nasal)	4-Way Long Acting	
	Neo-Synephrine II	
	Otrivin	
	Rhinall Long Acting	
	Sine-Off Once-A-Day	
	Sinex Long-Acting	
	Sinutab Long Acting	
	Sinus Spray	

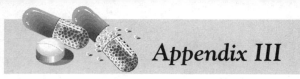

Adverse Interactions Between Drugs

Drug	Interaction	Explanation of Interaction
Aminoglycosides		
Cephaloridine	Increased nephrotoxicity	Not established
Cephalothin	Increased nephrotoxicity Potentiated resp. depression	Not established
Ethacrynic acid	Increased ototoxicity	Additive
Polymyxins	Increased nephrotoxicity	Additive
Ampicillin		
Contraceptives, oral	Decreased contraceptive effect	Not established
Anesthetics, general		
Antihypertensive drugs	Hypotension	Usually additive
Antacids		
Digoxin	Decreased drug levels	Decreased digoxin absorption
Indomethacin	Decreased drug levels	Decreased indomethacin absorption
Isoniazid	Decreased isoniazid effect with aluminum antacids	Decreased absorption of isoniazid
Quinolones	Decreased drug absorption with aluminum- and magnesium- containing antacids	Decreased quinolone absorption
Salicylates	Decreased salicylate levels	Increased renal clearance
Tetracyclines oral	Decreased tetracycline levels	Decreased tetracycline absorption
Anticoagulants, oral		
Anabolic and androgenic steroids	Increased anticoagulant effect	Not established
Barbiturates	Decreased anticoagulant effect	Induction of microsomal enzymes
Bile acid binding resins	Reduced hypoprothrombinemic response	Binding in the GI tract
Carbamazepine	Decreased anticoagulant effect	Induction of microsomal enzymes
Cimetidine	Increased anticoagulant effect	Inhibition of microsomal enzymes
Contraceptives, oral	Decreased anticoagulant effect	Increased factor VII and X (prothrombin may decrease)
Dextrothyroxine	Increased anticoagulant effect	Not established
Hypoglycemics	Increased sulfonylurea hypoglycemia	Inhibition of microsomal enzymes
Indomethacin	Increased bleeding risk	Inhibition of platelet function

Drug	Interaction	Proposed Mechanism
Metronidazole	Increased anticoagulant effect	Inhibition of microsomal enzymes
Miconazole	Increased anticoagulant effect	Not established
Phenylbutazone or oxyphenbutazone	Increased anticoagulant effect	Displacement from binding sites; inhibition of microsomal enzymes
Phenytoin	Increased phenytoin toxicity with dicumarol	Inhibition of microsomal enzymes
	Decreased hypoprothrombinemic response (transient)	Protein binding displacement
	Decreased hypoprothrombinemic response (delayed)	Inhibition of microsomal enzymes
Rifampin	Decreased anticoagulant effect	Induction of microsomal enzymes
Salicylates (>2 g/day)	Increased bleeding time	Inhibition of platelet function
	Increased hypoprothrombinemic effect	Reduction in plasma prothrombin
Sulfinpyrazone	Increased anticoagulant effect	Not established
Sulfonamides	Increased anticoagulant effect	Inhibition of microsomal enzymes; displacement from binding sites
Thyroid hormones	Increased anticoagulant effect	Increased clotting factor catabolism
Barbiturates		
β-Adrenergic blockers	Decreased β-blocker effect	Induction of microsomal enzymes
Anticoagulants, oral	Decreased anticoagulant effect	Induction of microsomal enzymes
Antidepressants, tricyclic	Decreased antidepressant effect	Induction of microsomal enzymes
Chloramphenicol	Increased barbiturate effect	Inhibition of microsomal enzymes
Contraceptives, oral	Decreased contraceptive effect	Induction of microsomal enzymes
Corticosteroids	Decreased steroid effect	Induction of microsomal enzymes
Digitoxin	Decreased digitoxin effect	Induction of microsomal enzymes
Doxycycline	Decreased doxycycline effect	Induction of microsomal enzymes
Meperidine	Increased CNS depression	Increased meperidine metabolites

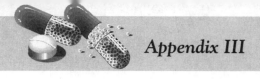

Drug	Interaction	Proposed Mechanism
Phenothiazines	Decreased phenothiazine effect	Induction of microsomal enzymes
Rifampin	Decreased barbiturate effect	Induction of microsomal enzymes
Valproic acid	Increased phenobarbital effect	Decreased phenobarbital metabolism
Benzodiazepines		
Cimetidine	Increased effect of chlordiazepoxide and diazepam	Inhibition of microsomal enzymes
β-Adrenergic blockers (see sympathomimetic amines)		
Calcium channel blockers (nifedipine, verapamil)	Decreased antihypertensive effects	Induction of microsomal enzymes
Cephaloridine		
Aminoglycoside antibiotics	Increased nephrotoxicity	Not established
Ethacrynic acid	Increased nephrotoxicity	Additive
Furosemide	Increased nephrotoxicity	Additive
Cephalothin		
Aminoglycoside antibiotics	Increased nephrotoxicity	Not established
Chloramphenicol		
Barbiturates	Increased barbiturate effect	Inhibition of microsomal enzymes
Phenytoin	Increased phenytoin toxicity	Inhibition of microsomal enzymes
Cimetidine		
Anticoagulants, oral	Increased anticoagulant effect	Inhibition of microsomal enzymes
Benzodiazepines	Increased effect of chlordiazepoxide	Inhibition of microsomal enzymes
Theophylline	Increased theophylline toxicity	Inhibition of microsomal enzymes
Contraceptives, oral		
Ampicillin	Decreased contraceptive effect	Induction of microsomal enzymes
Anticoagulants, oral	Decreased anticoagulant effect	Increased factor VII and X (prothrombin may decrease)
Barbiturates	Decreased contraceptive effect	Induction of microsomal enzymes
Carbamazepine	Decreased contraceptive effect	Induction of microsomal enzymes

Drug	Interaction	Proposed Mechanism
Hypoglycemics, oral	Increased glucose levels	Increased glucose tolerance
Phenytoin	Decreased contraceptive effect	Induction of microsomal enzymes
Primidone	Decreased contraceptive effect	Induction of microsomal enzymes
Tetracyclines	Decreased contraceptive effect	Not established
Diazepam	Slower diazepam elimination	Impaired metabolism
Corticosteroids		
Barbiturates	Decreased corticosteroid effect	Induction of microsomal enzymes
Diuretics (except spironolactone and triamterene)	Increased potassium loss	Additive enzymes
Estrogens	Usually increased cortico-steroid effect	Increased protein binding
Phenytoin	Decreased corticosteroid effect	Induction of microsomal enzymes
Rifampin	Decreased corticosteroid effect	Induction of microsomal enzymes
Danazol		
Estrogens	Decreased estrogen effects	Inhibition of gonadotropins
Diazoxide		
Anesthetics, general	Hypotension	Usually additive
Phenytoin	Decreased anticonvulsant effect	Not established (enhanced phenytoin metabolism)
Sympathomimetic amines	Decreased antihypertensive effect	Pharmacologic antagonism
Digoxin		
Antacids, oral	Decreased digoxin effect	Decreased digoxin absorption
Bile acid binding resins	Decreased digoxin levels	Decreased digoxin absorption binding in the gut
Diuretics (except potassium sparing)	Increased digoxin toxicity	Hypokalemia
Quinidine	Increases serum digoxin	Decreased renal clearance of digoxin
Sympathomimetic amines	Increased tendency to cardiac arrhythmia	Additive
Ergot alkaloids (ergotamine, ergotrate, cafergot and similar agents)		
Ephedrine	Postpartum hypertension	Additive
Methoxamine	Postpartum hypertension, headaches	Additive

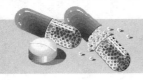

Appendix III

Drug	Interaction	Proposed Mechanism
Propranolol	Headaches, vasoconstriction	Additive
Sympathomimetics	Hypertension, headaches	Additive
Estrogens		
Anticoagulants	Usually decreased anticoagulant effect	Increased coagulation factors
Corticosteroids	Potentiation of corticosteroid (esp. anti-inflammatory) effects, esp. with hydrocortisone	Possibly due to increased steroid being protein bound
Hypoglycemics	Increased blood glucose levels	Decreased glucose tolerance
Oxytocin	Increased uterine contractility	Not established
Phenobarbital	Decreased drug levels	Induction of microsomal enzymes
Vitamins	Decreased folate levels	Not established
Furosemide		
Cephaloridine	Increased nephrotoxicity	Additive
Corticosteroids	Increased potassium loss	Additive
Digitalis drugs	Increased digitalis toxicity	Hypokalemia
Indomethacin	Decreased antihypertensive and natriuretic effects	Prostaglandin inhibition
Lithium	Increased lithium toxicity	Decreased renal lithium clearance
Phenytoin	Reduced diuresis	Not established
Propranolol	Increased β-blockade	Not established
Heparin		
Aspirin	Increased bleeding risk	Inhibition of platelet function
Hydralazine		
Anesthetics, general	Hypotension	Usually additive
Sympathomimetic amines	Decreased antihypertensive effect	Pharmacologic antagonism
Hypoglycemics, oral		
Contraceptives, oral	Increased blood glucose levels	Decreased glucose tolerance
Dicumarol	Increased hypoglycemia	Inhibition of microsomal enzymes
Propranolol	Prolonged hypoglycemia	Reduced glycogenolysis
	Masks tachycardia and tremor	β-Receptor blockade
	Hypertension during hypoglycemia	Blocked β effects of epinephrine
Rifampin	Decreased hypoglycemic effect	Induction of microsomal enzymes
Salicylates	Increased hypoglycemia, esp. with chlorpropamide	Displacement from binding sites; additive

Drug	Interaction	Proposed Mechanism
Indomethacin		
Antacids, oral	Decreased indomethacin effect	Decreased indomethacin absorption
Anticoagulants, oral	Increased bleeding risk	Inhibition of platelet function
β-Adrenergic blockers	Decreased antihypertensive effect	Possibly by prostaglandin inhibition
Diuretics	Decreased antihypertensive and natriuretic effects of thiazides and furosemide	Possibly by prostaglandin inhibition
Lithium	Increased lithium toxicity	Decreased renal lithium clearance
Influenza vaccine		
Theophylline	Increased theophylline effect	Decreased theophylline metabolism
Insulin		
Corticosteroids	Increased glucose levels	Antagonism
Diuretics (thiazide)	Increased glucose levels	Antagonism
Oral contraceptives	Increased glucose levels	Decreased glucose tolerance
Phentolamine	Increased insulin secretion	Blockade of adrenergic suppression of insulin secretion
Propranolol	Increased insulin activity, hypoglycemia	Pharmacologic action
Salicylates	Decreased glucose levels	Decreased protein binding
Sulfonamides	Decreased glucose levels	Decreased protein binding
Iron, oral		
Tetracyclines	Decreased tetracycline effect	Decreased tetracycline absorption
Isoniazid		
Aluminum antacids	Decreased isoniazid effect	Inhibition of isoniazid absorption
Phenytoin	Increased phenytoin toxicity	Inhibition of microsomal enzymes
Lithium		
Diruetics (except spironolactone and triamterene)	Increased lithium toxicity	Decreased renal lithium clearance
Indomethacin	Increased lithium toxicity	Decreased renal lithium clearance
Methyldopa	Increased lithium toxicity	Not established
Phenothiazines	Decreased phenothiazine levels	Not established
Meperidine		
Barbiturates	Increased CNS depression	Increased meperidine metabolites

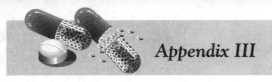

Drug	Interaction	Proposed Mechanism
MAO Inhibitors	Hypertension; hypotension and coma	Not established
Methadone		
Curariform drugs	Increased respiratory depression	Additive
Rifampin	Methadone withdrawal symptoms	Induction of microsomal enzymes
Methyldopa		
Anesthetics, general	Hypotension	Usually additive
Sympathomimetic amines	Decreased antihypertensive effect	Pharmacologic antagonism
Tolbutamide	Increased hypoglycemia	Inhibition of microsomal enzymes
Metronidazole		
Alcohol	Increased alcohol toxicity	Inhibition of aldehyde dehydrogenase
Anticoagulants, oral	Increased anticoagulant effect	Inhibition of microsomal enzymes
Miconazole		
Amphotericin B	Decreased anticandidal effect	Not established
Anticoagulants, oral	Increased anticoagulant effect	Not established
Oxytocics		
Ephedrine	Severe hypertension	Additive
Estrogens	Increased uterine contractility	Not established
Sympathomimetic amines	Severe hypertension, vasoconstriction, migraine headache	Additive
Phenothiazines		
Barbiturates	Decreased phenothiazine effect	Induction of microsomal enzymes
Phenytoin		
Antidepressants, tricyclic	Increased phenytoin toxicity with imipramine	Not established
Contraceptives, oral	Decreased contraceptive effect	Induction of microsomal enzymes
Corticosteroids	Decreased corticosteroid effect	Induction of microsomal enzymes
Doxycycline	Decreased doxycycline effect	Induction of microsomal enzymes
Furosemide	Decreased diuresis	Decreased furosemide absorption

Drug	Interaction	Proposed Mechanism
Isoniazid	Increased phenytoin toxicity	Inhibition of microsomal enzymes
Phenylbutazone	Increased phenytoin toxicity	Inhibition of microsomal enzymes
Potassium-sparing diuretics-ACE inhibitors	Increased potassium-retaining effects	Additive

Primidone

Contraceptives, oral	Decreased contraceptive effect	Induction of microsomal enzymes

Progesterone and similar agents

Phenobarbital	Decreased drug effect	Induction of microsomal enzymes
Phenothiazines	Increased phenothiazine effect	Inhibition of microsomal enzymes
Phenylbutazone	Increased progestin effects	Inhibition of microsomal enzymes
Rifampin	Decreased progestin effect	Induction of microsomal enzymes

Propranolol

Anesthetics, general	Hypotension	Usually additive
Barbiturates	Decreased β-blocker effect	Induction of microsomal enzymes
Chlorpromazine	Increased effects of both drugs	Inhibition of metabolism of both drugs
Ergots	Headaches, vasoconstriction	Additive
Hypoglycemics, oral	Prolonged hypoglycemia	Decreased glycogenolysis
	Masks tachycardia and tremor	β-Receptor blockade
	Hypertension during hypoglycemia	Blocked β effects of epinephrine
Indomethacin	Decreased antihypertensive effect	Possibly by prostaglandin inhibition
Lidocaine	Increased lidocaine effect	Decreased lidocaine clearance
Sympathomimetic amines	Decreased antihypertensive effect	Pharmacologic antagonism
	Hypertension with epinephrine, possibly others	Unopposed α-adrenergic stimulation
Theophylline	Increased theophylline effect with propranolol	Decreased theophylline clearance

Ritodrine

Anesthetics (general)	Hypotension	Vasodilitation
Corticosteroids	Pulmonary edema	Increased diastolic pressure
Digitalis	Cardiac arrhythmias	Increased conduction velocities
Hypoglycemics	Increased glucose levels	Pharmacologic effect

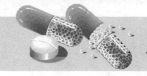

Drug	Interaction	Proposed Mechanism
Propranolol	Antagonism	Pharmacologic antagonism
Salicylates		
Antacids	Decreased salicylate levels	Increased renal clearance
Anticoagulants, oral	Possible increased bleeding risk with aspirin	Inhibition of platelet function
	Increased hypoprothrombinemic effect (more than 2 g/day of salicylates)	Reduction of plasma prothrombin
Heparin	Increased bleeding risk	Inhibition of platelet function
Hypoglycemics	Increased hypoglycemia	Displacement from binding sites; additive
Sulfamethoxazole-trimethoprim	Same as sulfonamides	
Sulfonamides		
Anticoagulants, oral	Increased anticoagulant effect	Displacement from binding sites
Hypoglycemics	Increased sulfonylurea hypoglycemia	Not established
Sympathomimetic amines		
Antihypertensive drugs	Decreased antihypertensive effect	Inhibition of norepinephrine uptake by neurons
β-Adrenergic blockers (non-selective)	Hypertension with epinephrine, possibly with others	Unopposed α-adrenergic stimulation
Digitalis drugs	Increased tendency to cardiac arrhythmias	Additive
Tetracyclines		
Antacids, oral	Decreased tetracycline effect	Decreased tetracycline absorption
Barbiturates	Decreased doxycycline effect	Induction of microsomal enzymes
Carbamazepine	Decreased doxycycline effect	Induction of microsomal enzymes
Contraceptives, oral	Decreased contraceptive effect	Not established
Iron, oral	Decreased tetracycline effect	Decreased tetracycline absorption
Phenytoin	Decreased doxycycline effect	Induction of microsomal enzymes

Drug	Interaction	Proposed Mechanism
Theophylline		
Cimetidine	Increased theophylline toxicity	Inhibition of microsomal enzymes
Erythromycin	Increased theophylline effect	Inhibition of theophylline metabolism
Influenza vaccine	Increased theophylline effect	Inhibition of theophylline metabolism
Propranolol	Increased theophylline effect	Decreased theophylline clearance
Smoking (tobacco and marijuana)	Decreased theophylline effect	Increased metabolism
Thiazide diuretics		
Corticosteroids	Increased potassium loss	Additive
Digitalis drugs	Increased digitalis toxicity	Hypokalemia
Indomethacin	Decreased antihypertensive and natriuretic effects	Possibly by prostaglandin inhibition
Salicylates	Increased CNS toxicity with acetazolamide	Increased plasma nonionized salicylate with increased CNS levels
Thyroid hormones		
Anticoagulants	Increased anticoagulant effects	Increased clotting factor catabolism
Vitamin K		
Antibiotics	Decreased clotting factor synthesis	Inhibition of bacterial production of vitamin K due to antibiotic usage
Mineral oil	Decreased clotting factor	Decreased absorption of

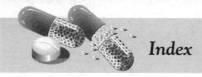

Index

Page references followed by the letter t refer to tables.

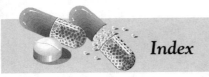

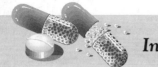

Index

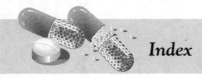